ON CALL
NEUROLOGY

Be on call with confidence!

Successfully managing on-call situations requires a masterful combination of speed, skills, and knowledge. Rise to the occasion **with W.B. SAUNDERS COMPANY'S On Call Series!** These pocket-size resources provide you with immediate access to the vital, step-by-step information you need to succeed!

Other titles in the On Call series

ON CALL
NEUROLOGY

RANDOLPH S. MARSHALL, MD

Assistant Professor of Neurology
Columbia University College of Physicians and Surgeons
Co-Director, Cerebral Localization Laboratory
Assistant Attending Neurologist
Presbyterian Hospital in the City of New York

STEPHAN A. MAYER, MD

Assistant Professor of Neurology (in Neurosurgery)
Columbia University College of Physicians and Surgeons
Director, Neurological Intensive Care Unit
Assistant Attending Neurologist
Presbyterian Hospital in the City of New York

W.B. SAUNDERS COMPANY
A Division of Harcourt Brace & Company
Philadelphia London Toronto Montreal Sydney Tokyo

W.B. SAUNDERS COMPANY
A Division of Harcourt Brace & Company

The Curtis Center
Independence Square West
Philadelphia, Pennsylvania 19106

Library of Congress Cataloging-in-Publication Data

Marshall, Randolph S.

On call neurology / Randolph S. Marshall, Stephan A. Mayer.

p.   cm.

Includes index.

ISBN 0–7216–6523–3

1. Neurology—Handbooks, manuals, etc. I. Mayer, Stephan A. II. Title.
    [DNLM: 1. Nervous System Diseases—therapy.   2. Emergencies.
    3. Nervous System Diseases—diagnosis.   4. Neurology—methods.
    WL 140 M369o 1997]

RC355.M37 1997

616.8—dc21

DNLM/DLC   96–36902

Cover illustration is *OPUS 1971*, enamel on steel, by Virgil Cantini, PhD, from the private collection of the artist.

On Call Neurology   ISBN 0–7216–6523–3

Printed in the United States of America.

Last digit is the print number: 9   8   7   6   5   4   3   2   1

To our wives, Rebecca and Elizabeth

PREFACE

This book is meant to serve as a pocket reference for medical students, house officers, and nonneurologist physicians who care for patients in the hospital. Neurologic problems are common and by their nature complex. The goal of *On Call Neurology* is to provide the reader with accessible, highly structured protocols for the assessment and management of neurologic disorders that present in the emergency room, intensive care unit, hospital floor, or clinic. We have tried to emphasize treatment and have attempted to simulate the focused and goal-directed thought processes of an experienced clinical neurologist.

On Call Neurology is designed to be comprehensive in scope but is admittedly limited in depth. We acknowledge that much of the content reflects "our way" of doing things. It is our hope that the protocols presented in this book will stimulate the student of neurology (whether a medical student or an attending neurologist) to research the literature, analyze the available data, and reach independent conclusions about optimal patient care. In short, we have intended this book to serve as a starting point for clinical problems in neurology, rather than as a definitive reference.

We are grateful to our patients, colleagues, and teachers at The Neurological Institute of New York at Columbia-Presbyterian Medical Center, who taught us most of what we know about neurology. In particular, we would like to thank J.P. Mohr, John Brust, Matthew Fink, and Lewis P. Rowland. Their voices can be heard in many of the pages of this text, and their dedication to teaching and education has served as an inspiration to generations of young physicians like us.

Stephan A. Mayer

Randolph S. Marshall

NOTICE

Neurology is an ever-changing field. Standard safety precautions must be followed, but as new research and clinical experience broaden our knowledge, changes in treatment and drug therapy become necessary or appropriate. The editors of this work have carefully checked the generic and trade drug names and verified drug dosages to ensure that the dosage information in this work is accurate and in accord with the standards accepted at the time of publication. Readers are advised, however, to check the product information currently provided by the manufacturer of each drug to be administered to be certain that changes have not been made in the recommended dose or in the contraindications for administration. This is of particular importance in regard to new or infrequently used drugs. It is the responsibility of the treating physician, relying on experience and knowledge of the patient, to determine dosages and the best treatment for the patient. The editors cannot be responsible for misuse or misapplication of the material in this work.

THE PUBLISHER

STRUCTURE OF THE BOOK

This book is divided into four main sections:

The first section, Introduction, provides an overview of the clinical approach to the neurologic patient, including the neurologic examination, neuroanatomic localization, and neurodiagnostic testing.

The second section, Patient-Related Problems: The Common Calls, is a symptom-oriented approach to chief complaints that frequently require neurologic consultation in the emergency room, clinic, or hospital floor. Each problem is approached from its inception, beginning with relevant questions that should be asked over the phone, temporary orders that should be given, and the major life-threatening disorders that should be considered as one approaches the bedside:

■ PHONE CALL

Questions

Pertinent questions to assess the urgency of the situation.

Orders

Urgent orders to stabilize the patient and gain additional information before you arrive at the bedside.

Inform RN

RN to be informed of the time the housestaff anticipates arrival at the bedside.

■ ELEVATOR THOUGHTS

The differential diagnoses to be considered while the housestaff is on the way to assess the patient (i.e., while in the elevator).

■ MAJOR THREAT TO LIFE

Neurologic emergencies that can lead to death or neurologic devastation unless immediate action is taken.

■ BEDSIDE

Quick Look Test

The quick look test is a rapid visual assessment to place the patient into one of three categories: well, sick, or critical. This helps determine the necessity of immediate intervention.

Vital Signs

Selective History and Chart Review

Including pertinent negatives and neurologic review of systems.

Selective Physical and Neurologic Examination

A rapid, focused neurologic examination designed to assess the extent and degree of neurologic dysfunction.

■ MANAGEMENT

Provides guidelines for neurodiagnostic testing and gives access to indicated medications and dosages. When applicable, checklists and specific management protocols are provided.

The third section, Selected Neurologic Disorders, provides an overview of important neurologic diseases and their management not covered comprehensively in the "common calls" section, such as CNS infections, multiple sclerosis, neuromuscular diseases, movement disorders, and brain tumors.

The fourth section, the Appendices, provides neuroanatomic references and other materials helpful for managing neurologic patients.

The On-Call Formulary is a compendium of medications commonly used to treat neurologic disorders. Drug indications, mechanisms of action, dosages, routes of administration, side effects, and comments for optimal use are provided.

COMMONLY USED ABBREVIATIONS

ABG	arterial blood gas
ACA	anterior cerebral artery
ACE	angiotensin converting enzyme
ACTH	adrenocorticotropic hormone
AFB	acid-fast bacillus
AIDS	acquired immunodeficiency syndrome
AION	anterior ischemic optic neuropathy
ALS	amyotrophic lateral sclerosis
AMN	adrenomyeloneuropathy
ANA	antinuclear antibody
ANCA	antineutrophil cytoplasmic antibody
APD	afferent pupillary defect
aPTT	activated partial thromboplastin time
AV	arteriovenous
AVM	arteriovenous malformation
BAER	brainstem auditory evoked response
bid	two times a day
BP	blood pressure
BUN	blood urea nitrogen
CAA	cerebral amyloid angiopathy
CBC	complete blood count
CBF	cerebral blood flow
CHF	congestive heart failure
CIDP	chronic inflammatory demyelinating polyneuropathy
CMAP	compound muscle action potential
CMV	cytomegalovirus
CN	cranial nerve
CNS	central nervous system

CPAP	continuous positive airway pressure
CPK	creatine phosphokinase
CPP	cerebral perfusion pressure
CPR	cardiopulmonary resuscitation
CRAO	central retinal artery occlusion
CSF	cerebrospinal fluid
CT	computed tomography
DDAVP	desmopressin acetate
DIC	disseminated intravascular coagulation
D5W	5% dextrose in water
D5WNS	5% dextrose in normal saline
D50W	50% dextrose in water
DVT	deep vein thrombosis
DWI	diffusion-weighted imaging
EBV	Epstein-Barr virus
ECG	electrocardiogram
EEG	electroencephalogram
EMG	electromyography
EP	electrophysiologic
ER	emergency room
ESR	erythrocyte sedimentation rate
EtOH	ethanol
FDA	Food and Drug Administration
FFP	fresh frozen plasma
FNF	finger-nose-finger
GBM	glioblastoma multiforme
GBS	Guillain-Barré syndrome
GCS	Glasgow Coma scale
GI	gastrointestinal
GU	genitourinary
HCG	human chorionic gonadotropin
HEENT	head, eyes, ears, nose, throat

HIV	human immunodeficiency virus
HKS	heel-knee-shin
HR	heart rate
HSE	herpes simplex encephalitis
HSV-1	herpes simplex virus 1
HTLV-1	human T-cell lymphotropic virus type I
Hz	Hertz
ICA	internal carotid artery
ICH	intracerebral hemorrhage
ICP	intracranial pressure
ICU	intensive care unit
IgG	immunoglobulin G
IM	intramuscular
IMV	intermittent mandatory ventilation
INO	internuclear ophthalmoplegia
INR	international normalized ratio
ION	ischemic optic neuropathy
IV	intravenous
IVIG	intravenous immune globulin
IVP	intravenous push
KVO	keep the vein open
LFT	liver function test
LCM	lymphocytic choriomeningitis
LP	lumbar puncture
MABP	mean arterial blood pressure
MAO	monoamine oxidase
MCA	middle cerebral artery
MELAS	mitochondrial encephalomyopathy, lactic acidosis, and stroke
MI	myocardial infarction
MLD	metachromatic leukodystrophy
MLF	median longitudinal fasciculus

MMN	multifocal motor neuropathy
MMSE	Mini Mental State Examination
MRI	magnetic resonance imaging
MS	multiple sclerosis
MSA	multiple-system atrophy
NCS	nerve conduction study
NCV	nerve conduction velocity
NPO	"nil per os" (nothing by mouth)
NS	normal saline
NSAID	nonsteroidal anti-inflammatory drug
OCB	oligoclonal band
OKN	opticokinetic nystagmus
ON	optic neuritis
PCA	posterior cerebral artery
PCNSL	primary central nervous system lymphoma
Pco_2	partial pressure of carbon dioxide
PCR	polymerase chain reaction
PE	pulmonary embolism
PEEP	positive end-expiratory pressure
PET	positron emission tomography
PLED	periodic lateralizing epileptiform discharge
PML	progressive multifocal leukoencephalopathy
PNET	primitive neuroectodermal tumor
PO	"per os" (by mouth)
Po_2	partial pressure of oxygen
PPD	purified protein derivative
PPRF	paramedian pontine reticular formation
PRN	as needed
PT	prothrombin time
PTT	partial thromboplastin time
PVS	persistent vegetative state
qd	every day
qhs	every day at nighttime

qid	four times a day
RA	rheumatoid arthritis
RAM	rapid alternating movements
RBC	red blood cell
RF	rheumatoid factor
RPR	rapid plasmin reagin
SAH	subarachnoid hemorrhage
SBP	systolic blood pressure
SC	subcutaneous
SFEMG	single-fiber electromyogram
SIADH	syndrome of inappropriate antidiuretic hormone
SIMV	synchronized intermittent mandatory ventilation
SL	sublingual
SLE	systemic lupus erythematosus
SMA	spinal muscular atrophy
SMP	sympathetically maintained pain
SPECT	single photon emission computed tomography
SPEP	serum protein electrophoresis
SSEP	somatosensory evoked potential
SSPE	subacute sclerosing panencephalitis
t-PA	tissue plasminogen activator
TCA	tricyclic antidepressant
TCD	transcranial Doppler
TENS	transcutaneous electric nerve stimulation
TFTs	thyroid function tests
TGA	transient global amnesia
TIA	transient ischemic attack
tid	three times a day
TMB	transient monocular blindness
VDRL	Veneral Disease Research Laboratory
VEP	visual evoked potential
VER	visual evoked response
WBC	white blood cell

CONTRIBUTORS

Casilda Balmaceda, MD
Assistant Professor of Clinical
  Neurology and
  Neurosurgery
Columbia University College
  of Physicians and Surgeons
Assistant Attending
  Neurologist
Presbyterian Hospital in the
  City of New York
New York, New York
  *Neoplasms of the Central
    Nervous System*

J. Torres Gluck, MD
Attending Neurosurgeon
Our Lady of Mercy Medical
  Center
New York, New York
  *Neoplasms of the Central
    Nervous System*

Elan D. Louis, MD
Assistant Professor of
  Neurology
Columbia University College
  of Physicians and Surgeons
Assistant Attending
  Neurologist
Presbyterian Hospital in the
  City of New York
New York, New York
  Movement Disorders

Timothy Lynch, MB, MRCPI
Assistant Professor of
  Neurology
Columbia University College
  of Physicians and Surgeons
Assistant Attending
  Neurologist
Presbyterian Hospital in the
  City of New York
New York, New York
  *Demyelinating and
    Inflammatory Disorders of
    the Central Nervous System*

Louis H. Weimer, MD
Assistant Professor of
  Neurology
Columbia University College
  of Physicians and Surgeons
Assistant Attending
  Neurologist
Presbyterian Hospital in the
  City of New York
New York, New York
  Nerve and Muscle Diseases

CONTENTS

SELECTED NEUROLOGIC DISORDERS

APPENDICES

INTRODUCTION

APPROACH TO THE NEUROLOGIC
PATIENT ON CALL

It's in the early morning hours. You get a call from a resident in the emergency room (ER). A 49-year-old woman with rheumatoid arthritis developed double vision after midnight and is having difficulty holding her head up. She is short of breath. How do you proceed? What do you tell the ER resident? What tests should be ordered? How urgent is this situation?

Neurology, perhaps more than any other field in medicine, demands familiarity with a wide spectrum of anatomic details and diagnostic studies. Electrophysiologic, serologic, genetic, pathologic, and a host of imaging techniques have enabled diagnoses to be made with a higher degree of accuracy and certainty than ever before. Yet all diagnostic puzzles, simple or complex, begin with the presentation of a symptom by a patient to a doctor.

It is often said that 90% of the neurologic diagnosis comes from the patient's history. Indeed, it is the exception when a diagnosis is stumbled upon after a "shotgun" approach of ordering diagnostic studies unguided by the patient's initial complaints. In the type of encounter for which this book was written, namely, a rapid response to an acute complaint, the single most important factor in the encounter is the initial interview with the patient. This book aims to guide you through a logical, focused, and effective approach to diagnosis and management of your patient's acute problem. After a discussion of general principles of managing patients on call, some key points about neurologic history taking are covered in this chapter. The neurologic physical examination is outlined in Chapter 2. Differential diagnosis and anatomic localization are discussed in Chapter 3. The basics of the most important initial diagnostic studies are covered in Chapter 4.

■ PRINCIPLES OF MANAGING PATIENTS
WHEN ON CALL

1. **Obtain adequate information from the initial phone contact.**

    Whether the initial telephone contact is with a floor nurse, an emergency room physician, or a neurology colleague, your success at initiating the correct diagnostic and management algorithm depends on obtaining sufficient and appropriate information from the outset. During the initial phone conversation you should establish the nature of the complaint, understand its acuteness and its severity, and learn what has been done so far (e.g., Have vital signs been checked? Has any labwork been sent?). With this baseline information, you will be in a position to ascertain the urgency of the situation, give appropriate orders, and inform the caller how soon you will arrive at the bedside. Specific recommendations for the questions to be asked and orders to be given are outlined under the heading **Phone Call.**

2. **Establish a working differential diagnosis before you see the patient.**

One principle in evaluating a specific complaint in an on-call situation is to establish a reasonable set of diagnoses to consider as you head to the bedside. Some preparatory thought will produce a more efficient and directed interview and examination of the patient. Each chapter presents a limited differential diagnosis under the heading **Elevator Thoughts.**

3. **Prioritize your diagnoses by placing the most potentially dangerous diagnoses at the top of the list.**

Your investigation of the patient's complaint will follow a logical and informed algorithm, with the goal of arriving at a probable diagnosis and at specific management recommendations. Your priority when you are addressing an acute problem on call, however, is to ensure the immediate safety of the patient. After establishing a working differential diagnosis, you should be clear about which diagnoses are predictive of major morbidity or mortality. In this book, we will help you prioritize your differential diagnosis under the heading **Major Threat to Life.**

4. **Be focused in your bedside assessment.**

Unlike the comprehensive examination that you perform when admitting a patient to the hospital or when seeing a patient for the first time in the clinic, your history taking and examination of the patient when you are on call needs to be focused and efficient. Your assessment will begin with the **Quick Look Test.** Is your patient comfortable, in some distress, or about to die? Some situations will call for immediate action, such as the administration of an anticonvulsant for a patient in status epilepticus or the intubation of a myasthenic patient in neuromuscular respiratory failure. Other situations will call for an initial physical assessment, such as a search for signs of trauma or drug intoxication. In most on-call settings, however, once the immediate safety of the patient is ensured, you will embark on a **Selective History** or a **Selective Chart Review.** The physical examination needs to be limited, at least initially. A **Selective Physical Examination** will be outlined in each chapter, with the pertinent elements highlighted for each specific complaint. The focused history and examination is covered in each chapter under the heading **Bedside.**

5. **Know when to call for additional consultation.**

   Most of the complaints covered in this book will be within your realm of knowledge as a neurology resident. In many settings, however, input from other services may be helpful in making the diagnosis or may be necessary to embark on treatment. For example, an ophthalmologic consultation may be crucial to assist with the differential diagnosis of branch retinal artery occlusion versus anterior ischemic optic neuropathy. A neurosurgeon may be needed to place an intracranial pressure monitor or to evaluate for evacuation of a subdural hematoma. If there is any doubt about your course of action, it is always better to obtain the opinion of another specialist or a more experienced clinician.

6. **Make your management recommendations specific and immediate.**

   Most of the calls you will receive while on call will be for an acute neurologic complaint. Although it will be your responsibility to solve the clinical problem as completely as possible, many times you will be unable to make a diagnosis or complete a treatment during the time you are involved with the patient. A crucial diagnostic study may not be available at night, for instance, or the treatment protocol you recommend may extend over the ensuing days or weeks. Reaching a particular step in the diagnostic algorithm may even not be possible until some other piece of information is obtained by the patient's primary team of doctors. Keep in mind that as an on-call neurologist, your primary goal is to establish a diagnosis that is as accurate as possible and to make specific and immediate recommendations for the management of the complaint you are addressing. Such recommendations are discussed under the heading **Management.**

7. **Be accurate and concise in your documentation of the encounter.**

   In most on-call situations you will be asked to see a patient for whom you are not the primary physician. As a result, in addition to your having minimal information at the beginning of the encounter, the assessment you make and the recommendations you give are likely to be followed up by a physician other than you the next morning. The family member or caretaker who provides the initial information may not be available when the primary team takes charge of the patient the next day. You must therefore document the patient's history and physical examination as precisely as possible. Make sure you date and time your note.

If there was a delay in arriving at the bedside because of another emergency, document this. Include relevant laboratory data in your note. Your evaluation and formulation of the problem should be well integrated and transparent. The recommendations for treatment should be stated clearly and should be concordant with what was written in the orders. If discussions with family members took place, the content and outcome of the discussions should be documented.

■ PRINCIPLES OF HISTORY TAKING IN NEUROLOGY

Key features of the neurologic history include the following:

1. **Patient's age**

   Even within the adult neurologic patient population, age is often crucial in the initial consideration of the differential diagnosis. Disorders causing ataxia, for instance, would include multiple sclerosis and viral cerebellitis in patients under 45 years of age, whereas cerebral infarction and alcoholic cerebellar degeneration would be high on the differential diagnosis list for the same syndrome in older patients. Likewise, acute visual loss may result from temporal arteritis in an elderly person, but optic neuritis would be much less likely in that population. Hereditary myopathies rarely present after early adulthood, but myopathy due to polymyositis is a common diagnosis in the elderly.

2. **Patient's gender**

   Aside from some genetic conditions such as X-linked hereditary disorders, most neurologic diseases affect men and women equally. However, some diseases have a predominance in one sex. Benign intracranial hypertension and multiple sclerosis, for example, are more common in women.

3. **Other demographic factors**

   Race, ethnicity, and socioeconomic status are emerging as factors in differential diagnosis as epidemiology and population genetics have become more sophisticated. Although stating the patient's race, ethnicity, socioeconomic status, and sexual orientation may be unnecessary for all presentations, under certain circumstances, these factors may assist in arriving at a diagnosis. For example, in African-American and Hispanic patients, intracranial atherosclerosis is more likely to be the cause for ischemic stroke, whereas in Caucasians, extracranial atherosclerosis tends to develop with higher frequency.

4. **Temporal course of the disease**

   The temporal pattern of your patient's symptoms is one of the most important pieces of history that you will obtain. Many neurologic disorders can be differentiated by their temporal course. Precipitous onset suggests a vascular or epileptic etiology across a wide spectrum of complaints. Onset over minutes to hours suggests a toxic or infectious cause. Subacute or chronic progression of symptoms prompts investigation of metabolic, neoplastic, or degenerative disorders.

The subsequent pattern of symptoms is also important. Symptoms that follow a paroxysmal course lead to a limited differential diagnosis: transient ischemic attack, migraine, and seizure are often considered when paroxysmal episodes are relatively short lived. Myasthenia gravis, multiple sclerosis, and periodic paralysis have a fluctuating or recurrent course as well, but typically with less rapid cycles.

5. Characterization of the symptoms

It may seem excessive or inefficient to obtain a detailed description of your patient's symptoms, yet the initial disqualification of untenable diagnoses can be accomplished with confidence only when you are sure of the symptoms being reported. The patient's explanatory model of the illness may be quite different from your own understanding of pathophysiology. It is not uncommon, for example, for a patient to attribute an unfamiliar symptom to an event or factor in his or her life. Even though you know a brain stem stroke was unlikely to have been caused by "that bad fish I had last night," your therapeutic alliance with the patient, not to mention your ability to elicit a helpful history, relies on your ability to understand the differences between your algorithm for establishing the correct diagnosis and the patient's understanding of the illness. The mode of onset, prior occurrences, surrounding events, and character of the complaint—including what makes it better or worse—are important in establishing an initial differential diagnosis. You may need to ask more than once or use alternative terminology to elicit the details of a particular symptom. Notoriously ambiguous symptom descriptions in neurology include "heavy," which may mean weak, numb, or clumsy; "numb," which may mean decreased sensation or paresthesias; "dizzy," which may mean vertiginous, lightheaded, or confused; and "confused," which may mean disoriented, agitated, aphasic, or even sleepy. Be wary also of actual diagnoses that are presented in lieu of symptoms. The patient who keeps getting "seizures" in the arm or the one who presents with "trauma" should be redirected to a vocabulary of symptoms alone.

6. Medical history

Although a detailed medical history is not necessary in every interview, you will need to obtain information about any disease that could contribute to the patient's present complaint. For example, it is crucial to be aware of cerebro-vascular risk factors including cardiac disease, hypertension, diabetes mellitus, and smoking if stroke is in the differential diagnosis. A history of carcinoma would be important if metastasis or paraneoplastic disease is being considered. Some systemic illnesses, such as sarcoidosis, systemic lupus erythematosus, and diabetes mellitus, may be associated with a spectrum of neurologic complaints. Information regarding current medications should be elicited in every case. Travel and occupational history may be relevant, for example, when toxic and infectious etiologies are under consideration. If the patient cannot provide the necessary information, you may need to interview a family member or caretaker or review the patient's medical record.

7. **Review of systems**

Whereas a complete review of systems may be helpful in the office setting or when a student is learning neurology, the yield of such a "survey" approach is low when you are called to the bedside for a specific complaint. Instead, we advocate a focused questioning of the patient on the basis of a preliminary differential diagnosis. The differential diagnosis should get more restricted as the interview proceeds. The iterative approach to the differential diagnosis is further discussed in Chapter 3.

2

THE NEUROLOGIC EXAMINATION

Clinical examination is of primary importance in the practice of neurology, even with the availability of advanced neuroimaging techniques. **This is because the neurologic examination provides critical information that no other test can provide: it tells you whether the patient's nervous system is working normally.** Unfortunately, many clinicians never master the neurologic examination because it is taught in a way that makes it seem time-consuming, excessively complicated, and sometimes of questionable relevance. In real on-call situations, however, expert neurologists almost never perform the type of comprehensive, top-to-bottom examination that is taught in medical school; rather, they focus on the problem at hand, eliminate those parts of the examination that are not relevant, and actively test hypotheses suggested by the history.

The intent of this chapter is to acquaint (or reacquaint) the physician with the basic components of the neurologic examination. Suggested problem-oriented examinations for specific clinical presentations (e.g., coma, back pain, or acute weakness) are provided in later chapters.

■ THE NEUROLOGIC EXAMINATION

The components of the neurologic examination are shown in Box 2–1.

Box 2–1. COMPONENTS OF THE NEUROLOGIC EXAMINATION

For the beginner, even remembering all of the components of the neurologic exam can be difficult. Memorizing the first letter of the seven main sections of the exam (M C M C R S G) may be helpful for avoiding omissions when first learning the examination:

Mental status
Cranial nerves
Motor
Coordination
Reflexes
Sensory
Gait and station

Mental Status

The importance of the mental status examination cannot be overemphasized. In patients with suspected intracranial pathology (for instance, in those experiencing sudden severe headache), a change in mental status signals that the problem is more than just one of pain: it indicates that the brain is not working correctly. The implications for further workup and management are significant.

Human mentation is extraordinarily complex, and students of neurology frequently have difficulty with the mental status examination because they are taught to evaluate a "laundry-list" of mental functions (Table 2–1) without emphasis on how to integrate the findings. To simplify the mental status examination, we advocate a five-step approach that emphasizes five basic elements: (1) alertness and attention, (2) confusion, disorientation, or abnormal behavior, (3) language, (4) memory, and (5) other higher cortical functions.

- **Step One: Examination of level of consciousness, attention, and concentration**

As illustrated schematically in Figure 2–1, the brain's arousal and attention mechanism (mediated by the diffuse cortical projections of the reticular activating system of the brain stem) serves as the foundation of all higher cognitive function. Level of consciousness, attention, and mental concentration can be conceptualized as three levels of a pyramid, because dysfunction at a more basic level (depressed level of consciousness) almost guarantees that functions at the top of the pyramid (attention and concentration) will be abnormal. Similarly, if a patient cannot remain alert or attend or concentrate, normal functioning of memory, language, or other higher functions cannot be expected. *Delirium* is characterized by severe attentional deficits in a patient with relatively preserved alertness (mildly lethargic to hyperalert).

   1. **Level of consciousness.** *Is the patient alert, lethargic, stuporous, or comatose? Lethargy* resembles sleepiness but with one important difference: the patient cannot be fully and permanently awakened. *Stupor* can be operationally defined by the requirement for painful stimuli to obtain the patient's best verbal or motor response. *Coma* indicates lack of responsiveness even to painful stimuli.

   2. **Attention.** *Is the patient attentive to you?* Global attention is impaired in patients who are lethargic or encephalopathic. A normally attentive patient looks at you and responds to questions and commands immediately. Inattention is characterized by impaired visual fixation and pursuit, delayed verbal responses requiring multiple

Table 2–1 □ MENTAL STATUS: EMOTIONAL AND HIGHER COGNITIVE FUNCTIONS

Behavior	Is the patient's behavior appropriate, hostile, or bizarre?
Abstract reasoning	Can the patient judge similarities and interpret proverbs? Poor abstract reasoning results in "concrete thinking."
Insight	Does the patient have an appropriate understanding of the current medical problem?
Judgment	Is the patient's judgment impaired? Ask what the patient would do if he or she found a wallet or smelled smoke in a theater.
Calculations	Can the patient add, subtract, and multiply?
Visuospatial ability	Can the patient copy figures, draw a clock face, or bisect a line?
Praxis	Does the patient have *apraxia*—the inability to execute motor tasks (whistle or blow out a match) in response to a verbal command (ideational apraxia) or in imitation (ideomotor apraxia) in the absence of a comprehension, sensory, or motor deficit?
Affect	Is the patient's affect (an immediately expressed and observed emotion) depressed, euphoric, restricted, flat, or inappropriate?
Mood	What is the patient's long-term emotional disposition?
Thought form	Does the patient display loosening of associations, flight of ideas, tangentiality, circumstantiality, or incoherence? When seen in the absence of impaired level of consciousness, attention, memory, or language, thought disorders are characteristic of psychiatric illness.
Thought content	Is the patient's thought content characterized by paranoia, delusions, suicidal or homicidal ideation, compulsions, obsessions, phobias, or derealization?
Perceptions	Does the patient have hallucinations or illusions?

prompts, and motor impersistence. *Spatial hemineglect* results from large hemispheric lesions and is almost always associated with impaired global attention as well.

3. **Concentration.** *Can the patient count from 20 to 1 and recite the months in reverse?* These are relatively overlearned tasks and are less susceptible to the effects of prior education than are serial sevens. Abnormal responses include long pauses, omissions, and reversals.

- **Step Two: Assessment for disorientation, confusion, or a behavioral abnormality**

This step is initially based on observation during history

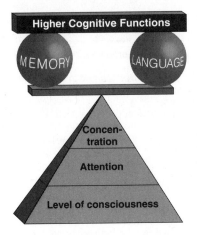

Figure 2–1 □ Schematic representation of the basic elements of human cognition. Arousal mechanisms (level of consciousness, attention, and concentration) serve as the foundation of all mental activity. Language and memory are anatomically localized, highly developed basic cognitive modalities. All other higher cognitive functions depend on normal function of these three basic elements.

taking. *Behavior* should be assessed in terms of psychomotor activity (agitation versus abulia) and emotional responses (elation, sadness, anger, or flattening).

1. **Formally test orientation to name, place, time (date, day of week, month, and year), and situation.** Disorientation reflects abnormal *integrative functioning* of the brain. Unlike abnormalities of arousal, memory, or language, disorientation has no implications with regard to anatomic localization—there is no "orientation center" in the brain. *Remember that disorientation typically follows a sequential pattern, first involving situation, then time, place, and name.* Hence, a patient who is oriented to time and place but who does not know his or her own name probably has a psychiatric problem.

- **Step Three: Language testing**

Focal lesions of the dominant hemisphere may lead to *aphasia*, defined as abnormal language production or comprehension. Four essential components of language should always be tested:

1. **Fluency.** *Is the rate and flow of the patient's speech production normal?* Dysfluency is defined by reduction in the rate of speech production. Speaking with effort, finding words with difficulty, losing normal grammar and syntax, making perseverative responses, and making spontaneous paraphasic errors are characteristic.

2. **Comprehension.** *Can the patient perform one- and two-step commands?* If the patient is attentive, inability to follow commands implies impaired auditory comprehension.

3. **Naming.** *Can the patient name a watch, a pen, and glasses?* Check for *anomia* and *paraphasic errors*. Listen for *phone-*

mic paraphasias (substitution of one phoneme for another, e.g., "tadle" for "table") and *semantic paraphasias* (substitution of one semantically related word for another, e.g., "door" for "window").

4. **Repetition.** *Can the patient repeat "The train was an hour late" and "Today is a sunny day"?* Intact repetition in the presence of serious deficits in fluency or comprehension is diagnostic of *transcortical aphasia,* which implies a good prognosis for recovery.

With the above information—fluency, comprehension, naming, and repetition—you can diagnose and classify any aphasia (Table 2–2). Asking the patient to read aloud is also a sensitive screening test for aphasia and alexia. *Broca's aphasia* (localized to the dorsolateral dominant frontal lobe) results in nonfluent, effortful speech and is usually associated with hemiparesis. *Wernicke's aphasia* (localized to the posterior superior temporal lobe) leads to fluent, nonsensical speech with impaired comprehension, and in most cases, the patient is unaware of the problem (anosognosia). If an aphasia is present and more precise characterization of the deficit is desired, check reading and writing in detail. Don't confuse aphasia with *dysarthria,* which is a motor disorder.

- **Step Four: Memory testing**

  Memory is classified as **immediate, short term,** and **long term.** In neurologic patients, impaired immediate recall is usually due to attentional deficits rather than to pure amnesia. Short-term memory can be tested by asking the patient to recall three words (e.g., "Jane, red, elephant") in 3 to 5 minutes. Long-term (remote) memory is best tested by asking about famous politicians (e.g., Richard M. Nixon or John F.

Table 2–2 □ CLASSIFICATION OF APHASIAS

	Fluency	Compre-hension	Naming	Repetition
Broca's aphasia (motor)	Abnormal	Normal	Abnormal	Abnormal
Wernicke's aphasia (sensory)	Normal	Abnormal	Abnormal	Abnormal
Transcortical motor aphasia	Abnormal	Normal	Abnormal	Normal
Transcortical sensory aphasia	Normal	Abnormal	Abnormal	Normal
Global aphasia	Abnormal	Abnormal	Abnormal	Abnormal
Conduction aphasia	Normal	Normal	Normal	Abnormal
Anomic aphasia	Normal	Normal	Abnormal	Normal

Kennedy), twentieth-century historical events (the Watergate crisis or World War II), or sports figures. *Confabulatory (incorrect)* responses occur with severe amnestic disorders.

- **Step Five: Testing for emotional and higher cognitive functions**

    These components of the mental status exam are listed in Table 2–1 and are usually not anatomically localizable and not essential to test in all cases. They are primarily of value for identifying complex cognitive and neuropsychiatric disorders.

Cranial Nerves

CN 1   **Olfactory nerve**

         Testing for olfactory nerve function is rarely needed and is usually omitted.

CN 2   **Optic nerve**

         1. Fundus

            Check for papilledema, optic disk pallor or atrophy, retinal hemorrhages or exudates, spontaneous venous pulsations, and hypertensive microvascular changes (arteriovenous [AV] nicking and copper wiring) (Fig. 2–2).

         2. Visual fields

            Stand facing the patient, instruct him or her to look at your nose, and have the patient count fingers in all four quadrants (Fig. 2–3). Test each

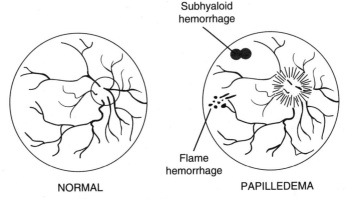

Subhyaloid
hemorrhage

Flame
hemorrhage

NORMAL   PAPILLEDEMA

Figure 2–2 □ Common abnormalities found on examination of the optic fundus. Papilledema is characterized by optic disk congestion and the loss of distinct vessels crossing the blurred disk margin.

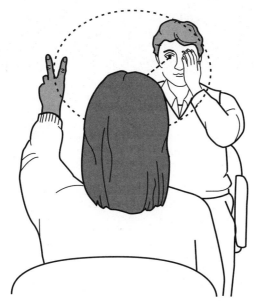

Figure 2–3 □ Technique for visual field testing.

eye separately. Check lateralized blink to threat if the patient is inattentive.
3. Visual acuity
    Test acuity with eyeglasses, one eye at a time, using a "near card."
4. Color vision
    This is usually tested only by an ophthalmologist. Color desaturation occurs with optic nerve disorders.

CN 3,
CN 4,
CN 6

Oculomotor, trochlear, and abducens nerves
1. Eyelids
    Check for *ptosis,* defined as a drooping eyelid that does not clear the upper margin of the pupil. Ptosis occurs with oculomotor nerve (CN 3) injury or with *Horner's syndrome* (ptosis, miosis, facial anhidrosis), which results from injury to central or peripheral sympathetic nerve pathways.
2. Pupils
    Check for shape, symmetry, reactivity to light, and accommodation. *Anisocoria* (pupillary asymmetry) can result from *miosis* (an abnormally small pupil) or *mydriasis* (an abnormally large pu-

pil), and in some cases, examination in both light and dark conditions is necessary to determine which pupil is abnormal.

An *afferent pupillary defect* (APD, or Marcus Gunn pupil) results from a lesion of the optic nerve (e.g., optic neuritis in multiple sclerosis). It is elicited using the swinging flashlight test: as the light swings from one eye to the other at 3-second intervals, the abnormal pupil will *dilate* rather than constrict when the light shines on it.

3. Extraocular movements

Ask the patient to fixate on and follow your finger in all directions of gaze. Unilateral impairment of ocular motility usually results from an isolated cranial nerve deficit. Besides checking for limitations of eye movement, look for abnormalities of *fixation* (square wave jerks, nystagmus, opsoclonus), *smooth pursuit* (saccadic pursuit), and *saccadic eye movements* (hypometric saccades, ocular dysmetria). Test saccades by asking the patient to rapidly switch fixation from one hand to the other.

Opticokinetic nystagmus (OKN) is a normal physiologic nystagmus that occurs when the patient is asked to fixate on a series of moving visual stimuli (e.g., striped OKN tape). Asymmetric loss of OKN results from frontal or parietal lobe lesions on the side to which the tape is moving.

CN 5   **Trigeminal nerve**

Sensory function of V1, V2, and V3 is evaluated by testing for deficits to light touch, pinprick, and temperature on the forehead, cheek, and chin, respectively (Fig. 2–4). Motor function can be tested by palpating the masseters when the teeth are clenched and by checking for asymmetry of lateral jaw movements. Lateral pterygoid muscle weakness results in ipsilateral deviation on jaw opening and weakness of lateral movement to the opposite side.

The *corneal reflex* (mediated by V1) is elicited by lightly touching the cornea with a cotton wisp, which results in contraction of the orbicularis oculi (CN 7). It usually needs to be tested only in comatose patients, or if focal brain stem or cranial nerve pathology (e.g., an acoustic neuroma) is suspected.

CN 7   **Facial nerve**

A *widened palpebral fissure* and *flattened nasolabial fold* are indicative of facial weakness. Ask the patient to grin and raise the eyebrows, and check the strength

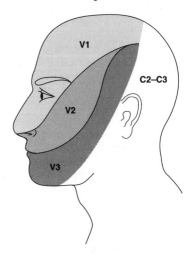

Figure 2–4 □ Sensory distribution of the trigeminal nerve.

of eye and lip closure against active resistance. Upper motor neuron facial weakness tends to spare the contralateral forehead because it has bilateral upper motor neuron innervation, whereas the lower portion of the face does not.

Taste usually requires testing only when there is evidence of facial weakness. Dip a wet cotton swab in sugar or salt and apply it to the tip and side of the tongue with the tongue kept protruded. Absence of taste confirms a peripheral CN 7 lesion proximal to the junction of the chorda tympani.

CN 8   **Vestibulocochlear nerve**
Auditory deficits can be screened for by testing appreciation of *finger rub* in each ear. If unilateral hearing loss is present, sensorineural and conduction deafness can be differentiated using a 512-Hz tuning fork:

- *Weber's test* is performed by striking the tuning fork and placing it against the middle of the forehead. Ask the patient if the tone is equal in both ears. Diminution in the affected ear indicates sensorineural hearing loss. A louder tone in the affected ear results from *conduction deafness* (disease of the ossicles in the middle ear). In conduction deafness, a pure tone transmitted through the skull is appreciated in the affected ear, whereas the tone sounds softer in the normal ear because of competing ambient noise transmitted via the tympanic membrane and ossicles.

- *The Rinne test* is performed to confirm the presence of conduction deafness in the affected ear. Strike the tuning fork, place it on the mastoid process, and ask the patient when the tone can no longer be heard. Then place it over the external auditory meatus—normally, the patient will hear the tone again; if not, conduction deafness is present.

CN 9, CN 10 **Glossopharyngeal and vagus nerves**
Ask the patient to say "ah," check for symmetry and adequacy of soft palate elevation, and listen for hoarseness or nasal speech (all motor functions of CN 10). The gag reflex, tested by lightly touching the posterior oropharynx with a cotton swab (CN 9 sensory, CN 10 motor), is often absent or depressed in older patients. *Dysphagia* and risk for aspiration are best screened for by asking the patient to swallow a small quantity of water (3 oz); coughing indicates aspiration and inability to protect the airway.

CN 11 **Spinal accessory nerve**
Have the patient flex and turn the head to each side against resistance (tests the sternocleidomastoid muscle). Contraction of the left sternocleidomastoid muscle turns the head to the right and vice versa. Have the patient shrug the shoulders against resistance to test the trapezius muscle.

CN 12 **Glossopharyngeal nerve**
Have the patient stick out the tongue and push it into each cheek. Unilateral CN 12 dysfunction results in deviation of the tongue to the weak side upon protrusion and in inability to push the tongue into the opposite cheek.

Motor

1. **Inspection**
Look for *muscle wasting* (atrophy), *facsiculations,* and *adventitious movements*. Preferential spontaneous movement of the limbs on one side suggests paresis of the unused limbs. If the patient is comatose, check for a preferential localizing response to sternal rub.
Tremor should be evaluated at rest (rest tremor), with sustained posture (postural tremor), and with active movement (action or intention tremor).

2. **Tone**
Have the patient relax; check muscle tone by passively moving the elbows, wrists, and knees.

a. **Hypotonia** occurs with acute paralysis, lower motor neuron disease, ipsilateral cerebellar lesions, and chorea.
b. **Hypertonia** comes in three varieties:
   (1) **Spasticity** develops as a consequence of upper motor neuron lesions. It is generally characterized by a sudden increase in tone (a "catch") as the limb is passively flexed or extended. The clasp-knife phenomenon is a particular form of spasticity sometimes encountered in the legs; muscle tone is greatest at the beginning of movement and slowly decreases until there is a sudden loss of resistance.
   (2) **Rigidity** occurs with disease of the basal ganglia. Increased resistance is present throughout the full range of motion. *Cogwheel rigidity,* characterized by a regular ratchet-like loss of resistance, is especially characteristic of parkinsonism. Cogwheel rigidity at the wrist can often be accentuated if the patient is asked to repeatedly open and close the opposite hand.
   (3) **Gegenhalten** (holding against), or paratonia, occurs with dementia and frontal lobe syndromes. It is characterized by a variably and inconsistently increased tone that alternates with relaxation.
3. **Screening tests for hemiparesis**
   In many instances, cerebral lesions lead to subtle hemiparesis with normal strength against resistance. Check the following to screen for subtle indications of hemiparesis (Fig. 2–5):

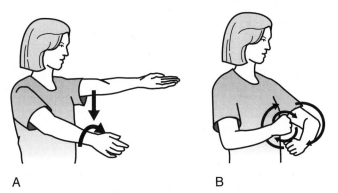

A   B

Figure 2–5 □ Screening procedures for mild hemiparesis. *A,* Pronator drift: the weaker right arm drifts downward and pronates. *B,* Arm-rolling test: the stronger left arm tends to "orbit" the weaker right arm.

a. **Pronator drift**
   Have the patient hold both arms forward, palms up, with eyes closed. Check for pronation and downward drift.
b. **Rapid finger taps**
   Check thumb and forefinger taps in each hand separately. Although often considered a sign of cerebellar dysfunction, slowing of fine rapid finger movements also occurs with corticospinal tract lesions.
c. **Arm-rolling test**
   Have the patient make fists and rotate the forearms around each other. With hemiparesis, the normal arm will tend to orbit the weaker arm.
4. **Power**
   Detailed testing of strength against active resistance in multiple individual muscle groups is usually unnecessary unless a peripheral cause of weakness is suspected. *For screening purposes, testing of strength at the shoulders, wrists, hips, and ankles will often suffice.* Be aware that estimates of lower extremity strength in bedridden patients are often unreliable and that walking is the best way to screen for leg weakness.
   By convention, muscle strength is graded using the following scale:

   0   No muscle contraction detected
   1   A barely detectable flicker or trace of contraction
   2   Movement occurs only in the plane of gravity
   3   Active movement against gravity but not against resistance
   4   Active movement against resistance but less than normal strength (may be graded as 4+, 4, or 4−)
   5   Normal strength

Coordination

Disease of the cerebellar hemispheres leads to limb ataxia, whereas midline cerebellar lesions lead to gait ataxia. The following tests can be used to detect incoordination and ataxia.
1. **Finger-to-nose test**
   Have the patient alternately touch a fingertip to his or her nose and your finger. Check for intention tremor (irregular chaotic movements as the target is approached) and past pointing (often easier to elicit when the eyes are closed).
2. **Rapid rhythmic alternating movements**
   Have the patient touch each of the fingers to the thumb in rapid succession, turn the hand over and back (pronation-supination) as fast as possible, and touch the toe and the heel to the floor in rapid succession. With cerebellar disease, these movements are slow and awkward (*dysdiadochokinesis*).

3. **Heel-to-shin test**
   Have the patient slide the heel up and down the front of the shin. Limb ataxia results in a side-to-side "tremor" as the test is performed.

Reflexes

1. **Deep tendon reflexes**
   Striking the muscle tendon with a reflex hammer normally leads to a reflex muscle contraction mediated by the lower motor neuron reflex arc. *Hyperreflexia* results from upper motor neuron lesions as a result of release from normal descending inhibition, whereas *hyporeflexia* results from lesions of the lower motor neuron. The principal deep tendon reflexes and their corresponding spinal roots are listed in Table 2–3. Severe hyperreflexia results in *clonus*—repeated rhythmic contraction elicited by striking a tendon or dorsiflexing the ankle.
   By convention, deep tendon reflexes are graded as follows:

0	Absent
1+	Diminished
2+	Normal
3+	Increased (may spread to adjacent muscles)
4+	Unsustained clonus (a few beats)
5+	Sustained clonus

2. **Plantar reflex**
   Firmly stroke the sole of the patient's foot with the handle end of your reflex hammer, beginning at the heel and following up the lateral margin and across the ball of the foot to the base of the big toe. Flexion of the big toe at the metatarsophalangeal joint is the normal response; extension (*Babinski's sign*) occurs with upper motor neuron lesions. If the patient is sensitive, lightly stroking the lateral heel alone is often enough to elicit a normal response.

Table 2–3 □ DEEP TENDON REFLEXES

Reflex	Segments
Jaw jerk	Trigeminal nerve (CN 5)
Biceps reflex	C5 and C6
Brachioradialis reflex	C5 and C6
Triceps reflex	C7 and C8
Finger flexion reflex (Hoffman's reflex)	C8 and T1
Knee reflex	L2, L3, and L4
Ankle reflex	S1

3. **Cutaneous reflexes**

These reflexes do not require routine testing, but their testing is useful when a spinal cord or a cauda equina lesion is suspected. They are frequently absent in otherwise normal elderly or obese individuals. The presence of these reflexes implies normal function of the spinal cord and corresponding sensory and motor nerves:

a. **Abdominal reflexes**

Use a key, wooden stick, or reflex hammer handle to lightly stroke from the lateral to the medial section of the abdomen above (T8–T9) and below (T11–T12) the umbilicus. The normal response is local contraction of the ipsilateral rectus abdominis muscle.

b. **Cremasteric reflex**

Striking the medial thigh (L1–L2) results in ipsilateral retraction of the scrotum (S1).

c. **Bulbocavernosus reflex and anal wink**

Squeezing the head of the penis (S2–S3) or stroking the perianal skin (S3–S4) results in reflex contraction of the external anal sphincter (S3–S4).

4. **Frontal release signs**

These primitive reflexes are typically seen with dementia or frontal lobe disease, but they may also occur in normal individuals.

a. **Snout, suck, and root reflexes**

These reflexes are elicited by lightly tapping the upper lip or the side of the mouth.

b. **Palmomental reflex**

Lightly stroking the palm results in ipsilateral contraction of the mentalis muscle. A unilateral palmomental contraction implies contralateral frontal lobe disease.

c. **Grasp reflex**

Placing two fingers in the palm results in involuntary grasping.

d. **Glabellar reflex**

Obligatory blinking occurs each time the glabellar area between the eyes is tapped.

Sensory

Sensory testing, because of its subjectivity, is the most difficult and least reliable part of the neurologic examination. In patients with depressed level of consciousness or severe inattention, sensory testing usually provides little useful information and should be omitted. In most cases, testing for signs of sensory loss is unnecessary unless the patient has symptoms of sensory loss. **The key to a successful and efficient sensory exam is to know**

what you're looking for. Sensory loss typically occurs in specific patterns, which you should try to rule in or rule out:

- Hemisensory loss (cortical lesions)
- Stocking-glove sensory loss (neuropathy)
- Spinal level and Brown-Séquard's syndrome (spinal cord lesions)
- Dermatomal sensory loss (nerve root lesions)
- Peripheral nerve sensory loss (mononeuropathy)
- Saddle anesthesia (lesion in cauda equina or conus medullaris)

A few simple rules can help make the sensory examination easier:

Box 2–2. RULES FOR SENSORY EXAMINATION

1. *Don't ask leading questions.*
     When testing for hemisensory loss, ask "Does this feel the same on both sides?" If you ask "Which side feels sharper?", you are likely to get inconsistent (and insignificant) lateralizing responses.
2. *When mapping a region of sensory loss, move from the affected into the normal region.*
     Patients are better able to detect when a pinprick turns sharp than when it becomes dull.
3. *Beware of fatigue.*
     Cooperation in the sensory examination takes concentration, and patients may become fatigued. Rather than taking a thorough, top-to-bottom approach, start your sensory examination by getting right to the point.

---

1. **Primary sensory modalities**
    Sensation is mediated by two pathways: the dorsal columns, which mediate vibration and joint position, and the spinothalamic tracts, which mediate pain and temperature. Touch is mediated by both sensory pathways and is thus usually the last modality to be affected.
    a. **Light touch**
        Test by lightly touching with fingertips or cotton wool.
    b. **Pinprick**
        Use a clean safety pin. *Hyperalgesia* refers to an exaggerated painful sensation; *hyperpathia* refers to an abnormal painful sensation (e.g., burning, tingling).
    c. **Temperature**
        Test with the handle of a reflex hammer or tuning fork submerged under cold tap water.

d. **Vibration**

Apply a 128-Hz tuning fork to the toes, medial malleolus, patella, fingers, wrist, and elbow, and ask when the sensation stops. In the elderly, vibration is commonly absent or reduced in the feet.

e. **Joint position (proprioception)**

Grasp the sides of the digit and ask the patient to identify small (5 to 10 degrees), random, up or down movements. Remember that even with complete proprioceptive loss, 50% of responses will be correct!

2. **Cortical sensory modalities**

If the primary sensory modalities are intact, disturbances of these modalities imply dysfunction of the contralateral parietal lobe. *The main utility of cortical sensory testing is for the detection of subtle hemisensory neglect.*

a. **Double simultaneous stimulation (face-hand test)**

Have the patient close the eyes; quickly touch one cheek and the contralateral hand at the same time. *Extinction* refers to consistent neglect of the hand stimulus on one side and implies a lesion of the contralateral parietal lobe. *Caudal neglect* refers to the tendency to consistently neglect the hand stimulus on either side; it occurs with dementia and frontal lobe disease.

b. **Graphesthesia**

Have the patient close the eyes and identify a number traced on the palm.

c. **Stereognosis**

Ask the patient to close the eyes and identify a key, coin, paperclip, or similar object placed in the palm.

Gait and Station

Disturbances of gait can result from dysfunction in one of many neurologic subsystems, including the motor cortex, corticospinal tracts, basal ganglia, cerebellum, vestibular system, peripheral nerves, muscles, and visual and proprioceptive afferent tracts. **Hence, gait testing is an excellent screening procedure, and many practitioners make it the first part of the neurologic examination.**

Specific components of gait analysis include *posture, width of stance, length of stride, arm swing,* and *balance.* Specific types of gait disturbance are listed in Table 2–4. Test the following:

- Natural gait

  Tandem gait

  Have the patient walk a straight line, touching toe to heel.
- Toe walking
- Heel walking

Table 2–4 □ SOME ABNORMALITIES OF GAIT

Gait	Features
Hemiparetic	Patient drags or circumducts the affected leg (moves stiffly in a circular motion outward and forward) and has a reduced ipsilateral arm swing
Ataxic	Patient has a wide-based stance with a veering and staggering gait; patient may consistently fall to the same side as the affected cerebellum
Parkinsonian	Patient has a stooped posture, takes small steps (festination), hestitates and freezes, and turns "en bloc"
Steppage	Patient lifts the knee high off the ground because of inability to dorsiflex at the ankle; patient has foot slap (results from peripheral neuropathy)
Waddling	Patient's pelvis drops on non–weight-bearing side with each step (results from myopathy with hip girdle weakness)
Scissor	Patient's gait is stiff, with short steps that cross forward on each other (results from spastic paraparesis)
Apraxic	Patient's gait is slow and unsteady; patient has trouble initiating steps, and the feet barely elevate off the floor (i.e., "magnetic gait") (results from hydrocephalus or frontal lobe disease)
Hysterical	Patient has a bizarre, wild, careening gait but never falls; patient shows excellent balance

- Sitting to standing

  To assess proximal leg strength, have the patient stand up from a chair with the arms folded.

- Romberg's test

  Have the patient stand with eyes open and feet together. If the patient cannot do so, suspect a severe cerebellar or vestibular disturbance. *If substantial instability or falling occurs only after the patient closes the eyes, Romberg's test is positive.* A positive test indicates either *proprioceptive* (i.e., neuropathy or dorsal column disease) or *vestibular* dysfunction.

- Pull test

  Stand behind the patient and pull back on the shoulders. Normally, the patient should be able to regain balance after one step. Falling or retropulsion (many backward steps) suggests *impaired postural reflexes,* as occurs with parkinsonism.

3

DIFFERENTIAL DIAGNOSIS AND
ANATOMIC LOCALIZATION

The classic approach to differential diagnosis is to obtain the history and to perform the physical examination in a more or less blinded fashion, and then to compile a list of all possible diagnoses from which each diagnosis is rated reasonable, unlikely, or untenable. Such an approach may be useful in didactic sessions in which both time and textbooks are abundant. The approach we will take in this book, however, and the approach used most often in the clinical setting is to establish a list of possible diagnoses based on preliminary information from an initial telephone contact, and then to narrow the differential diagnosis list iteratively after proceeding through the history, chart review, and examination of the patient. The end result will be a short list of diagnoses—one or two common disorders, one or two conditions that could be life-threatening or dangerous, and one or two rare conditions that could become important considerations once the most common and the most dangerous possibilities have been eliminated. Each chapter in the **Patient-Related Problems** section of this book will prompt you to ask the proper questions to establish the initial differential diagnosis and will then guide you through a focused history and examination to narrow your list to the appropriate final diagnosis.

■ ESTABLISHING THE INITIAL DIFFERENTIAL DIAGNOSIS

Neurologic complaints lend themselves to categorization of the differential diagnosis based on **anatomic localization.** Acute visual dysfunction, for example, may be divided into unilateral loss of vision (suggesting pathology in the retina or optic nerve), binocular visual field defects (implying disease in the optic tracts or radiations), or diplopia (suggesting either neuromuscular or brain stem dysfunction). Other neurologic complaints are best categorized initially by the **rate of onset.** The likely diagnoses related to acute ataxia, for instance, are different from those associated with chronic or subacute gait failure. The differential diagnosis for many neurologic complaints, however, contains a wide variety of disorders that are not easily sorted until more information is obtained from the history and physical examination. For these complaints, we suggest that you develop a stan-

Table 3–1 □ **MNEMONIC FOR THE DIFFERENTIAL DIAGNOSIS OF NEUROLOGIC DISORDERS**

V:	Vascular
I:	Infectious
T:	Traumatic
A:	Autoimmune
M:	Metabolic/toxic
I:	Iatrogenic, Idiopathic/hereditary
N:	Neoplastic
S:	Seizure, pSychiatric, Structural

dard method of considering the differential diagnosis. One mnemonic, which appears in many of our patient complaint chapters, may be useful: VITAMINS. Some categories related to this mnemonic are unique to neurologic differential diagnosis, but others may overlap with other mnemonics you have used in the past. Some neurologic complaints require consideration of many diagnoses in one category and few or none in others, but we have tried to present the differential diagnosis in the VITAMINS format whenever possible in this book. The categories represented are outined in Table 3–1. The differential diagnosis appears under the heading **Elevator Thoughts** in each chapter to emphasize the approach of beginning with a broad view and then rapidly focusing on the few most important diagnoses as the encounter with the patient proceeds.

■ **ANATOMIC LOCALIZATION**

The neurologic examination is presented in Chapter 2. Certain principles of anatomic localization warrant emphasis here, because establishing the correct diagnosis in neurology is often dependent on localization of the lesion. Listed here in tabular form are general principles of localization of lesions from the brain to the periphery. Most of these localizations are discussed within the pertinent **Patient-Related Problems** chapters.

Localization in the Upper Motor Neuron (Pyramidal) System

Principle: Tone is increased, causing spasticity and hyperreflexia.

Site	Symptoms	Signs
Cortex	• Differential weakness of limbs and face • Sensory symptoms • Language, visual, or attentional alterations	• Fractionated weakness (e.g., arm greater than face and leg) • Aphasia, hemianopia, or hemineglect • Cortical and primary sensory loss • Cognitive dysfunction
Corona radiata	• Differential weakness of limbs and face	• Fractionated weakness • Primary sensory loss
Internal capsule	• Weakness only	• Face, arm, and leg affected equally and densely
Brain stem	• Unilateral or bilateral weakness • Diplopia, vertigo, dysarthria, or dysphagia	• Dense hemiparesis • Ocular or oropharyngeal weakness
Spinal cord	• Difficulty with gait • Difficulty walking • Urinary incontinence	• No face involvement • Spastic quadriparesis (cervical) or paraparesis (thoracic) • Sensory level

Localization in the Lower Motor Neuron System

Principle: Tone is decreased, causing flaccidity and hyporeflexia.

Site	Symptoms	Signs
Anterior horn	• Progressive flaccid weakness	• Wasting, weakness, fasciculations • No sensory loss
Root/plexus	• Single limb weakness and sensory loss • Pain in the neck, back, or limb	• Weakness in radicular/plexus distribution • Electromyogram (EMG) shows denervation in affected muscles

Nerve	• Focal weakness (mononeuritis) • Distal weakness (polyneuropathy)	• Focal or distal weakness • Atrophy in affected distribution • Fasciculations • Hyporeflexia • Slowing or low amplitude on conduction studies; denervation on EMG
Neuromuscular junction	• Fluctuating weakness • Diplopia	• Positive edrophonium test • Decremental response with repetitive stimulation on EMG
Muscle	• Proximal weakness • Difficulty climbing stairs and brushing hair • Muscle aches	• Proximal weakness • Normal nerve conduction • Polyphasic, low-amplitude motor units on EMG

Localization Within the Brain Stem

Principle: Specific cranial nerve involvement guides localization (Fig. 3–1).

Site   **Signs and symptoms**

Midbrain
- Impaired vertical gaze
- **CN 3 palsy** (plus contralateral abduction nystagmus suggests ipsilateral internuclear ophthalmoplegia [INO])
- **CN 4 palsy**
- Contralateral motor signs (hemiparesis suggests Weber's syndrome; ataxia suggests Claude's syndrome; tremor or chorea suggests Benedikt's syndrome)
- Alterations in consciousness, perception, or behavior (peduncular hallucinosis)

Pons
- Dysarthria and dysphagia
- Contralateral hemiparesis or hemisensory loss
- Ipsilateral facial sensory loss **(CN 5)**
- Ipsilateral gaze palsy (paramedian pontine reticular formation [PPRF]) or one-and-a-half

syndrome (PPRF and median longitudinal fasciculus [MLF])
- Locked-in syndrome (bilateral basis pontis; associated with ocular bobbing)
- Horizontal nystagmus (often brachium pontis)
- Ataxia

Pontomedullary junction	• Vertigo **(CN 8)** • Dysarthria • Horizontal or vertical nystagmus • Contralateral hemisensory loss and hemiparesis
Lateral medulla (Wallenberg syndrome)	• Ipsilateral Horner's syndrome • Ipsilateral limb ataxia • Ipsilateral face and contralateral body numbness • Gait ataxia • Vertigo, dizziness **(CN 8)** • Dysphagia **(CN 9, CN 10, and CN 12 palsies)**
Medial medulla (rare)	• Hemiplegia • Contralateral posterior column sensory loss • Ipsilateral tongue weakness **(CN 12 palsy)**

Localization in the Spinal Cord

Principle: Localization is assisted by the combination of tracts involved.

Site	Signs and symptoms	Common causes
Hemicord (Brown-Séquard's syndrome)	• Ipsilateral hemiparesis • Contralateral spinothalamic sensory loss • Ipsilateral dorsal column sensory loss • Sphincter dysfunction	• Penetrating trauma • Extrinsic cord compression
Anterior cord	• Upper and lower motor paralysis • Spinothalamic sensory loss • Sphincter dysfunction • Sparing of posterior columns	• Anterior spinal artery infarction (often involves T4 to T8)

Central cord	• Paraparesis • Lower motor paralysis; wasting and fasciculations in arms • Sensory loss in "shawl" distribution (if in cervical region)	• Syringomyelia • Neck flexion-extension injury • Intrinsic tumor
Posterior cord	• Proprioceptive and vibratory sensory loss • Segmental tingling and numbness • Sensation of constricting "bands"	• Vitamin B_{12} deficiency • Demyelination (multiple sclerosis) • Extrinsic compression
Foramen magnum	• Spastic quadriparesis • Neck pain and stiffness • C2 to C4 and upper facial numbness • Ipsilateral Horner's syndrome • Ipsilateral tongue and trapezius muscle weakness	• Tumor (meningioma, chordoma) • Atlantoaxial subluxation
Conus medullaris	• Lower sacral saddle sensory loss (S2 to S5) • Sphincter dysfunction; impotence • Aching back or rectal pain • L5 and S1 motor deficits (ankle and foot weakness)	• Intrinsic tumor • Extrinsic cord compression
Cauda equina	• Sphincter dysfunction • Paraparesis with weakness in the distribution of multiple roots • Sensory loss in multiple bilateral dermatomes	• Extrinsic tumor • Carcinomatous meningitis • Arachnoiditis • Spinal stenosis

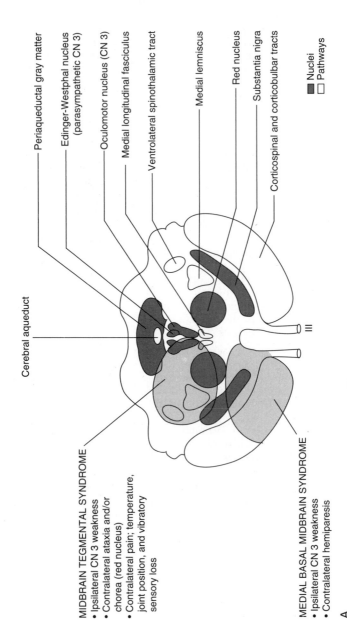

Periaqueductal gray matter

Edinger-Westphal nucleus (parasympathetic CN 3)

Oculomotor nucleus (CN 3)

Medial longitudinal fasciculus

Ventrolateral spinothalamic tract

Medial lemniscus

Red nucleus

Substantia nigra

Corticospinal and corticobulbar tracts

■ Nuclei
□ Pathways

Cerebral aqueduct

MIDBRAIN TEGMENTAL SYNDROME
• Ipsilateral CN 3 weakness
• Contralateral ataxia and/or chorea (red nucleus)
• Contralateral pain; temperature, joint position, and vibratory sensory loss

MEDIAL BASAL MIDBRAIN SYNDROME
• Ipsilateral CN 3 weakness
• Contralateral hemiparesis

A

III

Figure 3–1 □ Brain stem sections at the level of the midbrain (*A*), pons (*B*), and medulla (*C*).

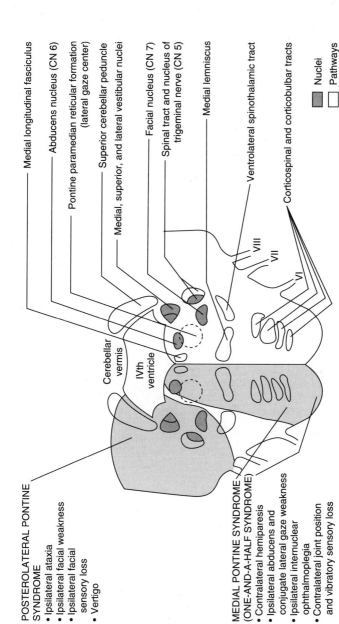

Medial longitudinal fasciculus

Abducens nucleus (CN 6)

Pontine paramedian reticular formation (lateral gaze center)

Superior cerebellar peduncle

Medial, superior, and lateral vestibular nuclei

Facial nucleus (CN 7)

Spinal tract and nucleus of trigeminal nerve (CN 5)

Medial lemniscus

Ventrolateral spinothalamic tract

Corticospinal and corticobulbar tracts

Nuclei

Pathways

Cerebellar vermis

IVth ventricle

VIII

VII

VI

POSTEROLATERAL PONTINE SYNDROME
- Ipsilateral ataxia
- Ipsilateral facial weakness
- Ipsilateral facial sensory loss
- Vertigo

MEDIAL PONTINE SYNDROME (ONE-AND-A-HALF SYNDROME)
- Contralateral hemiparesis
- Ipsilateral abducens and conjugate lateral gaze weakness
- Ipsilateral internuclear ophthalmoplegia
- Contralateral joint position and vibratory sensory loss

B

Figure 3–1 □ Continued

33

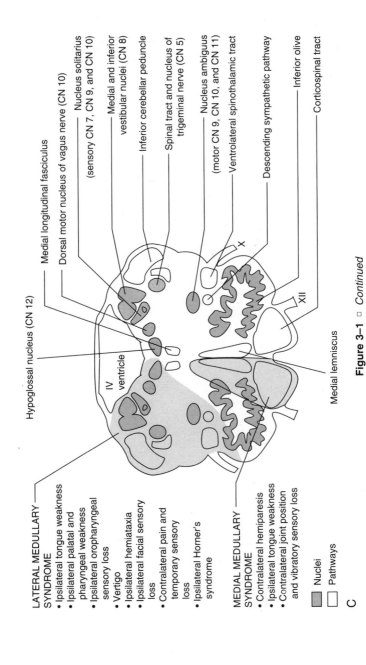

Hypoglossal nucleus (CN 12)

Medial longitudinal fasciculus

Dorsal motor nucleus of vagus nerve (CN 10)

Nucleus solitarius
(sensory CN 7, CN 9, and CN 10)

Medial and inferior
vestibular nuclei (CN 8)

Inferior cerebellar peduncle

Spinal tract and nucleus of
trigeminal nerve (CN 5)

Nucleus ambiguus
(motor CN 9, CN 10, and CN 11)

Ventrolateral spinothalamic tract

Descending sympathetic pathway

Inferior olive

Corticospinal tract

IV ventricle

X

XII

Medial lemniscus

LATERAL MEDULLARY
SYNDROME
• Ipsilateral tongue weakness
• Ipsilateral palatal and
  pharyngeal weakness
• Ipsilateral oropharyngeal
  sensory loss
• Vertigo
• Ipsilateral hemiataxia
• Ipsilateral facial sensory
  loss
• Contralateral pain and
  temporary sensory
  loss
• Ipsilateral Horner's
  syndrome

MEDIAL MEDULLARY
SYNDROME
• Contralateral hemiparesis
• Ipsilateral tongue weakness
• Contralateral joint position
  and vibratory sensory loss

■ Nuclei
□ Pathways

C

Figure 3–1 □ *Continued*

4

DIAGNOSTIC STUDIES

A thorough history and examination should enable you to localize the disease process and generate a differential diagnosis. Confirmation of the diagnosis will usually require neurodiagnostic testing. When any of the tests described below are performed, it is essential to know what you're looking for and to understand the sensitivity (likelihood of a true positive result if the disease is present) and specificity (likelihood of a true negative result if the disease is absent) of each test for diagnosing the disease in question. Risks, benefits, and cost must also be considered.

■ LUMBAR PUNCTURE

Examination of the cerebrospinal fluid (CSF) by lumbar puncture (LP) is essential for diagnosing meningitis and subarachnoid hemorrhage when computed tomography (CT) is negative. It can also be helpful in evaluating peripheral neuropathy, carcinomatous meningitis, pseudotumor cerebri, multiple sclerosis (MS), and a variety of other inflammatory disorders.

- **Technique of LP**

    Proper positioning is the key to success (Fig. 4–1). Have the patient's back right up to the edge of the bed, the head flexed, and the legs curled up in the fetal position. Place a pillow under the head; it may be helpful to place another pillow between the legs. *Ensure that the shoulders and hips are parallel to each other and perpendicular to the bed* (i.e., not tilted forward). Locate the interspace between L4 and L5, which lies at the intercristal line (across the tops of the iliac crests), and insert the needle one level above, between L3 and L4. After sterilizing the area and locally injecting xylocaine, insert a 20- or 22-gauge needle, parallel to the bed and tilted slightly cephalad. As you enter the subarachnoid space, you will feel a slight "pop." Measure the opening pressure and collect the CSF.

- **Examination of the CSF**

    This should always include a cell count (2 ml), protein and glucose analysis (2 ml), a Gram stain and culture (2 ml), and a CSF Venereal Disease Research Laboratory (VDRL) test (1 ml). Additional CSF tests are listed in Table 4–1. If red blood cells (RBCs) are encountered, check for xanthochromia, a yellowish tinge that differentiates true subarachnoid hemor-

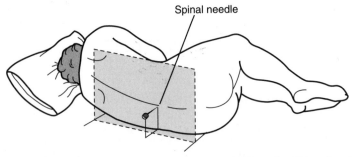

Spinal needle

Figure 4–1 □ Positioning for lumbar puncture. A pillow should be placed beneath the head. Hips and shoulders should be parallel to each other and perpendicular to the bed. The spinal needle should be parallel to the bed.

rhage (>12 hours old) from a traumatic tap. To evaluate the significance of white blood cells (WBCs) in a traumatic tap, recall that the normal ratio of WBCs to RBCs in peripheral blood is 1:700.

- **Complications of LP**

The most frequent complication (in approximately 5% of patients) of LP is *spinal headache,* which results from persistent leakage of CSF from the entry site, leading to low intracranial pressure (ICP) and traction on the pain-sensitive intracranial

Table 4–1 □ CSF TESTS

- Cell count
- Protein and glucose levels
- Gram stain and culture
- VDRL test
- India ink test (for *Cryptococcus neoformans*)
- Wet smear (for fungi and amebae)
- Stain and culture for AFB (for tuberculosis)
- Cryptococcal antigen titers
- pH and lactate levels (abnormal in MELAS)
- Oligoclonal bands (abnormal in multiple sclerosis)
- IgG index (intrathecal IgG production)
- Bacterial antigen tests (for pneumococcus, meningococcus, and *Haemophilus influenzae*)
- Viral isolation studies
- Cytology (requires fixation in formalin)
- Lyme disease antibody titers (compare with serum titers)
- Polymerase chain reaction for Lyme disease, tuberculosis, HSV-1 infection, cytomegalovirus infection, and others

AFB = acid-fast bacteria; CSF = cerebrospinal fluid; HSV-1 = herpes simplex virus 1; IgG = immunoglobulin G; MELAS = mitochondrial encephalomyopathy, lactic acidosis, and stroke; VDRL = Venereal Disease Research Laboratory.

dura when the patient is upright. The risk is minimized by keeping the patient supine for 3 to 6 hours after the procedure. Other complications are rare and occur only in patients with predisposing conditions: (1) *meningitis* can result if the needle is passed through infected tissue (e.g., cellulitis) before penetrating the dura, (2) *epidural hematoma* with compression of the cauda equina can result in patients with coagulopathy, (3) *tentorial herniation* can result in patients who have space-occupying lesions or severe basilar meningitis, and (4) *complete spinal block* and cord compression can result in patients who have a partial spinal block. These predisposing conditions are relative (not absolute) contraindications to LP, and the risk/benefit ratio of performing or not performing the procedure needs to be considered in each case.

■ COMPUTED TOMOGRAPHY

CT provides "slice" images of the brain by sending axial x-ray beams through the head. The amount of radiation involved is essentially harmless. Tissues are differentiated by the degree to which they attenuate the x-ray beams:

Low attenuation (appears **black**):	Air (darkest)
	Fat
	CSF and water
Medium attenuation (appears **gray**):	Edematous or infarcted brain
	Normal brain
	Subacute hemorrhage (5 to 14 days old)
High attenuation (appears **white**):	Hemorrhage
	Intravenous contrast material
	Bone or metal (brightest)

- **Intravenous contrast material**
  When injected, contrast is normally confined to the cerebral vessels. Hence, *contrast enhancement detects the presence of a disrupted blood-brain barrier.* Contrast is useful in patients with suspected neoplasm, abscess, vascular malformation, or new-onset seizures.

■ MAGNETIC RESONANCE IMAGING

Magnetic resonance imaging (MRI) provides greater resolution and detail than does CT but takes longer to perform. MRI is superior to CT for evaluating the brain stem and posterior fossa and is superior to myelography for identifying intramedullary spinal cord lesions. Because it uses a powerful magnetic field, there is no exposure to radiation. However, MRI is contraindicated in patients with implanted ferromagnetic objects such as pacemakers, orthopedic pins, and older aneurysm clips.

- **T1 images**

  T1 images are best for showing *anatomy*. CSF and bone appear black, normal brain appears gray, fat and subacute hemorrhage (>48 hours old) appear white. Most pathologic processes (e.g., infarction or tumor) are associated with increased water content and hence appear darker than normal brain.

- **T2 images**

  T2 images are best for showing *pathology*. CSF and brain edema appear white (high signal, long T2), normal brain is gray, and bone appears black. Most pathologic processes (e.g., infarction, tumor) lead to bright high-signal (white) changes on T2 images. Blood on a T2 image varies in signal intensity according to the age of the hemorrhage, as depicted in Table 4–2.

- **Flow voids**

  Flow voids appear black on both T1 and T2 images and represent high-velocity blood flow (e.g., normal cerebral vessels or arteriovenous malformations [AVMs]).

- **Proton density images**

  Proton density images are partway between T1 and T2 images. Their main utility is for differentiating periventricular pathology (e.g., white matter demyelination) from CSF.

- **MR angiography**

  MR angiography produces images of the extracranial and intracranial cerebral circulation with the brain and skull images erased. The resolution is adequate for the evaluation of

Table 4–2 □ EVOLUTION OF APPEARANCE OF HEMORRHAGE ON MRI

Feature	T1 Image	T2 Image	Metabolic Change
Blood			
4–6 hours	No change	○	Intact RBC with oxyhemoglobin
7–72 hours	No change	●	Intact RBC with deoxyhemoglobin
4–7 days	○	●	Intact RBC with methemoglobin
1–4 weeks	○	○	Free methemoglobin
Months	●	●	Hemosiderin with macrophages
Edema	●	○	Increased water content

● = low signal, appears dark; ○ = high signal, appears bright; MRI = magnetic resonance imaging; RBC = red blood cell.

large-scale lesions (e.g., internal carotid artery stenosis) but is inferior to standard angiography for evaluating small intracranial lesions (e.g., aneurysm).
- **MR venography**
  MR venography provides subtraction images of the major venous sinuses. It can be useful for diagnosing dural sinus thrombosis but may be less sensitive than angiography.

■ MYELOGRAPHY

Myelography consists of injecting radiopaque dye into the spinal canal via either a lumbar or a suboccipital approach. After the patient is tilted, x-rays and axial CT slices allow visualization of the spinal subarachnoid space and can reveal extradural compressive lesions, ruptured intervertebral disks, and vascular malformations on the surface of the cord. In recent years, this test has been largely supplanted by MRI; however, myelography can still be useful if MRI is equivocal, and it remains essential for ruling out cord compression if MRI is not available. Complications are generally the same as those associated with LP.

■ DOPPLER ULTRASONOGRAPHY

- **Carotid duplex Doppler ultrasonography**
  This imaging technique can provide an accurate and noninvasive estimate of the degree of stenosis of the extracranial internal carotid arteries. B-mode ultrasonography gives a graphic image of the arterial wall and can detect plaques, whereas pulsed Doppler ultrasonography analyzes velocity and turbulence related to stenosis. Results are generally classified as (1) normal, (2) <40% stenosis, (3) 40 to 60% stenosis, (4) 60 to 80% stenosis, (5) 80 to 99% stenosis, and (6) occlusion. If carotid Doppler scans suggest occlusion, confirmation with angiography is required, because high-grade stenosis cannot be ruled out in all cases. Positioning of the transducer over the posterior neck can also differentiate normal, high-resistance, and absent flow in the proximal vertebral arteries.
- **Transcranial Doppler (TCD) ultrasonography**
  This technique measures the velocity of blood flow in the intracranial proximal cerebral arteries (internal carotid artery [ICA] siphon, middle cerebral artery [MCA], anterior cerebral artery [ACA], posterior cerebral artery [PCA], ophthalmic, basilar, and vertebral). The main parameters obtained by TCD ultrasonography are blood flow velocity and pulsatility. TCD ultrasonography can be useful for the following:

1. Diagnosing intracranial stenosis or occlusion
2. Evaluating the hemodynamic significance of carotid stenosis or occlusion (look for blunted poststenotic flow and reversed collateral flow in the ACA or ophthalmic artery)
3. Assessing vasospasm in patients with subarachnoid hemorrhage (high-velocity flow)
4. Screening for arteriovenous malformations (high-velocity flow, very low pulsatility)
5. Identifying severely increased ICP (low-velocity flow, high pulsatility)
6. Diagnosing brain death (systolic spikes with absent diastolic flow)

■ ANGIOGRAPHY

Cerebral angiography provides high-resolution images of the extracranial and intracranial cerebral vasculature (Fig. 4–2). The procedure is performed by threading a small catheter into the cerebral vessels via the femoral artery. Angiography is useful for identifying the following:

1. Occluded or stenotic vessels
2. Arterial dissections
3. Aneurysms
4. Arteriovenous malformations
5. Vasculitic narrowing ("beading")
6. Dural venous sinus thrombosis

- **Complications**
  Although infection or bleeding at the puncture site can occur, the most important complication (in 1 to 2% of patients) is stroke, which results from emboli generated by the catheter and which occurs most frequently in older patients with atherosclerotic disease.

■ ELECTROMYOGRAPHY AND NERVE CONDUCTION STUDIES

Electromyography (EMG) and nerve conduction studies assess the integrity and function of muscle and nerve, respectively, and essentially serve as extensions of the clinical examination.

- **EMG**
  This test can help distinguish neuropathic from myopathic disease, define the precise distribution of muscle involvement, and aid in the diagnosis of specific muscle disorders with unique features (e.g., myotonia). The procedure is performed by inserting a needle electrode into a muscle and analyzing motor unit potentials, both at rest (spontaneous

Diagnostic Studies **41**

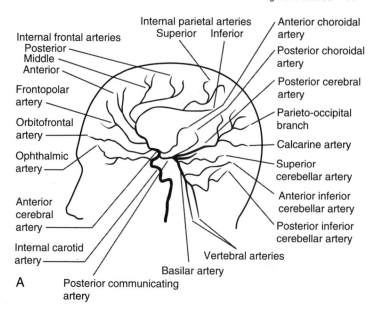

A

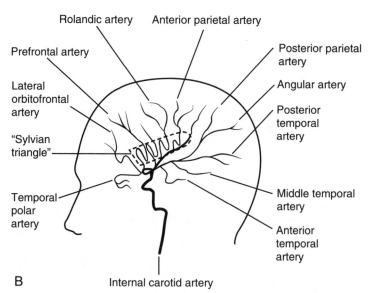

B

Figure 4–2 □ Diagram of a lateral cerebral angiogram. *A,* Anterior cerebral and posterior cerebral arteries. *B,* Middle cerebral artery.

activity) and with varying degrees of muscle contraction. The following parameters are analyzed:

1. **Insertional activity.** Excessive insertional activity is seen in both neuropathic and myopathic disease and hence is nonspecific.

2. **Spontaneous activity.** Normal muscle is electrically silent. Spontaneous muscle fiber contractions (*fibrillation potentials* and *positive sharp waves*) and spontaneous motor unit discharges (*fibrillations*) usually signify muscle denervation. After an acute nerve injury (e.g., disk herniation and nerve root compression), spontaneous activity usually takes 2 weeks to appear. *Paraspinal muscle denervation* implies nerve root injury as opposed to more distal lesions of the plexus or peripheral nerve. *Myotonia* is a special form of continuous motor unit activity characterized by high-frequency waxing and waning discharges, producing a "dive bomber" sound.

3. **Motor unit potential.** This parameter can differentiate myopathy from denervation. Neuropathic features reflect reinnervation of previously denervated motor units, resulting in *high-amplitude, polyphasic potentials.* Myopathic features reflect loss of muscle fiber mass, resulting in *low-amplitude, polyphasic potentials of short duration.*

4. **Recruitment pattern.** Voluntary muscle contraction leads to progressive recruitment of motor units and to a dense interference pattern that completely obliterates the baseline. In neuropathic disease, there are fewer motor units in the affected muscle, resulting in a *reduced* or *discrete recruitment* of motor units. Myopathic disease, with random loss of muscle fibers, leads to *early recruitment* and a *low-amplitude interference pattern.*

5. **Single-fiber EMG (SFEMG).** This technique examines the temporal relationship between firing of single muscle fibers innervated by the same motor neuron. Impaired neuromuscular transmission (e.g., in myasthenia gravis) results in a varying interval, referred to as a "jitter."

- **Nerve conduction studies**

    Nerve conduction studies can be performed on motor or sensory nerves. The procedure is performed by applying electrical stimulation to skin sites overlying a peripheral nerve and recording the speed of conduction and amplitude of the "downstream" action potential. The following parameters are analyzed:

    1. **Conduction velocity.** Conduction velocity is generally reduced ($<60\%$ of normal) in demyelinating neuropathy. *Conduction block* reflects focal demyelination and is identified when nerve stimulation proximal to the block

leads to a compound muscle action potential (CMAP) amplitude that is less than 50% of that obtained by stimulating distal to the block.

2. **Amplitude.** The amplitude of the CMAP correlates with the number of muscle fibers activated by stimulation of the peripheral nerve. In general, reduced CMAP amplitude with relatively preserved conduction velocity is characteristic of *axonal neuropathy.*

3. **Late responses.** *F waves* result from antidromic conduction followed by orthodromic conduction in the same nerve. Delayed or absent F waves, in combination with normal peripheral nerve conduction, implies disease of the proximal nerve (e.g., root compression, early Guillain-Barré syndrome). The *H reflex* is the electrical counterpart of the ankle jerk and can be performed to assess the integrity of the S1 root; the antidromic potential travels down a sensory nerve, synapses in the spinal cord, and then travels orthodromically down a motor nerve.

4. **Repetitive stimulation.** Muscle responses to repetitive stimulation are useful for assessing neuromuscular junction disease. In myasthenia gravis (see Chapter 16), repetitive stimulation at 2 to 3 Hz produces a characteristic *decremental response* (>10% drop in amplitude between the first and the fifth CMAP).

■ ELECTROENCEPHALOGRAPHY

Electroencephalography (EEG) provides a multichannel recording of the surface electrical activity of the brain. Background rhythms (Fig. 4–3) are analyzed with regard to amplitude and

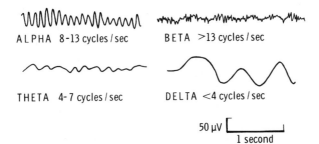

ALPHA 8-13 cycles / sec   BETA >13 cycles / sec

THETA 4-7 cycles / sec   DELTA <4 cycles / sec

50 μV

1 second

Figure 4–3 □ Basic EEG rhythms. (From Solomon GE, Kutt H, Plum F: Clinical Management of Seizures, 2nd ed. Philadelphia, WB Saunders Co, 1983.)

frequency (delta waves, <4 Hz; theta waves, 4 to 7 Hz; alpha waves, 8 to 13 Hz, and beta waves, >13 Hz). In the awake, normal adult, a posterior dominant alpha rhythm is detected when the eyes are closed and the patient is in a relaxed state. Sleep results in characteristic sequential changes (progressive slowing, vertex transients, sleep spindles, and K complexes) that reflect highly organized synchronous activity. The primary utility of EEG is for evaluating epileptiform disorders and causes of diffuse encephalopathy.

■ **Seizure disorders**

The main value of EEG in patients with seizures is for detecting *interictal epileptiform activity* (spikes and sharp waves). Focal epileptiform activity reflects a single irritative focus and corresponds with partial-onset seizures, whereas paroxysmal spike-and-wave discharges of diffuse origin correspond with generalized-onset seizures (Fig. 4–4). Occasionally an *electrographic seizure* will be recorded by chance during

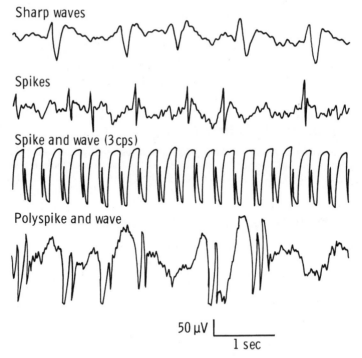

Figure 4–4 □ Paroxysmal EEG patterns seen in patients with epilepsy. (From Solomon GE, Kutt H, Plum F: Clinical Management of Seizures, 2nd ed. Philadelphia, WB Saunders Co, 1983.)

the examination. The absence of epileptiform discharges does not imply the absence of a seizure disorder, however, since 20 to 40% of EEG recordings in patients with epilepsy appear normal. *Sleep, sleep deprivation, hyperventilation,* and *photostimulation* can be used to elicit epileptiform activity or absence seizures, and they are collectively referred to as activation procedures. EEG can also be used to identify *nonconvulsive status epilepticus* (complex-partial or absence status) in patients with prolonged postictal or otherwise unexplained impairment of consciousness.

- **Diffuse encephalopathy**

    Diffuse background slowing (in the range of theta and delta waves) is an almost universal finding in patients with impaired level of consciousness of any cause. In patients with focal lesions (e.g., stroke or brain tumor), the slowing is usually more pronounced in the ipsilateral hemisphere. In most patients in whom the cause of encephalopathy is readily identified (e.g., drug overdose, head trauma), EEG is not helpful. However, in some instances, unique patterns that can point to a specific diagnosis are identified:

    1. **Periodic lateralizing epileptiform discharges (PLEDs).** These can occur with large destructive lesions of any type and do not always correspond with clinical seizure activity. In patients with encephalitis, bilateral PLEDs are highly suggestive of herpes simplex infection.
    2. **Triphasic waves.** Triphasic waves are nonspecific but can occur with high frequency in patients with metabolic encephalopathy (e.g., in hepatic, renal, and pulmonary failure).
    3. **Beta activity.** Beta activity combined with diffuse slowing suggests intoxication with barbiturates, benzodiazepines, or other sedative-hypnotic drugs.
    4. **Periodic discharges.** Periodic discharges consisting of bisynchronous bursts of high-amplitude, sharp waves are characteristic of subacute sclerosing panencephalitis (SSPE) and Jakob-Creutzfeldt disease.

- **Prognosis in coma**

    In hypoxic-ischemic coma, prognosis for recovery of consciousness is related to the severity of slowing and attenuation of the background rhythm. A *burst-suppression pattern* implies an extremely poor prognosis. Keep in mind, however, that prognosis is usually related more to the cause of coma than to the depth of coma. *Alpha coma* and *spindle coma patterns* tend to occur with brain stem coma, but they do not have important prognostic significance.

- **Brain death**

    Electrocerebral silence can be used as a confirmatory test for brain death (see Chapter 20).

■ EVOKED POTENTIALS

Evoked potentials provide a recording of electrical activity in central sensory pathways produced by visual, auditory, or sensory stimulation. Signals are recorded by placing electrodes over the scalp or the spine and using a computer to average and amplify the signal, which results in a characteristic pattern of waveform peaks that have approximate anatomic correlates. There are three types of evoked potential studies:

- **Visual evoked responses (VER)**
  The visual stimulus is delivered as an alternating checkerboard pattern or a stroboscopic flash; the waveform corresponds with stimulation of the occipital cortex.
- **Brain stem auditory evoked responses (BAER)**
  Auditory signals are delivered by clicks through earphones. The waveform corresponds with stimulation of CN 8, the cochlear nucleus, pons, and inferior colliculus.
- **Somatosensory evoked potentials (SSEP)**
  Electrical stimuli are delivered to peripheral nerves. The waveform corresponds with stimulation of the lumbosacral or the brachial plexus, the cervicomedullary dorsal column nuclei, and the sensory cortex.

  The uses of evoked potentials in clinical practice are as follows:
  1. **Multiple sclerosis.** Evoked potentials can be used to support the diagnosis in a patient with a single symptom by identifying subclinical demyelination at a different anatomic site (e.g., abnormal VERs in a patient with transverse myelitis).
  2. **Brain stem lesions.** Brain stem lesions can be verified and localized with BAER.
  3. **Acoustic neuroma.** BAER can be used to verify CN 8 injury.
  4. **Spinal cord injury.** SSEP can be used for prognosis by differentiating complete from partial injury.
  5. **Hypoxic coma.** Absence of cortical potentials by SSEP implies that consciousness will not be regained.

■ MUSCLE AND NERVE BIOPSY

Muscle and nerve biopsy specimens are extremely fragile, and the procedure should be performed only by an experienced surgeon with adequate neuropathology backup for processing and analysis. The sural nerve and gastrocnemius muscle are often examined together, although biopsy of almost any muscle can be performed. Muscle biopsy is essential for diagnosing causes of myopathy such as polymyositis, genetic biochemical deficiencies, mitochondrial disease, sarcoidosis, and infection (e.g., trichinosis). The causes of neuropathy that can be diagnosed by nerve biopsy are listed in Table 21–4.

■ BRAIN BIOPSY

Brain biopsy can be performed either as an open procedure, usually of the anterior nondominant temporal lobe, or by using stereotactic needle localization. Although stereotactic biopsy is often necessary for deep lesions, the diagnostic yield is better with the open procedure because more tissue can be obtained. The main complication is hemorrhage (in approximately 1% of cases). Brain biopsy is of value for diagnosing brain tumors or abscess, central nervous system (CNS) vasculitis, neurosarcoidosis, and encephalitis.

PATIENT-RELATED PROBLEMS: THE COMMON CALLS

5

SEIZURES

Seizures are dramatic and frightening for all who witness the event—patients, families, and staff—and tend to induce panic, rather than rational thought, even on a neurology service. It is your job to proceed in a logical and thorough manner to identify the cause of the seizure and to halt it if it persists.

Clinical seizures are caused by an excessive, synchronous, abnormal discharge of cortical neurons that produces a sudden change in neurologic function. Seizures are classified as *simple* if there is no impairment of consciousness or as *complex* if an alteration in consciousness occurs (Table 5–1). Seizures may be *focal*, involving a single brain region and causing limited dysfunction, such as clonic movements of a single limb, paresthesias, or abnormal speech or behavior; or they may be *generalized*, involving the whole brain and producing loss of consciousness and convulsions. Most seizures last seconds to minutes. *Status epilepticus* is defined as seizures lasting longer than 30 minutes or repetitive seizures over 30 minutes between which the patient does not return to a baseline neurologic level.

■ PHONE CALL

Questions

1. **Is the patient still seizing? If yes, how long has it been going on?**

   Any patient seizing on admission to the emergency room (ER) should be considered to be in status epilepticus until the course of the seizure is known.

2. **What is the patient's level of consciousness?**

   A patient may have a decreased level of consciousness if the seizure is still occurring (nonconvulsive status epilepticus) or if the patient is postictal. The two states can be difficult to differentiate without an electroencephalogram (EEG).

3. **Is this the first known seizure for this patient?**

   If the patient has a known history of epilepsy, there may be records available regarding anticonvulsants that have worked or failed in the past. Other information regarding past seizures will be gained from taking the patient's history.

4. **Is the patient on anticonvulsant medication?**

   Anticonvulsant levels need to be checked for any seizure

Table 5–1 □ **INTERNATIONAL CLASSIFICATION OF EPILEPTIC SEIZURES**

1. Partial (focal, local) seizures
   a. Simple partial seizures (no impairment of consciousness)
      (1) With motor symptoms
      (2) With sensory symptoms
      (3) With autonomic symptoms
      (4) With psychic symptoms
   b. Complex partial seizures (impairment of consciousness)
      (1) Beginning as simple partial seizures and progressing to impairment of consciousness
         (a) With no other features
         (b) With features as in simple partial seizures
         (c) With automatisms
      (2) With impairment of consciousness at onset
         (a) With no other features
         (b) With features as in simple partial seizures
         (c) With automatisms
   c. Partial seizures evolving to secondarily generalized (convulsive or nonconvulsive) seizures
      (1) Simple partial seizures evolving to generalized seizures
      (2) Complex partial seizures evolving to generalized seizures
      (3) Simple partial seizures evolving to complex partial seizures, then evolving to generalized seizures
2. Generalized seizures (convulsive or nonconvulsive)
   a. Absence (petit mal) seizures
   b. Myoclonic seizures
   c. Clonic seizures
   d. Tonic seizures
   e. Tonic-clonic seizures
   f. Atonic seizures
3. Unclassified epileptic seizures (unclassified because of inadequate or incomplete information, e.g., neonatal rhythmic eye movements)

patient on medication. Many anticonvulsants are epileptogenic at toxic levels.

5. Is the patient diabetic?

Focal or generalized seizures may be caused by hyper- or hypoglycemia.

6. Is the patient immunocompromised?

Additional elements in the differential diagnosis need to be considered in immunocompromised patients, particularly opportunistic infections such as toxoplasmosis, fungal meningitides, and tubercular meningitis.

Orders

If the patient is still seizing:

1. Have two intravenous (IV) setups ready at the bedside.

2. Have oral airway and Ambu bag available at the bedside.
3. Have diazepam 10 mg ready at the bedside.
4. Clear any sharp or hard objects from the bed, put the side rails up, and pad the side rails.
5. Perform a finger stick glucose test.

If the patient has stopped seizing:
1. Have an oral airway ready at bedside.
2. Perform a finger stick glucose test.

Inform RN

"Will arrive at the bedside in . . . minutes."

If the patient is still seizing, it must be considered a medical emergency. If the patient has stopped seizing, another seizure may occur within a few minutes.

■ ELEVATOR THOUGHTS (DIFFERENTIAL DIAGNOSIS OF SEIZURES)

On your way to the bedside, you should generate a list of probable diagnoses based on the initial information you obtained from your telephone conversation with the nurse.

V (vascular): Intracranial hemorrhage, acute or chronic ischemic infarction, subarachnoid hemorrhage, arteriovenous malformation, venous sinus thrombosis, or amyloid angiopathy

I (infectious): meningitis (bacterial, viral, fungal), meningoencephalitis (herpes simplex encephalitis), or abscess (bacterial, fungal, or parasitic)

T (traumatic): new head injury (e.g., from a fall) or old head injury with subdural hematoma

A (autoimmune): systemic lupus erythematosus, central nervous system (CNS) vasculitis, or multiple sclerosis

M (metabolic/toxic): hypo- or hypernatremia, hypo- or hypercalcemia, hypo- or hyperglycemia, hypomagnesemia, hyperthyroidism, uremia, hyperammonemia, ethanol (EtOH) toxicity or EtOH withdrawal, other drugs including cocaine, phencyclidine, and amphetamines

I (idiopathic/iatrogenic): idiopathic epilepsy or medications (Table 5–2 lists common medications that can cause seizures)

N (neoplastic): brain metastasis or primary CNS tumor

S (structural): congenital structural defects (rare in adults)

Paroxysmal conditions that may mimic seizures: hypoglycemia, syncope, asterixis, stroke/transient ischemic attack, myoclonus, dystonia, tremor, narcolepsy, complicated migraine, panic attack, hyperventilation, malingering

Table 5–2 □ **COMMON MEDICATIONS THAT MAY CAUSE SEIZURES**

Antidepressants	Antimicrobial agents
Imipramine	Penicillin, ampicillin
Amitriptyline	Synthetic penicillins
Nortriptyline	Cephalosporins
Bupropion	Metronidazole
Antipsychotic agents	Isoniazid
Chlorpromazine	Pyrimethamine
Thioridazine	Antineoplastic agents
Trifluoperazine	Vincristine
Perphenazine	Chlorambucil
Haloperidol	Methotrexate
Analgesics	Carmustine (BCNU)
Fentanyl	Cytosine arabinoside
Meperidine	Bronchodilators
Pentazocine	Aminophylline
Propoxyphene	Theophylline
Local anesthetics	Others
Lidocaine	Insulin
Procaine	Antihistamines
Sympathomimetics	Anticholinergics
Terbutaline	Atenolol
Ephedrine	Baclofen
Phenylpropanolamine	

■ **MAJOR THREAT TO LIFE**

- Aspiration of gastric contents if the airway is not protected
- Head injury
- Lactic acidosis, hypoxia, or hypotension from a prolonged seizure

These conditions may produce permanent brain injury.

Measures to prevent aspiration and subsequent injury to the patient are described in Management I. The patient should be positioned in the lateral decubitus position to prevent aspiration of gastric contents. All hard or sharp objects should be removed from the bed, the side rails should be up, and the side rails should be padded. Procedures for aborting an ongoing seizure are described below.

■ **BEDSIDE**

Quick Look Test

Is the patient still seizing?

Most seizures will have stopped by the time you arrive at the bedside. If there is still seizure activity, prepare to treat it.

If the patient has stopped seizing, assess the patient's level of consciousness.

Is the patient awake and alert? Is he or she interactive and conversing?

A period of lethargy or stupor may follow a generalized seizure. Focal deficits such as a hemiparesis may also be apparent from a quick look.

Does the patient look comfortable? Is there any sign of respiratory distress or agitation or any complaint of headache?

Management I

Treatment of an Ongoing Seizure

1. **Keep calm.** It is likely that others in the room are reacting with fear or panic. Ask family members to leave the room. Tell them you will speak with them as soon as the situation is evaluated and under control.
2. **Ensure that all measures have been taken to protect the patient from physical injury and aspiration of gastric contents.** Have one or two people maintain the patient in a lateral decubitus position (Fig. 5–1).
3. **Administer oxygen by nasal cannula or face mask,** particularly if the patient is older or has a history of cardiac disease.
4. **Watch and wait for 3 minutes.** A majority of seizures will stop spontaneously within a short time. There is no immediate risk to the patient, provided the risks of aspiration and physical injury have been addressed. During the waiting period, do the following:
   - Check the **finger stick glucose** level. If there is significant hypo- or hyperglycemia, this may be the first condition to treat.
   - Make sure there are **two IV setups available,** at least one with 0.9% normal saline (NS). If the patient has no IV access, an IV line will need to be started. If the seizures stop within 3 minutes, however, IV insertion and blood drawing will be much easier.
   - Draw **diazepam 10 mg** in a 10-ml syringe.
   - **Elicit any further history** not obtained in the initial phone call. Is this a first-ever seizure? Is the patient on anticonvulsants? What is the patient's admitting diagnosis? Is the patient diabetic? Is the patient immunocompromised? Has the patient been febrile in the last 24 hours? Ask for the chart to be brought to the bedside.
   - **Observe the seizure type.** Generalized seizures, in which both sides of the body are involved and in which there is altered level of consciousness, are potentially the most dangerous if the seizures persist for longer than 30 min-

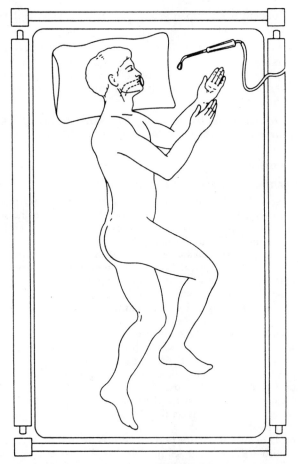

Figure 5–1 □ Positioning of the patient to prevent aspiration of gastric contents. (From Marshall SA, Ruedy J: On Call: Principles and Protocols, 2nd ed. Philadelphia, WB Saunders Co, 1993, p 223.)

utes. A partial seizure, in which a single limb or side of the body is involved, may suggest a structural lesion.

5. **If the seizure has not remitted in 3 minutes,** ensure that an IV line is available. If the patient has no IV access, have one or two people hold the forearm while the most experienced person available inserts two IV lines and draws blood. Avoid the antecubital area because convulsions may cause flexion of the arm and block off the IV site.

6. Order the following **blood tests:** complete blood count

(CBC), electrolytes, glucose, magnesium (Mg), calcium (Ca), ammonia, EtOH level, toxicology screen, and anticonvulsant level (if applicable).

7. If the patient is hypoglycemic, give **glucose (50 ml of D50W)** by slow, direct injection. If there is any history or suspicion of alcoholism, administer **thiamine 100 mg by slow, direct injection over 3 to 5 minutes.** The administration of thiamine will prevent susceptible patients from developing Wernicke's encephalopathy. If hypoglycemia is the cause of the seizure, the seizure should stop, and the patient should wake up soon after the glucose administration.

8. If glucose levels are normal or after glucose has been given, administer **diazepam 5 to 10 mg by IV push over 2 to 3 minutes.**

   Diazepam is best given in NS to avoid precipitation. An Ambu bag with face mask should be at the bedside because benzodiazepines can cause respiratory depression. Alternatives to diazepam include **lorazepam 2 to 4 mg.** Lorazepam may be given intramuscularly (IM) and may be helpful if no peripheral IV access can be achieved.

9. If the seizure persists, a **5-mg dose of diazepam may be repeated every 5 minutes up to a maximum of 20 mg.** Watch for respiratory depression.

Treatment of Status Epilepticus

1. If the seizure has not stopped with two doses of the benzodiazepine, administer **fosphenytoin** (the prodrug of phenytoin) **15 to 20 mg/kg as a slow IV push or IV infusion.** (This loading dose corresponds to approximately 1500 mg in a 70-kg patient.) The rate of administration should not exceed 200 mg/min because fosphenytoin can cause cardiac arrhythmias, prolongation of the QT interval, and hypotension. The electrocardiogram (ECG) should be monitored continuously, and the blood pressure should be checked each minute during the infusion. The rate of administration should be slowed if ECG changes or hypotension occurs. The usual protocol is to give **500 mg with a slow IV push over 5 minutes, and then repeat twice.** If IV access is unavailable, fosphenytoin can also be given IM. If the patient is known to be on phenytoin already and is suspected to have subtherapeutic levels, **a load of 10 mg/kg bolus** may be given. Fosphenytoin, like most anticonvulsants, may be epileptogenic at high concentrations.

2. Approximately 80% of prolonged seizures will be brought under control with a combination of diazepam and fosphenytoin, but if the seizure lasts longer than 30 minutes, transfer the patient to an intensive care unit (ICU) for probable intubation. Prolonged status epilepticus may require active

treatment of hypoxia, hypotension, cardiac arrhythmias, cardiac failure, lactic acidosis, hyperpyrexia, electrolyte disturbances, or rhabdomyolysis.

3. Once the patient is in the ICU, if the patient is continuing to seize despite a full fosphenytoin load, the next step is to administer barbiturates. **Phenobarbital should be infused IV at a rate of 100 mg/min and should be stopped at a loading dose of 15 to 20 mg/kg.** Intubation, if not already done, is likely to be required at this point. Continue monitoring the blood pressure and ECG.

4. If there is no response to phenobarbital, consider the seizure to be refractory status epilepticus. As the next step, administer **pentobarbital 5 to 20 mg/kg loading dose and then 1 to 3 mg/kg per hour as a maintenance dose.** Monitor the EEG continuously to keep the patient in a burst suppression pattern. Hypotension is nearly always encountered with pentobarbital, and pressors may be required. General anesthesia with halothane and neuromuscular blockade has been used in some cases to avoid rhabdomyolysis, but this eliminates the ability to follow the neurologic examination.

5. Although nearly all seizures may be brought under control with anticonvulsant therapy, continued control may be impossible until the underlying cause is identified and treated.

Evaluation and Initial Management If the Seizure Has Stopped

A single first seizure that has stopped often does not need to be treated. Anticonvulsant therapy should be reserved for patients who have had more than one seizure or who have risk factors that make another seizure more likely. The potential danger to the patient is not over, however. A patient who has had one seizure may have another seizure within a few minutes. Order "seizure precautions" for the patient (Table 5–3). Remember also that a seizure is a symptom, not a disease. Your primary job now should be to identify the cause of the seizure and to treat the underlying condition.

1. **Draw blood and order the following tests:** CBC, electro-

Table 5–3 □ SEIZURE PRECAUTIONS

Bed should be at the lowest position
Side rails should be up
Side rails should be padded
Patient should ambulate to bathroom only with supervision
Only axillary temperatures should be measured
Patient should be supervised when using sharp objects
Oral airway, oxygen, and suction should be at bedside

lytes, glucose, Mg, Ca, ammonia, EtOH level, toxicology screen, and anticonvulsant level.

2. **Ensure that there is intravenous access.** Start an IV running to keep the vein open with 0.9% NS.

3. **Ask for the chart** to be brought to the bedside while you perform a selective physical examination.

Selective Physical Examination

Initial physical examination of a patient who has had a seizure should take no more than 5 minutes. Important clues to the etiology of the seizure may emerge. Pay particular attention to unilateral focal deficits that could indicate a structural lesion.

Vital signs: Fever could be a clue to an infectious cause, although a prolonged seizure may cause hyperpyrexia. Dyspnea may suggest hypoxia. Cardiac arrhythmia or tachycardia could suggest a cardioembolic or syncopal event. Hypertensive encephalopathy may present with seizures.

HEENT: Look for evidence of bites on the tongue, lips, or buccal mucosa. Look for any evidence of new or old head injury. Check the fundi for papilledema.

Neck: Look for neck stiffness (meningismus).

Skin: Look for cafe au lait spots or port-wine stains as a sign of neurocutaneous disorders (e.g., neurofibromatosis or Sturge-Weber syndrome). Hematomas, lacerations, or even fractures may have been produced as a consequence of the seizure.

Chest: Focal decreased breath sounds or rales may be a clue to aspiration. Cardiac murmur or arrhythmia may suggest a cardioembolic event.

GU: Incontinence, particularly urinary, may accompany a generalized seizure.

Neurologic examination: Assess for new or residual focal deficits:

The *level of consciousness* may be decreased after a seizure. A period of lethargy, stupor, or inattentiveness may follow a generalized seizure. If the patient is awake, have him or her count backward from 20 to 1 as a screening test for attentiveness.

Aphasia has been partially screened for by asking the patient to count backwards from 20 to 1. If the patient is unable to do this task, he or she may be either too inattentive, in which case aphasia testing will be futile, or aphasic. Ask the patient to show two fingers, then to repeat an unfamiliar phrase (e.g., "The spy fled to Greece").

Hemiparesis may be obvious, as evidenced by an inability to lift an arm or leg, or it may be subtle, as detected by a widened palpebral fissure, a flattened nasolabial fold, or a pronator drift when arms are extended with palms up.

Reflex asymmetry or a unilateral Babinski's sign may be indicative of a focal lesion.

Selective History and Chart Review

Reassess the timing, circumstances, and duration of the seizure. Try to establish with the patient or with witnesses whether this was indeed a seizure. An aura is often present at the onset of a seizure, which is thought to represent the beginning of the abnormal epileptic discharges. Auras are most commonly olfactory, gustatory, or other visceral sensations that precede motor or sensory activity. Were there rhythmic, synchronous movements of more than one body part? Identify a "focal signature" if present; that is, did the seizure begin in one part of the body and then progress or become generalized? Were there head and eye deviations at the beginning? A seizure that begins focally can aid in the localization of the underlying pathology. If both sides of the body were involved, did the patient lose consciousness, become incontinent, or bite the tongue or mouth?

From the chart, look for clues to the underlying cause. Check for the following:

1. Medications the patient is on that are potentially epileptogenic (see Table 5–2).
2. History of alcohol or drug use.
3. Underlying medical problems that could cause seizures, including hepatic or renal disease, prior head injury, cerebrovascular disease, connective tissue diseases, or carcinoma (lung, breast, and colon cancer are the most common tumors that metastasize to the brain).
4. HIV infection. Patients who are immunocompromised, particularly patients with acquired immunodeficiency syndrome (AIDS), are predisposed to opportunistic infections such as toxoplasmosis, tubercular meningitis, and cryptococcal meningitis and to CNS lymphoma.
5. Recent laboratory results: electrolyte, glucose, Ca and Mg levels, thyroid and liver function tests, toxicology screen, EtOH levels, and anticonvulsant levels.

■ MANAGEMENT II

Having accumulated information from the history, the physical examination, and the laboratory, a working differential diagnosis should be generated. As always, in an acute situation, the differential diagnosis should include the most dangerous diagnosis as well as the most likely. Management should proceed from the differential diagnosis.

1. If a **metabolic cause** is identified or suspected, the underlying cause should be treated appropriately.
2. If the examination reveals a focal deficit, if the onset of the seizure appeared to be focal, or if the patient has new-onset seizures, a **computed tomography (CT) or magnetic resonance imaging (MRI) scan** should be obtained. If there is no renal insufficiency, contrast should be administered. Keep in mind that a cerebral infarction may not be detectable by CT or MRI within the first 12 hours.
3. If no immediately treatable metabolic cause is identified or if a structural lesion is suspected, a loading dose of **fosphenytoin 15 to 20 mg/kg** should be given. If there is little concern of another seizure's occurring within a short period of time (as opposed to a patient with suspected alcohol or sedative withdrawal, HIV positivity, or a structural lesion, for example), the loading dose may be given orally.
4. If there is no evidence of a major mass effect or increased intracranial pressure on imaging, and, particularly, if an infectious etiology is suspected, a **lumbar puncture** may be performed so that antibiotic therapy, if warranted, may be targeted as specifically as possible. If infection is suspected, other supportive evidence should be sought as well, such as blood cultures, urine cultures, and chest x-ray.
5. If treatment was given to correct abnormal laboratory results, those tests should be repeated, including electrolytes, Mg, Ca, and glucose. If fosphenytoin was administered, a blood level should be ordered for the next morning.
6. An **EEG** should be obtained if the diagnosis of seizure is at all uncertain; it also serves the purpose of guiding long-term management. In most cases, an EEG is not helpful in the acute situation, except for cases of suspected nonconvulsive status epilepticus.
7. If **no underlying cause** for seizures is determined, idiopathic epilepsy may be the diagnosis. An EEG is often helpful in differentiating specific epileptic syndromes. Treatment with an appropriate anticonvulsant would then be indicated. Table 5–4 outlines some selected epilepsy syndromes. Table 5–5 lists some common anticonvulsants, their pharmacokinetics, and their side effects.

Table 5–4 □ SPECIAL EPILEPTIC SYNDROMES

1. Complex partial seizures (temporal lobe epilepsy)
   20% of all seizures
   Almost always adult onset
   Focal medial, temporal, or frontal discharges on EEG
   Alteration in consciousness; patient appears "dazed"
   Often begin with automatisms (chewing, lip smacking, picking at clothes) or psychiatric symptoms (e.g., abnormal affect, disturbed cognition, hallucinations, time distortion)
   Begin and end abruptly
   Treatment with carbamazepine, phenytoin, or valproate
2. Absence (petit mal) seizures
   Onset age 5–10 years
   Usually last 5 seconds
   No preceding aura, no postictal state
   Typical generalized 3-Hz spike and wave discharges on EEG
   Treatment with ethosuximide
3. Febrile convulsions
   May be single or recurrent
   Usually benign prognosis, particularly with onset between 6 months and 4 years and a normal EEG
   Single febrile convulsion usually not treated
   May treat with phenobarbital for recurrent seizures or if abnormal EEG
4. Infantile spasms (West's syndrome)
   Bilaterally symmetric tonic spasms
   "Hypsarrhythmia" on EEG
   75% associated with mental retardation
   Many progress to Lennox-Gastaut syndrome (multiple seizure types, slow-spike-and-wave EEG pattern, mental retardation)
   Seizures may be treated with adrenocorticotropic hormone or clonazepam, but treatment of seizures does not improve prognosis
5. Benign rolandic epilepsy
   Onset between ages 3 and 13 years
   Self-limited, rare after age 16
   Typically focal motor or sensory seizures, which may generalize
   Typical high-voltage midtemporal spikes on EEG
   Treat with carbamazepine to reduce seizure frequency
5. Juvenile myoclonic epilepsy
   Onset between 12 and 19 years
   Recurrent bilateral myoclonic jerks, typically on awakening, may generalize
   Bursts of 3- to 6-Hz spike-and-wave pattern on EEG
   Treatment with valproic acid generally effective

Table 5–5 □ SEIZURE MEDICATIONS

Drug	Target Serum Levels* (μg/ml)	Half-life (hours)	Side Effects/Toxicity
Phenytoin/fosphenytoin (Dilantin/Cerebyx)	10–20	24 ± 6	Nystagmus, ataxia, encephalopathy, hirsutism, gingival hyperplasia, peripheral neuropathy, megaloblastic anemia, hypocalcemia, systemic lupus erythematosus, exfoliative dermatitis
Carbamazepine (Tegretol)	4–12	20 ± 5	Drowsiness, dizziness, nausea, aplastic anemia, hyponatremia
Phenobarbital	15–30	96 ± 24	Drowsiness, depression, megaloblastic anemia, hyponatremia
Primidone (Mysoline)	8–12	6 ± 3	Ataxia, vertigo, drowsiness, nausea, megaloblastic anemia
Ethosuximide (Zarontin)	40–120	48 ± 12	Encephalopathy, systemic lupus erythematosus
Valproic acid (Depakene, Depakote)	50–100	10 ± 6	Weight gain, alopecia, menstrual irregularities, platelet dysfunction, hepatotoxicity, pancreatitis, hyperammonemia
Felbamate (Felbatol)	N/A	20 ± 6	Anorexia, vomiting, headache, somnolence
Gabapentin (Neurontin)	N/A	6 ± 2	Somnolence, dizziness, ataxia, fatigue, nystagmus, headache
Lamotrigine (Lamictal)	N/A	24 ± 5	Dizziness, headache, diplopia, ataxia, nausea, rash, blurred vision, somnolence

*Target level ranges may vary slightly among different laboratories.

6

STUPOR AND COMA

Stupor and coma refer, respectively, to moderate and severe depression of the level of consciousness. The acute onset of stupor or coma is a medical emergency. A wide variety of metabolic and structural disorders can produce this state. Management should focus on stabilizing the patient, establishing a diagnosis, and treating the underlying cause.

■ PHONE CALL

Questions

1. **What are the vital signs?**
2. **Is the airway protected?**
   Stuporous and comatose patients are at high risk for *aspiration*, because of impaired cough and gag reflexes, and *hypoxia*, which results from diminished respiratory drive. Endotracheal intubation is the most effective method for securing the airway and ensuring adequate oxygenation.
3. **Is there any history of trauma, drug use, or toxin exposure?**
   Obtain a quick description of recent events and pre-existing medical or neurologic conditions. Check the Emergency Medical Service sheet.
4. **Is someone available to provide further history?**
   Relatives, friends, ambulance personnel, or anyone else who has had recent contact with the patient should be identified and instructed to wait for further questioning.

Orders

1. **Call the anesthesiology service for intubation** if the patient is deeply comatose or exhibiting signs of respiratory compromise.
   In stuporous patients with normal respirations, give 100% oxygen via face mask until hypoxemia is ruled out.
2. **Order an intravenous line.**
3. **Order a finger stick glucose measurement.**
   This should always be checked immediately, because hypoglycemia is a rapidly treatable cause of stupor or coma that can coexist with other diagnoses (e.g., sepsis, cardiac arrest, or trauma).

4. **Order diagnostic blood tests.**
   - Serum chemistries (glucose, electrolytes, blood urea nitrogen [BUN], creatinine)
   - Complete blood count (CBC)
   - Arterial blood gas
   - Calcium, magnesium
   - Prothrombin time (PT)/partial thromboplastin time (PTT)
5. If the etiology of coma is unclear order toxicology screen, thyroid function tests, liver function tests, serum cortisol, and ammonia level.
6. **Insert a Foley catheter.**
7. **Order urinalysis, electrocardiogram (ECG), and chest x-ray.**
8. **Give emergency treatment.** These are often given "in the field," or whenever the cause of coma is unclear.
   - **Thiamine 100 mg intravenously (IV)**
     Thiamine reverses coma resulting from acute thiamine deficiency (Wernicke's encephalopathy). It must be given *before* dextrose because hyperglycemia can lead to consumption of thiamine and acute worsening of Wernicke's encephalopathy.
   - **50% dextrose 50 ml (1 ampule) IV**
   - **Naloxone (Narcan) 0.4 to 0.8 mg IV**
     Naloxone reverses coma caused by opiate intoxication. Up to 10 mg may be required to reverse severe intoxication.
   - **Flumazenil (Romazicon) 0.2 to 1.0 mg IV**
     Flumazenil reverses coma caused by benzodiazepine intoxication. Up to 3 mg may be required. *Do not give flumazenil if seizures have occurred, because flumazenil may precipitate further seizures.*

■ ELEVATOR THOUGHTS

What causes stupor or coma?

The causes of stupor and coma (Table 6–1) can be broadly grouped into three categories:

1. **Structural intracranial disorders (33%)**
   In most cases, these are diagnosed by positive brain imaging (computed tomography [CT] or magnetic resonance imaging [MRI]) or by lumbar puncture (LP).
2. **Toxic or metabolic disorders (66%)**
   Abnormal blood tests usually, but not always, confirm these disorders.
3. **Psychiatric disorders (1%)**

Stupor and coma result from diseases affecting either both of the cerebral hemispheres or the brain stem. As a rule, *unilateral hemispheric lesions* do not produce stupor or coma unless they are of a mass sufficient to compress either the

Table 6–1 □ CAUSES OF STUPOR AND COMA

1. **Structural intracranial disorders**
   a. Trauma
      (1) Epidural, subdural, intracerebral, or subarachnoid hemorrhage
      (2) Diffuse axonal injury
      (3) Concussion
   b. Cerebrovascular events
      (1) Intracerebral or subarachnoid hemorrhage
      (2) Hemispheric or brain stem infarction
      (3) Dural sinus thrombosis
      (4) Hypertensive encephalopathy
   c. Infection
      (1) Meningitis
      (2) Encephalitis
      (3) Abscess
   d. Inflammatory disorders
      (1) Autoimmune vasculitis or cerebritis
      (2) Demyelinating disease (e.g., multiple sclerosis)
   e. Neoplasm
   f. Hydrocephalus
2. **Toxic or metabolic disorders**
   a. Global hypoxia-ischemia
   b. Electrolyte or acid-base disorders
      (1) pH disturbances
      (2) Hyper- or hyponatremia
      (3) Hyper- or hypoglycemia
      (4) Hyper- or hypocalcemia
   c. Drug intoxication or withdrawal
   d. Temperature disorder (hyper- or hypothermia)
   e. Organ system dysfunction
      (1) Liver (hepatic encephalopathy)
      (2) Kidney (uremia)
      (3) Thyroid (myxedema, thyrotoxicosis)
      (4) Adrenal (hyper- or hypoadrenalism)
   f. Seizure and postictal states
   g. Thiamine or vitamin B_{12} deficiency
3. **Psychogenic coma**

contralateral hemisphere or the brain stem. *Focal brain stem lesions* produce coma by disrupting the reticular activating system. *Metabolic disorders* impair consciousness by diffuse effects on both the reticular formation and the cerebral cortex.

■ MAJOR THREAT TO LIFE

Three common and treatable causes of coma can rapidly lead to death:

- **Herniation and brain stem compression**
  Space-occupying mass lesions that produce coma are a neurosurgical emergency.

- **Increased intracranial pressure (ICP)**
    Increased ICP can lead to impaired cerebral perfusion and global hypoxic-ischemic injury (see Chapter 13).
- **Meningitis or encephalitis**
    Death from bacterial meningitis or herpes encephalitis can be prevented with early treatment (see Chapter 23).

■ BEDSIDE

Selective History

The cause of coma can frequently be determined by the history. Ask family, friends, ambulance personnel, or others who have had recent contact with the patient about the following:

1. Recent events
    When was the patient last seen? How was the patient discovered? Were there any preceding neurologic complaints? Was there any recent trauma or toxin exposure?
2. Medical history
3. Psychiatric history
4. Medications
5. Use of drugs or alcohol

Selective Physical Examination

With or without history, clues to the etiology of coma can be elicited from the physical examination.

Vital signs:	*Severe hypertension* suggests a structural central nervous system (CNS) lesion with increased ICP or hypertensive encephalopathy.
Skin:	Look for external signs of trauma, needle marks, rashes, cherry redness (suggests carbon monoxide poisoning), or jaundice.
Breath:	Alcohol, acetone, or fetor hepaticus (from liver failure) can lead to a pungent or "fruity" smell.
Head:	The skull should be inspected for fractures, hematomas, and lacerations.
Ear, nose, and throat:	*Cerebrospinal fluid (CSF) otorrhea or rhinorrhea* results from skull fracture with disruption of the dura (a positive dextrose stick test, indicating a high level of glucose, differentiates CSF from mucus). *Hemotympanum* is also highly suggestive of skull fracture. *Tongue biting* suggests an unwitnessed seizure.

Neck (do not manip-
    ulate the neck if
    there is suspicion
    of cervical spine
    fracture):

Stiffness suggests meningitis or subarachnoid hemorrhage.

Neurologic
    examination:

The goals of the neurologic examination
are (1) to determine the depth of coma
and (2) to localize the process leading
to coma.

1. **General appearance**

    Open eyelids and a slack jaw indicate deep coma. Head
    and gaze deviation suggest a large ipsilateral hemispheric
    lesion. Observe for *myoclonus* (which suggests a metabolic
    process), *rhythmic muscle twitching* (which is indicative of
    seizure activity), or *tetany* (spontaneous, prolonged muscle
    spasms).

2. **Level of consciousness**

    Many inexact terms are used to describe depressed level
    of consciousness (e.g., somnolent, clouded, drowsy, ob-
    tunded). Because of the lack of precision associated with
    these terms, it is much more useful to **document the re-
    sponse of the patient to a specific stimulus;** for example,
    "opens eyes temporarily and responds with brief phrases
    to repeated questioning," or "moans and localizes to sternal
    rub." Responses to verbal and noxious stimuli can be used
    to generate a **Glasgow Coma scale score** (Table 6–2), a repro-

Table 6–2. □ GLASGOW COMA SCALE

Parameter	Patient Response	Score
Eye opening	Spontaneous	4
	To voice	3
	To pain	2
	None	1
Best motor response	Obeys commands	6
	Localizes to pain	5
	Withdraws to pain	4
	Flexor posturing	3
	Extensor posturing	2
	None	1
Best verbal response	Conversant and oriented	5
	Conversant and disoriented	4
	Uses inappropriate words	3
	Makes incomprehensible sounds	2
	None	1
Total score		3–15

ducible and widely used method for quantifying level of consciousness. For the sake of simplicity, we advocate describing nonalert patients as *lethargic, stuporous,* or *comatose.*

a. **Lethargy**

Lethargy resembles sleepiness, except that the patient is incapable of becoming fully alert. These patients are conversant but inattentive and slow to respond. They are unable to adequately perform simple concentration tasks, such as counting from 20 to 1 or reciting the months in reverse.

b. **Stupor**

Stupor is characterized by incomplete arousal to painful stimuli. There is little or no response to verbal commands. Painful stimulation results in brief responses to questions, exclamations ("ouch"), or moaning. The patient may obey commands temporarily when aroused by noxious stimuli but more often only localizes to pain.

c. **Coma**

Coma is defined by the absence of verbal or complex motor responses to any stimulus. *A Glasgow Coma scale score of less than or equal to 8 is frequently used to define coma.*

3. **Respirations**

Abnormal respiratory patterns (Fig. 6–1) occur frequently with coma and can aid in localization. Respirations in intubated patients can be observed by briefly disconnecting the endotracheal tube from the ventilator.

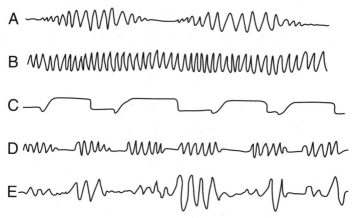

Figure 6–1 □ Abnormal respiratory patterns associated with coma. Tracings represent chest wall excursion; upward deflections represent inspiration. *A,* Cheyne-Stokes respiration. *B,* Central neurogenic hyperventilation. *C,* Apneustic breathing. *D,* Cluster breathing. *E,* Ataxic breathing.

   a. Patterns without localizing value
      (1) **Depressed respirations** can occur with severe coma of any cause.
      (2) **Cheyne-Stokes respiration** is characterized by alternating periods of hyperventilation and apnea. It usually occurs with bihemispheric lesions or metabolic encephalopathy. *Cheyne-Stokes respiration is a "stable" breathing pattern, in that it does not imply impending respiratory arrest.*
      (3) **Hyperventilation** in comatose patients is most often due to systemic disease. Hyperventilation associated with *metabolic acidosis* can result from lactic acidosis, ketoacidosis, uremia, or organic acid poisoning. An association with *respiratory alkalosis* can result from hypoxia or hepatic encephalopathy. **Central neurogenic hyperventilation** is sometimes associated with CNS lymphoma or brain stem damage from tentorial herniation.
   b. Patterns with localizing value
      (1) **Apneustic breathing** is characterized by a prolonged inspiratory phase (the inspiratory cramp) followed by apnea. It implies pontine damage.
      (2) **Cluster breathing** consists of brief cycles of shallow hyperventilation with periods of apnea. It has less of a crescendo-decrescendo quality than Cheyne-Stokes respiration and is often a sign of pontine or cerebellar damage.
      (3) **Ataxic (Biot's) breathing,** an irregular, chaotic breathing pattern, implies damage to the medullary respiratory centers and is usually seen in association with posterior fossa lesions. *Progression to apnea occurs frequently.*
4. **Visual fields**
   Visual fields should be tested with threatening movements, which normally evoke a blink. Asymmetry of this response implies hemianopia.
5. **Fundoscopy**
   Papilledema occurs after prolonged (>12 hours) elevation of ICP, and only rarely does it develop acutely. Thus, the absence of papilledema does not rule out increased ICP. *Spontaneous venous pulsations* are difficult to identify, but their presence implies normal ICP. *Subhyaloid hemorrhages* appear as globules of blood on the retinal surface and are commonly associated with subarachnoid hemorrhage.
6. **Pupils**
   The shape, size, and reactivity to light of the pupils should be noted.

a. **Symmetry and normal reactivity to light** implies structural integrity of the midbrain. *Reactive pupils in conjunction with absent corneal and oculocephalic responses are highly suggestive of metabolic coma.*

b. **Midposition (2 to 5 mm) fixed or irregular pupils** imply a focal midbrain lesion.

c. **Pinpoint reactive pupils** occur with pontine damage. Opiates and cholinergic intoxication (e.g., with pilocarpine) also produce small reactive pupils.

d. **A unilateral dilated and fixed pupil** usually occurs with CN 3 compression in the setting of uncal herniation. Ptosis and exodeviation of the eye are also seen. *An acutely "blown" pupil represents an immediate threat to life and requires urgent intervention.*

e. **Bilateral fixed and dilated pupils** can reflect central herniation, global hypoxia-ischemia, or poisoning with barbiturates, scopolamine, atropine, or glutethimide.

7. **Ocular movements**

Horizontal conjugate gaze is mediated by the *frontal eye fields* and the *pontine gaze centers.* The frontal eye fields, when activated, drive gaze to the opposite side. The pontine gaze centers, when activated, drive gaze to the same side. Vertical conjugate gaze is mediated by centers in the *midbrain tegmentum and lower diencephalon.* In unresponsive patients, conjugate eye movements can be actively elicited by testing the **oculocephalic and oculovestibular reflexes** (Fig. 6–2). Both reflexes are mediated by stimulating the semicircular canals, with CN 8 input to the vestibular nuclei and bilateral connections to the third, fourth, and sixth nuclei. *Thus, intact eye movements indicate brain stem integrity from the level of CN 3 to CN 8 (midbrain and pons).*

a. **The position of the eyes at rest** should be noted.

(1) **Gaze deviation away from the hemiparesis** results from hemispheric lesions contralateral to the hemiparesis.

(2) **Gaze deviation toward the hemiparesis** can result from the following:

(a) Pontine lesions contralateral to the hemiparesis

(b) "Wrong-way gaze" from thalamic lesions contralateral to the hemiparesis

(c) Seizure activity in the hemisphere contralateral to the hemiparesis

(3) **Forced downward eye deviation** results from lesions of the midbrain tectum. Association with impaired pupillary reactivity and refractory nystagmus is known as *Parinaud's syndrome.*

(4) **Slow roving eye movements** may be conjugate or dysconjugate and are not of localizing value. They

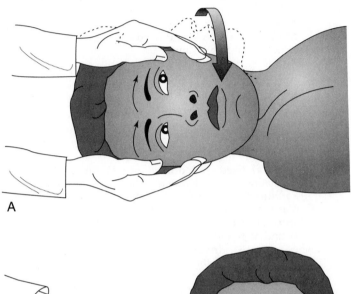

A

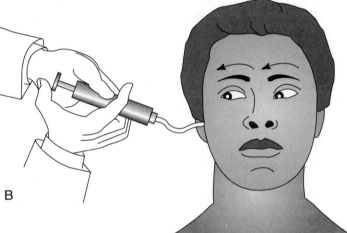

B

Figure 6–2 □ *A,* "Doll's eye" maneuver (oculocephalic reflex): with an intact brain stem (cranial nerves 3 through 8), the eyes move opposite to the direction of head turning. *B,* Cold caloric test (oculovestibular reflex): with an intact brain stem, injecting cold water in the auditory canal results in tonic conjugate eye deviation toward the cold ear.

are most frequently associated with bilateral hemispheric dysfunction and active oculocephalic reflexes.

(5) **Ocular bobbing** consists of fast downward "bobbing" with slow return to the primary position. It results from bilateral damage to the pontine horizontal gaze centers.

(6) **Saccadic (fast) eye movements** are not seen in coma and imply psychogenic unresponsiveness.

b. **The oculocephalic (doll's eye) reflex** should be noted.

This reflex is elicited by briskly turning the head side to side. In alert patients, supranuclear cortical inputs to the oculomotor nuclei control eye movement, and the response cannot be elicited. *An intact response consists of full conjugate eye movement opposite to the direction of head movement.*

A full and easy-to-elicit reflex ("ball-bearing eyes") implies bilateral cerebral hemisphere dysfunction and structural integrity of the brain stem, as seen with metabolic coma.

c. **The oculovestibular (cold caloric) reflex** should be tested.

This reflex is a more potent method for eliciting conjugate eye movements. The head is tilted 30 degrees above horizontal, and the ear is lavaged with 30 to 60 ml of ice water using butterfly tubing attached to a syringe. *A normal response consists of tonic eye deviation toward the cold ear and fast nystagmus away from the cold ear (mediated by the frontal lobe contralateral to the direction of the fast component).*

(1) **Tonic phase, bilaterally intact, with absent fast responses** suggests coma from bihemispheric dysfunction.

(2) **Conjugate gaze paresis** can result from unilateral hemispheric or pontine lesions.

(3) **Asymmetric eye weakness** implies a brain stem lesion. CN 3 paresis, CN 6 paresis, and intranuclear ophthalmoplegia are the most commonly identified abnormalities.

(4) **Absent oculovestibular responses** are seen with deep coma of any cause and imply severe depression of brain stem function.

8. **Corneal reflex**

Stroking the cornea with sterile gauze or cotton normally results in bilateral eye closure. The afferent limb of the reflex is mediated by CN 5, and the efferent limb by CN 7.

9. **Gag reflex**

In intubated patients, this reflex can be tested by gently manipulating the endotracheal tube.

10. **Motor responses**

Motor responses are the single best indicator of the depth and severity of coma.

a. **Spontaneous movements** should be observed for symmetry and purpose. Preferential movement on one side indicates weakness of the unused limbs.

b. **Limb tone** should be tested for symmetry.

Tone in the upper extremities is tested by passive motion at the elbow and wrist. Lower extremity tone is tested by a quick lifting motion under the thigh; if the heel elevates off the bed, tone is abnormally increased. *Bilaterally increased lower extremity tone is an important sign of herniation.*

c. **Induced movements** should be tested systematically by observing responses to stimuli of increasing intensity, in the following order:

(1) **Verbal command.** Ask the patient to open the eyes, protrude the tongue, raise one arm, and show two fingers. *Hand squeezing often occurs as an automatic response and, in isolation, should not be taken as evidence of the patient's following commands.*

(2) **Sternal rub.** Apply gentle pressure with fingertips. Proceed to deep knuckle pressure if there is no response.

(a) **Purposeful localizing responses** consist of precise hand movements and active attempts to ward off the examiner.

(b) **Gross localizing responses** are slower and less accurate. They occur with deepening coma or with nondominant hemispheric lesions causing impaired spatial discrimination.

(3) **Nailbed pressure.** Use the handle of the reflex hammer and gradually increase the pressure on each extremity.

(a) **Withdrawal** is mediated by the motor cortex. The movements are sudden, nonstereotyped, and variable in intensity.

(b) **Flexor (decorticate) posturing** (Fig. 6–3) results from damage to the corticospinal tracts at the level of the *deep hemisphere or upper midbrain.* The full response consists of flexion with adduction of the arms and extension of the legs.

(c) **Extensor (decerebrate) posturing** (see Fig. 6–3) consists of extension, adduction, and internal rotation of the arms and extension of the legs. It

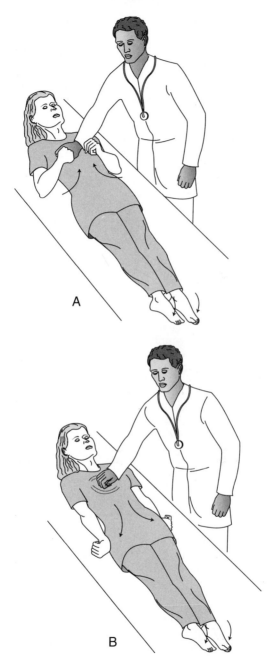

Figure 6–3 □ *A*, Decorticate (flexor) posturing. *B*, Decerebrate (extensor) posturing.

results from corticospinal tract damage at the level of the *pons or upper medulla.*

11. **Sensory responses**

Asymmetry of response to noxious stimulation suggests a lateralizing sensory deficit.

12. **Reflexes**

a. **Deep tendon reflexes**

Asymmetry indicates a lateralizing motor deficit caused by a structural lesion.

b. **Plantar reflexes**

Bilateral Babinski's responses can occur with structural or metabolic coma.

■ **DIAGNOSTIC TESTING**

Once the history and neurologic examination are completed, a differential diagnosis should be generated. Most patients in stupor or coma can be placed into one of three categories on the basis of neurologic findings:

1. **Nonfocal examination with brain stem intact**

This category is characterized by reactive pupils, full eye movements, and symmetric motor responses and suggests a toxic-metabolic etiology, CNS infection, or hydrocephalus.

2. **Focal hemispheric signs**

These are characterized by contralateral hemiparesis and gaze paresis and suggest a structural CNS lesion such as stroke, subdural hematoma, or neoplasm.

3. **Focal brain stem signs**

These are characterized by abnormal pupil reactivity, cranial nerve signs, and motor posturing and suggest a brain stem lesion or a space-occupying lesion associated with herniation or increased ICP.

Because it is important to quickly rule out life-threatening conditions in patients with coma, diagnostic testing should generally proceed in the following order in all patients until a diagnosis is established:

1. **Head CT (or MRI) scan**

Intravenous contrast should be given if a tumor or an abscess is suspected. Order bone windows if there is a history of trauma.

2. **Lumbar puncture**

LP should be performed to rule out meningitis, encephalitis, or subarachnoid hemorrhage if the diagnosis is not established by CT or MRI. *Never postpone treatment for meningitis or encephalitis if there is a delay in obtaining the CSF.*

3. **EEG**

An EEG may be necessary to rule out *nonconvulsive status*

epilepticus, a postictal state, or metabolic coma if the diagnosis is not established by CT and LP.

Pseudocoma states should be considered if the cause of coma remains unclear after diagnostic testing.

- **Psychogenic coma**

  Psychogenic coma occurs in patients who are physiologically awake but unresponsive. Clues to the diagnosis include negativistic behavior (active resistance to eye-opening or passive limb movement), avoidance behavior (the hand avoids the face when dropped from above the head), intact saccadic eye movements and nystagmus on cold caloric testing, and recovery of alertness in response to very painful stimuli.

- **Locked-in syndrome**

  Locked-in syndrome refers to bilateral pontine damage (usually from infarction) that renders the patient awake but completely paralyzed except for vertical eye movements. *Ocular bobbing* is a common finding.

- **Akinetic mutism**

  Akinetic mutism refers to states of extreme psychomotor retardation (abulia) resulting from extensive thalamic or frontal lobe damage. These patients appear awake but demonstrate reduced spontaneity and exhibit only limited responses after extremely long delays.

■ MANAGEMENT

Emergency Treatments for Patients in Coma

1. **Space-occupying lesions** require prompt neurosurgical evaluation because emergent decompression may be lifesaving.
2. **Increased intracranial pressure,** if suspected, should be treated immediately. Stepwise treatment includes
   a. *Head elevation*
   b. Intubation and *hyperventilation*
   c. *Sedation* if severe agitation is present (**midazolam 1 to 2 mg IV** is an effective, short-acting agent)
   d. *Osmotic diuresis* with **20% mannitol 1 g/kg via rapid IV infusion**

   These therapies can be used to "buy time" before definitive neurosurgical intervention. **Dexamethasone 10 mg IV every 6 hours** may also be of benefit for reducing edema associated with tumor or abscess. After these emergency treatments, an ICP monitor should be inserted to further guide management (see Chapter 13).
3. **Encephalitis** from herpesvirus infection, if suspected, should be treated empirically with **acyclovir 10 mg/kg IV every 8 hours.** Further diagnostic testing should proceed as outlined in Chapter 23.

4. **Meningitis,** if suspected, should be treated empirically. Cover with **ceftriaxone 1 g IV every 12 hours** and **ampicillin 1 g IV every 6 hours** pending CSF culture results.

General Care of the Comatose Patient

1. **Airway protection**

    Adequate oxygenation and ventilation and prevention of aspiration are the goals. Most patients will require endotracheal intubation and frequent orotracheal suctioning. *Nonintubated stuporous patients should always be made nothing by mouth (NPO).*

2. **Intravenous hydration**

    Use only isotonic fluids (e.g., normal saline) in patients with cerebral edema or increased ICP.

3. **Nutrition**

    Administer enteral feeds via a small-bore nasoduodenal tube. Nasogastric tubes impair the integrity of the upper and lower esophageal sphincters and increase the risk of gastroesophageal reflux and aspiration.

4. **Skin**

    Order that the patient be turned every 1 to 2 hours to prevent pressure sores. An inflatable or foam mattress and protective heel pads may also be beneficial.

5. **Eyes**

    Prevent corneal abrasion by taping the eyelids shut or by applying a lubricant.

6. **Bowel care**

    Constipation can be avoided by giving a stool softener **(docusate sodium 100 mg three times a day).** Intubation and steroids may predispose to gastric stress ulceration, and this should be prevented by giving an H_2 blocker **(ranitidine 50 mg IV every 8 hours).**

7. **Bladder care**

    Indwelling urinary catheters are a common source of infection and should be used judiciously. Use intermittent catheterization every 6 hours when possible.

8. **Joint mobility**

    Order daily passive range-of-motion exercises to prevent contractures.

9. **Deep vein thrombosis (DVT) prophylaxis**

    Immobility is a major risk factor for DVT and subsequent pulmonary embolism. Order heparin **5000 units subcutaneously (SC) every 12 hours,** external pneumatic compression stockings, or both.

■ PROGNOSIS

The prognosis for recovery from coma depends primarily on the cause, rather than on the depth, of coma. Coma from drug

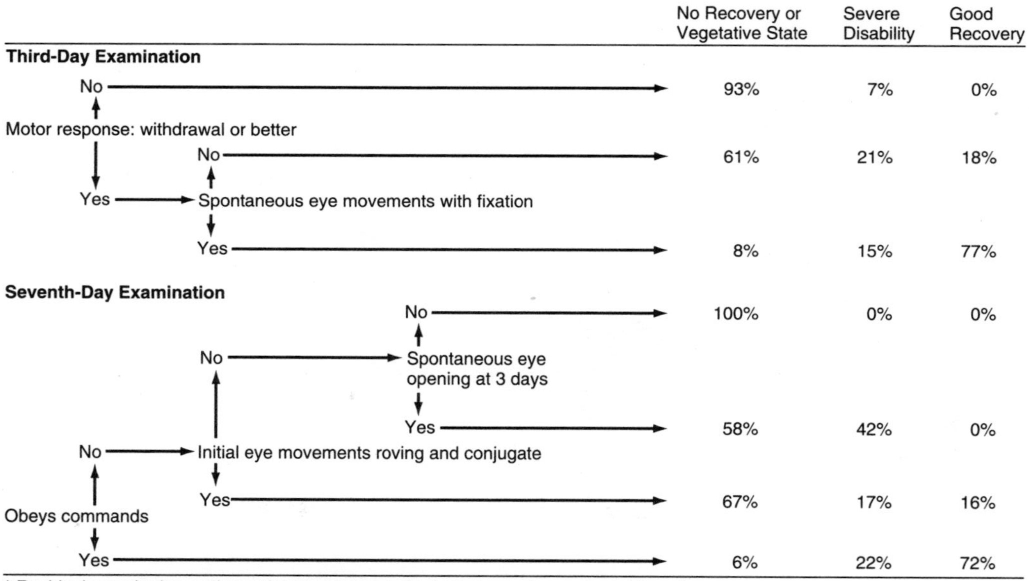

	No Recovery or Vegetative State	Severe Disability	Good Recovery
Third-Day Examination			
Motor response: withdrawal or better — No	93%	7%	0%
Spontaneous eye movements with fixation — No	61%	21%	18%
Spontaneous eye movements with fixation — Yes	8%	15%	77%
Seventh-Day Examination			
Spontaneous eye opening at 3 days — No	100%	0%	0%
Spontaneous eye opening at 3 days — Yes	58%	42%	0%
Obeys commands — No	67%	17%	16%
Obeys commands — Yes	6%	22%	72%

* Residual anesthetics, anticonvulsants, or metabolic derangements may be confounding.

Figure 6—4 □ Features predictive of recovery from hypoxic-ischemic coma. Outcomes refer to best functional state attained within the first year. (Modified from Levy DE, Caronna JJ, Singer BH), et al: Predicting outcome from hypoxic-ischemic coma. JAMA 1985;253:1420. Copyright 1985, American Medical Association.)

intoxication and metabolic causes carries the best prognosis; patients with coma from traumatic head injury fare better than those with coma from other structural causes; and coma from global hypoxia-ischemia carries the least favorable prognosis. Simple bedside testing can be used to prognosticate outcome as early as 3 days after hypoxic-ischemic coma (Fig. 6–4).

Persistent vegetative state (PVS) refers to a state of "eyes-open unresponsiveness" that is applied to patients in coma for 30 days or more. These patients assume normal sleep-wake cycles and display primitive responses to stimuli, such as chewing, sucking, and grasping, but demonstrate no evidence of conscious awareness. Prognostication is important, because this information may influence decisions to withhold life-sustaining measures such as cardiopulmonary resuscitation (CPR) or intensive care unit (ICU) care. Recovery of consciousness from PVS is generally defined as return of the ability to communicate or follow commands. By this criterion, 15% of patients with nontraumatic injury and 50% of patients with traumatic injury who are still in a vegetative state after 1 month will recover consciousness by 12 months. Recovery of consciousness after 12 months in a PVS is exceedingly rare.

7

ACUTE STROKE

Stroke should be suspected whenever a patient presents with the characteristic sudden onset of focal neurologic signs, such as hemiparesis, hemisensory loss, hemianopia, aphasia, or ataxia (Table 7–1). Time is of the essence for treating stroke, because the "therapeutic window" is only 3 to 6 hours. Because of the importance of early intervention in acute stroke, the emphasis of emergency room (ER) management should not be on identifying subtle, unusual, or interesting neurologic signs but on

1. **Stabilizing the patient**
2. **Obtaining blood tests, an electrocardiogram (ECG), and a chest x-ray**
3. **Establishing the diagnosis by history and physical examination**
4. **Obtaining a head computed tomography (CT) or magnetic resonance imaging (MRI) scan as soon as possible**

Further management of the patient, once the diagnosis has been established and the patient has left the ER, is discussed in Chapter 25.

■ PHONE CALL

Questions

1. **What were the presenting symptoms?**
2. **Exactly when did the symptoms begin?**
3. **What are the vital signs?**
4. **Does the patient have a history of hypertension, diabetes, or cardiac disease?**

Table 7–1 □ **PRESENTATIONS OF ACUTE STROKE**

Abrupt onset of facial or limb weakness (usually hemiparesis)
Sensory loss in one or more extremities
Sudden change in mental status (confusion, delirium, lethargy, stupor, or coma)
Aphasia (incoherent speech, lack of speech output, or difficulty understanding speech)
Dysarthria (slurred speech)
Loss of vision (hemianopia or monocular) or diplopia
Ataxia (truncal or limb)
Vertigo, nausea and vomiting, or headache

5. Is the patient taking aspirin or warfarin?

It is particularly important to perform an urgent CT scan in patients taking warfarin, in order to rule out intracerebral hemorrhage, because early treatment with fresh frozen plasma (FFP) can be lifesaving.

Orders

1. Establish an intravenous line with **0.9% normal saline (NS) at 20 ml/hour.**

   Hypotonic fluids such as D5W and half-normal saline aggravate cerebral edema.
2. Provide oxygen via a nasal cannula (if patient is tachypneic).
3. Keep the patient NPO (nothing by mouth).
4. Obtain an electrocardiogram (ECG).
5. Obtain a chest x-ray.
6. Obtain a stat noncontrast head CT scan.
7. Perform the following diagnostic blood tests:
   - Complete blood count (CBC) and platelets
   - Serum chemistries (glucose, electrolytes, blood urea nitrogen [BUN], creatinine)
   - Prothrombin time (PT)/partial thromboplastin time (PTT)
8. If indicated, perform the following tests:
   - Alcohol level
   - Liver function tests
   - Arterial blood gases
   - Toxicology screen

■ ELEVATOR THOUGHTS

What are the causes of stroke?
1. Infarction: causes 80% of all strokes
   a. Embolic
      (1) Cardiogenic embolism
         (a) Atrial fibrillation or other arrhythmia
         (b) Left ventricular mural thrombus
         (c) Mitral or aortic valve disease
         (d) Endocarditis (infectious or noninfectious)
      (2) Paradoxical embolism (patent foramen ovale)
      (3) Aortic arch embolism
   b. Atherothrombotic (large- or medium-vessel disease)
      (1) Extracranial disease
         (a) Internal carotid artery
         (b) Vertebral artery
      (2) Intracranial disease
         (a) Internal carotid artery

(b) Middle cerebral artery
(c) Basilar artery
  c. Lacunar (small penetrating artery occlusion)
2. Intracerebral hemorrhage (ICH): causes 15% of all strokes
  a. Hypertensive
  b. Arteriovenous malformation
  c. Amyloid angiopathy
3. Subarachnoid hemorrhage (SAH): causes 5% of all strokes
4. Miscellaneous causes (can lead to infarction or hemorrhage)
  a. Dural sinus thrombosis
  b. Carotid or vertebral artery dissection
  c. Central nervous system (CNS) vasculitis
  d. Moyamoya disease (progressive intracranial large artery occlusion)
  e. Migraine
  f. Hypercoagulable state
  g. Drug abuse (cocaine or amphetamines)
  h. Hematologic disorders (sickle cell anemia, polycythemia, or leukemia)
  i. MELAS (mitochondrial encephalopathy, lactic acidosis, and stroke)
  j. Atrial myxoma

■ MAJOR THREAT TO LIFE

- **Transtentorial herniation**
  Occurs primarily in the following presentations:
  1. Massive hemispheric infarction or hemorrhage
  2. Intraventricular extension of ICH or SAH
- **Cerebellar infarction or hemorrhage**
  All patients with large cerebellar lesions require neurosurgical evaluation because emergent decompression can be life-saving.
- **Aspiration**
  Aspiration pneumonia is a common cause of mortality in stroke patients. All patients should be considered to have impaired swallowing until proven otherwise.
- **Myocardial infarction (MI)**
  Acute MI complicates approximately 3% of acute ischemic strokes.

■ BEDSIDE

Quick Look Test

What is the patient's level of consciousness?
  The urgency of the situation can be immediately assessed by evaluating the level of consciousness. *Patients in stupor or coma*

are at the highest risk for further deterioration and are most likely to benefit from urgent intervention.

Airway and Vital Signs

Is the patient in respiratory distress?

If the patient's breathing appears labored, test for arterial blood gas levels and start oxygen. **Patients with severe dyspnea or depressed level of consciousness (stupor or coma) should be intubated prior to CT scanning.** Failure to control the airway in either setting can lead to massive aspiration or to respiratory arrest.

What is the blood pressure?

Hypertension occurs frequently after stroke as a nonspecific response to cerebral injury. In ischemic stroke, this response may be advantageous, because increased cerebral perfusion pressure improves blood flow in regions of marginally perfused brain (the ischemic penumbra) that have lost the capacity to autoregulate. As a result, *overly aggressive blood pressure (BP) reduction in acute ischemic stroke patients can lead to increased infarction and neurologic deterioration.* For this reason, only severe hypertension should be treated prior to CT scanning unless there is a nonneurologic indication (Box 7–1).

If the patient meets one of the criteria listed in Box 7–1 and needs urgent BP control, start with IV labetalol.

Box 7–1. GUIDELINES FOR ER TREATMENT OF HYPERTENSION IN ACUTE STROKE

Treat hypertension if a nonneurologic hypertensive emergency exists:

1. Acute myocardial ischemia
2. Cardiogenic pulmonary edema
3. Malignant hypertension (retinopathy)
4. Hypertensive nephropathy
5. Aortic dissection

Also treat hypertension if the BP is highly elevated on three repeated measurements 15 minutes apart:

1. Systolic BP >220 mm Hg
2. Diastolic BP >120 mm Hg

Otherwise, systolic BPs of 160 to 220 mm Hg should *not* be treated prior to CT scanning. If hemorrhage is identified by CT, reduction of the systolic BP to 150 to 180 mm Hg should be considered.

1. Order **100 mg of IV labetalol in a 20-ml syringe (5 mg/ ml)** to the bedside.
2. Order a labetalol drip to the bedside **(200 mg in 200 ml NS).**
3. **IV push 20 mg of labetalol over 2 minutes; repeat 40 to 80 mg at 10-minute intervals** until the desired BP is attained.
4. Once the desired BP is attained, start infusion of **2 mg/ min (120 ml/hour)** and titrate.

If labetalol fails to control hypertension and increased intracranial pressure (ICP) is not a concern, start **nitroprusside IV 50 mg/250 ml D5W (200 μg/ml) at 3 ml/hour (10 μg/min)** and titrate.

Low BP in acute stroke is unusual. Hypotension that is severe enough to precipitate cerebral infarction is rare but can occur in patients with severe carotid artery or intracranial artery stenosis.

What is the heart rate?

Rapid atrial fibrillation may require treatment with **digoxin 0.125 to 0.5 mg IV** or **verapamil 5 to 10 mg IV** for rate control prior to CT scanning.

What is the temperature?

The most common cause of fever in a stroke patient is aspiration pneumonia. If fever is present, order blood and urine cultures and consider administering antibiotics empirically **(cefoxitin 1 g IV every 6 hours** or **cefuroxime 750 mg IV every 8 hours).**

Selective History

If possible, obtain an eyewitness to corroborate the patient's account. Be sure to check the following:

1. **What time did the stroke begin?**

   Approximately 30% of strokes occur at night and present upon awakening.
2. **What were the initial symptoms?**

   A maximal deficit at onset in a fully alert patient supports cerebral infarction and suggests embolism, in particular. Loss of consciousness, headache, or vomiting supports intracerebral hemorrhage. Inquire specifically about the following:
   - Headache or neck pain (hemorrhage or dissection)
   - Loss of consciousness
   - Confused or slurred speech
   - Visual disturbances
   - Dizziness or vertigo (brain stem ischemia)
   - Weakness or clumsiness
   - Numbness or paresthesias
   - Gait instability

3. **Were there any antecedent attacks consistent with transient ischemic attack (TIA)?**
4. **Was any seizure activity observed?**
5. **What is the patient's medical history?**
6. **Has the patient used drugs or alcohol recently?**
   Cocaine can precipitate infarction or hemorrhage.
7. **What medications is the patient taking?**

Selective Physical Examination

A rapid screening examination should be directed toward the following:

Neck:	Auscultate for carotid bruits. Neck stiffness suggests subarachnoid hemorrhage.
Lungs:	Check for aspiration pneumonia or congestive heart failure.
Heart:	Murmurs suggest valvular heart disease and a possible source of embolism.
Neurologic examination:	Because time is of the essence, the initial neurologic examination needs to be systematic and efficient. The goal is to simply localize and characterize the severity of the deficit. An experienced examiner can accomplish this in 10 to 15 minutes; a more detailed examination should be carried out later.

- **Mental status**
  1. **Level of consciousness and attentiveness**
  2. **Concentration.** Ask the patient to count from 20 to 1 or to recite the months in reverse.
  3. **Orientation**
  4. **Aphasia.** Check the fluency of spontaneous speech, naming, repetition, and paraphasic errors (word or syllable substitutions).
  5. **Hemispatial neglect.** Forced head and gaze deviation implies a large hemispheric lesion.
- **Cranial nerves**
  1. **Fundus.** Check for papilledema.
  2. **Visual fields.** Ask the patient to count fingers in all four quadrants. Check the patient's blink-to-threat if the patient is inattentive.
  3. **Pupils**
  4. **Extraocular movements**
  5. **Face.** A widened palpebral fissure and flattened nasolabial fold are indicative of facial weakness.
  6. **Palate and tongue.** Check for symmetry and adequacy of the gag reflex.

- **Motor**
  1. **Spontaneous movements.** Preferential movement of the limbs on one side indicates paresis of the unused limbs. If the patient is unresponsive, check for a preferential localizing response to sternal rub.
  2. **Limb tone.** Increased tone occurs with deep lesions in the internal capsule or brain stem.
  3. **Arm (pronator) drift.** If the patient is unable to follow commands, passively elevate both arms and check whether one falls preferentially.
  4. **Power.** Check strength against active resistance at the shoulders, wrists, hips, and ankles.
- **Reflexes**
  1. **Deep tendon reflex**
  2. **Plantar reflex**

Proceed with the neurologic examination if the patient's level of consciousness allows:

- **Sensory**
  1. **Pinprick or pinch test** identifies a lateralizing deficit.
- **Coordination**
  1. **Finger-to-nose test** identifies intention tremor and past pointing.
  2. **Gait and station.** Check for reduced arm swing on the paretic side. A wide base is indicative of truncal ataxia.

■ MANAGEMENT I: ACUTE MANAGEMENT

Once the history and examination are completed, you should be able to localize the lesion clinically. **The main differential diagnoses are infarction and hemorrhage, which can be accurately diagnosed only by CT.** Hence, all further management decisions (anticoagulation, BP management, or further workup) will depend on the results of the head CT.

Hemorrhage

Radiographic Assessment

Blood is readily identified by the presence of a high-density (bright) signal (Fig. 7–1*A*). If ICH is present, be sure to check for the following radiographic findings:

- *Subarachnoid hemorrhage* (Fig. 7–1*B*) in association with intraparenchymal hemorrhage suggests a ruptured aneurysm and requires angiography.
- *Intraventricular hemorrhage* (Fig. 7–1*C*) in association with ventricular enlargement requires neurosurgical evaluation for possible emergent ventriculostomy.

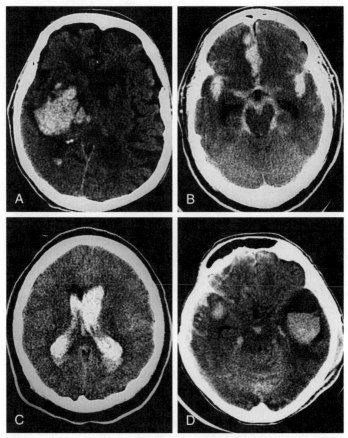

Figure 7–1 □ CT scans of brain hemorrhage. *A*, Intracerebral hemorrhage. *B*, Subarachnoid hemorrhage. *C*, Intraventricular hemorrhage. *D*, Acute hemorrhage with fluid/fluid level, indicative of a clotting disturbance.

- *Fluid/fluid levels* within a hematoma (Fig. 7–1D) result from separation of red cells and plasma and are indicative of a coagulopathy.
- *Edema and mass effect* usually lead to delayed neurologic deterioration when associated with a large hemorrhage (>30 ml). An abnormally large or an irregular amount of edema associated with hemorrhage suggests (1) hemorrhagic infarction, (2) bleeding associated with neoplasm, or (3) venous infarction from dural sinus thrombosis.

Checklist for Acute Management

1. **Rule out coagulopathy.**

   Confirm that the PT and PTT are normal. If the PT is elevated, give **FFP 4 to 8 units IV every 4 hours** and **vitamin K 15 mg IV push, then subcutaneously (SC) three times a day** until the PT is normalized. Reverse heparin anticoagulation with **protamine sulfate 10 to 50 mg slow IV push** (1 mg reverses approximately 100 units of heparin).

2. **Control severe hypertension.**

   In contrast to the approach taken with acute cerebral infarction, a somewhat more aggressive approach to BP control is suggested for patients with acute ICH, because high levels may lead to worsening of perilesional edema. Although the optimal management has yet to be established, we advocate reduction of systolic BPs that are higher than 180 mm Hg to levels between 150 and 180 mm Hg using a labetalol drip (see Airway and Vital Signs).

3. **Obtain a neurosurgical evaluation.**

   The criteria for emergent evacuation of intracerebral hemorrhage are controversial. Surgery can be lifesaving if the patient is deteriorating and signs of herniation appear. Consideration should also be given to inserting a *ventricular drain* in patients with intraventricular hemorrhage or a *parenchymal ICP monitor* in patients with large, deep hemorrhages who are not candidates for surgery.

4. **Consider angiography** to rule out an aneurysm or arteriovenous malformation (AVM). This is particularly important in young (less than 50 years of age), nonhypertensive patients.

5. **Consider mannitol (1 g/kg IV)** for deepening coma or if clinical signs of brain stem compression are evident (see Chapter 13 for further details).

   Steroids such as dexamethasone have not been shown to be effective in patients with ICH. We use **dexamethasone (10 mg IV every 6 hours)** only as a treatment of last resort for transtentorial herniation.

6. **Consider phenytoin loading (10 to 20 mg/kg IV or by mouth [PO])** in patients with large hemorrhages and depressed level of consciousness.

   In general, anticonvulsants can be withheld unless there is evidence of seizure activity. However, prophylactic treatment is reasonable if the patient's condition is critical enough to require intubation, treatment of increased ICP, or surgery.

Additional guidelines for the management of ICH or SAH are included in Chapter 25 and under Management II: General Care in this chapter.

Infarction

Radiographic Assessment

Infarction appears as a lucent (dark) signal on a CT scan but may not be apparent until 12 to 24 hours after onset. Early signs of infarction (Fig. 7–2) are important to recognize and include (1) loss of definition of the gray-white junction, (2) mild sulcal effacement, and (3) subtle, hazy lucency. The CT scan is frequently negative in patients with lacunar or brain stem infarction, and in these cases, MRI will frequently delineate the lesion. Newer MRI techniques such as diffusion-weighted imaging (DWI) may reveal ischemia or early infarction in the first few hours after stroke onset.

Affected Vascular Territory

Identification of the affected vascular territory can provide important information regarding the mechanism of the infarction. The topography of the major arterial territories of the brain are shown in Figure 7–3. Examples of the three main patterns of infarction, described below, are shown in Figure 7–4.

1. **Territorial infarction** respects the margins of an entire vascular territory or one of its branches. The cause is usually embolism, with infarction occurring in brain regions immediately distal to the site of occlusion.
2. **Border-zone infarction** may occur either (1) along the boundaries between different vascular territories (watershed infarction) or (2) in the deepest and least well-collateralized regions of a vascular territory (internal border-zone infarction). In either case, the cause is usually distal hemodynamic perfusion failure related to a more proximal stenosis or occlusion.

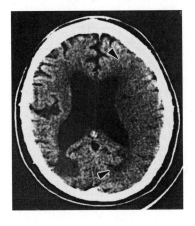

Figure 7–2 □ Early cerebral infarction, with loss of gray-white definition and sulcal effacement. (Arrowheads indicate anterior and posterior borders of the territory of the middle cerebral artery.)

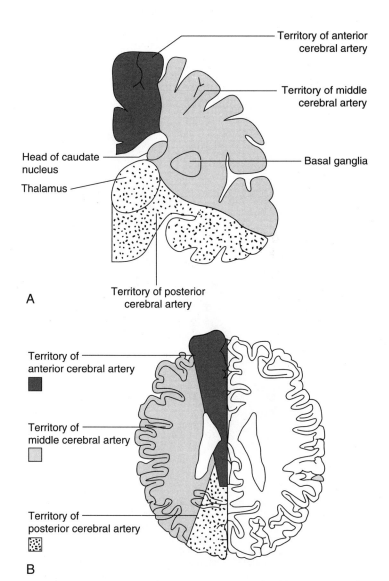

Figure 7–3 ◻ Coronal section *(A)* and axial section *(B)* at the level of the basal ganglia, showing the anatomic distribution of the major cerebral vascular territories.

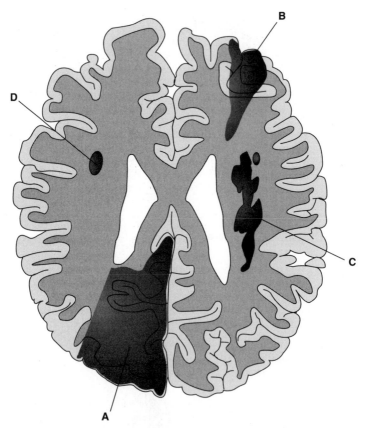

Figure 7–4 □ Schematic representation of different topographic patterns of cerebral infarction. A = territorial infarction (from posterior cerebral artery occlusion); B = watershed border-zone infarction (between the territories of the anterior cerebral artery and the middle cerebral artery); C = internal border-zone infarction (deep middle cerebral artery territory); D = lacunar infarction (lenticulostriate-penetrating artery occlusion).

3. **Lacunar infarction** appears as a small, deep infarction within the territory of a single, small penetrating artery. The mechanism is usually related to occlusion within the course of the small vessel (microatheroma or lipohyalinosis).

Goals of Management

1. **Limiting or reversing ongoing acute ischemia (3- to 6-hour window)**

    Thrombolysis with **tissue plasminogen activator (t-PA)** is the only currently approved treatment for reversing ischemia in acute stroke. It carries a 6% risk of significant bleeding and should be given only within 3 hours of onset and only if the head CT scan is normal. It should be administered by experienced clinicians only.

2. **Preventing neurologic deterioration related to an evolving stroke (72-hour window)**

    Stroke progression occurs in 20 to 40% of hospitalized patients with ischemic stroke, with the risk being highest in the first 24 hours. Clinical deterioration can result from one of three mechanisms:

    - **Progressive edema and infarct swelling.** This problem is generally limited to large infarcts. Brain edema generally peaks 3 to 5 days after onset and is rarely a problem within the first 24 hours.

        Approach: Treatment with mannitol is beneficial. Avoid hypotenic fluids. *Steroids are not effective.*

    - **Extension of ischemic territory.** This may result from either *progressive thrombosis within an occluded vessel* (i.e., progressive brain stem infarction in a patient with basilar artery thrombosis) or *distal perfusion failure related to a more proximal stenosis or occlusion* (i.e., enlargement of internal border-zone infarction in a patient with internal carotid artery [ICA] occlusion).

        Approach: Heparin may prevent progressive thrombosis, and optimization of volume status and blood pressure may mitigate perfusion failure.

    - **Hemorrhagic conversion.** This problem is frequently identified radiographically but rarely results in clinical symptoms. The three main risk factors are increased patient age, large infarct size, and acute hypertension.

        Approach: Defer anticoagulation of high-risk patients for 48 to 72 hours; treat severe hypertension.

3. **Preventing early recurrent stroke (30-day window)**

    Approximately 5% of patients hospitalized for ischemic stroke experience a second stroke within 30 days. This risk is highest (greater than 10%) in patients with severe carotid stenosis and cardioembolism and lowest (1%) in patients with lacunar infarction.

Approach: Early treatment with heparin may reduce the risk of early recurrent stroke in patients with cardioembolism but has not been proven to do so.

Checklist for Acute Management

1. **Consider IV t-PA (0.9 mg/kg IV over 1 hour with 10% of the dose given as an initial bolus; maximum of 90 mg)** if onset is definitely within 3 hours and CT shows no signs of widespread early infarction.

2. **Consider cardiac rhythm monitoring** for patients with evidence of arrhythmia or myocardial ischemia.

3. **Consider intensive care unit (ICU) observation** in patients with clinical or radiographic signs of massive hemispheric or cerebellar infarction, depressed level of consciousness, respiratory distress, or stroke-in-evolution.

4. **Obtain a neurosurgical evaluation** for possible decompressive surgery in patients with large cerebellar infarction.

5. **Consider MRI** in patients with posterior circulation strokes or if the infarction is not well delineated by CT.

6. **Consider IV heparin** (start at **800 units/hour, 20,000 units in 500 ml NS at 20 ml/hour)** in the following situations:
   - Suspected cardioembolic stroke
   - TIAs or infarction related to carotid artery stenosis
   - Stroke-in-evolution
   - Arterial dissection
   - Dural sinus thrombosis

   Keep in mind that heparin is relatively contraindicated in patients with large infarcts associated with mass effect or hemorrhagic conversion.

7. **Order a noninvasive neurovascular workup.**

   Proper decisions regarding the treatment of cerebral infarction are based on elucidation of the mechanism of the stroke.

   The following tests should be performed in every patient:
   - *Echocardiography* is an important technique for identifying cardiac sources of emboli. In many patients, transthoracic echocardiography is adequate. *Transesophageal echocardiography* provides more-detailed views of the left atrium and aortic arch and is a more sensitive test for detecting mural thrombi and valvular vegetations. An *agitated saline study* ("bubble study") is highly sensitive for detecting right-to-left atrial shunts, consistent with a patent foramen ovale.
   - *Carotid Doppler ultrasonography* is needed to rule out carotid stenosis that is symptomatic and greater than 70%, which is an indication for carotid endarterectomy.

The following tests should be performed in selected patients:

- *Transcranial Doppler ultrasonography* can be used to diagnose occlusion or stenosis of the major intracranial arteries. Abnormal intracranial waveforms and collateral flow patterns can also be used to determine whether a stenosis found in the neck is hemodynamically significant.
- *Magnetic resonance angiography* can be used to diagnose extracranial or intracranial stenosis or occlusion.
- *Holter monitoring* may be useful for detecting intermittent atrial fibrillation.

8. **Consider blood testing** to identify unusual causes of stroke, particularly in young patients.
   - *Blood cultures* if endocarditis is suspected.
   - *Procoagulant workup:* protein C activity, protein S activity, antithrombin III activity, lupus anticoagulant, anticardiolipin antibodies. *Note:* These tests should be obtained before anticoagulation is started.
   - *Vasculitis workup:* antinuclear antibody (ANA), rheumatoid factor (RF), rapid plasmin reagin (RPR), hepatitis virus serologies, erythrocyte sedimentation rate (ESR), serum protein electrophoresis (SPEP), cryoglobulins, and herpes simplex virus (HSV) serologies.
   - *Coagulation profile* to rule out disseminated intravascular coagulation (DIC).
   - *Beta-human chorionic gonadotropin (β-HCG)* testing to rule out pregnancy in young women with stroke.

Refer to Chapter 25 for further discussion of specific ischemic stroke syndromes, evaluation of TIAs, and the secondary prevention of ischemic stroke.

■ MANAGEMENT II: GENERAL CARE

Much of the morbidity and mortality associated with stroke is related to nonneurologic complications, which can be minimized by adherence to these guidelines:

1. **Fever**

   Fever exacerbates ischemic brain injury and should be treated aggressively with antipyretics (acetaminophen) or a cooling blanket, if necessary.

2. **Nutrition**

   Stroke patients are at high risk for aspiration. Patients with depressed level of consciousness, brain stem strokes, bilateral strokes, and large hemispheric strokes carry the highest risk. Formal assessment of swallowing ability by a speech pathologist or an ear, nose, and throat specialist should be completed before patients at risk are fed. Start enteral feeding via a nasoduodenal tube within 24 hours after the stroke if the patient cannot swallow safely.

3. **Intravenous hydration**

Hypovolemia is common among stroke patients and should be corrected with isotonic crystalloid. Avoiding volume depletion may be particularly important in patients with intracardiac thrombi (dehydration has been linked to progressive thrombus formation) or hemodynamic stroke. Hypotonic fluids (e.g., D5W and 0.45% saline) can aggravate cerebral edema and should be avoided.

4. **Glucose**

Hyperglycemia and hypoglycemia can lead to exacerbation of ischemic injury. Although the clinical relevance of these effects in humans is unclear, it seems prudent to prevent hyperglycemia (glucose level higher than 240 mg/dl) by avoiding administration of IV dextrose solutions and by treating with insulin, if needed.

5. **Pulmonary care**

Chest physical therapy (every 4 hours) should be ordered to prevent atelectasis in immobilized patients.

6. **Activity**

Patients with stroke should be mobilized and engaged in physical therapy as soon as possible. For immobilized patients, order patient turning every 2 hours (to prevent pressure sores) and joint range-of-motion exercises four times a day to prevent contractures. Heel splints to maintain the ankle in dorsiflexion can also prevent shortening of the Achilles tendon. Have the patient taken out of bed to a chair every day as soon as feasible.

7. **Prophylaxis for deep vein thrombosis (DVT)**

Ischemic stroke patients with significant immobility who are not on IV heparin should be treated with **heparin 5000 units every 12 hours** to prevent formation of DVT. This treatment can be started safely in patients with ICH after 72 hours.

8. **Bladder care**

Indwelling urinary catheters should be used judiciously; order intermittent catheterization every 6 hours when possible.

SPINAL CORD COMPRESSION

Spinal cord compression is one of the few true neurologic emergencies. The more severe the syndrome, the more acute the injury is likely to have been. Unlike the brain, which may have remarkable functional recovery, the spinal cord, once damaged, rarely recovers function. Patients with cord compression resulting from neoplastic disease of the spine who cannot walk before the onset of treatment will rarely walk again. Diagnosis of spinal cord injury depends on a clear understanding of the anatomy of the cord and the supportive structures.

■ PHONE CALL

This chapter will be most useful for patients in whom spinal cord compression is known or suspected. The response to such a call should focus on establishing the diagnosis and assessing the acuteness of the injury.

Questions

1. **What is the patient's general condition?**
2. **What are the vital signs? Is the patient in any respiratory distress?**
3. **Does the patient have back pain?**
4. **Is there history of trauma to the neck or back?**
5. **Does the patient have any known cancer or infection?**
    Back pain in a cancer patient is considered to result from a vertebral metastasis until it is proven otherwise.
6. **How long has the problem been going on?**

Orders

If trauma or an unstable spine is suspected, give the following orders:

1. **Immobilize the neck (back).**
    A Philadelphia collar or a backboard should be used to ensure adequate stability (Fig. 8–1). If such equipment is unavailable immediately, the cervical spine can be immobi-

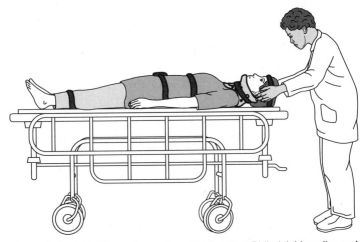

Figure 8–1 □ Stabilizing the neck and back with a Philadelphia collar and a backboard.

lized by holding the head firmly in a neutral position, using both hands.

2. **Check vital signs.**

Injury above the C5 level may compromise respiratory function. Cervical spinal injury, particularly with complete transection, may result in loss of sympathetic control, causing hypotension and bradycardia. Fever may point to an infectious process.

3. **Obtain plain x-rays of the neck (back) (anteroposterior and lateral).**

Flexion and extension views, if done carefully by an experienced staff, may be helpful. Even if there is no suspicion of trauma, the pattern of bony abnormality may suggest subluxation, unsuspected pathologic fracture from neoplasm, osteomyelitis, or other infection. In most circumstances, plain x-rays can provide quick information that can then be followed up by computed tomography (CT) or magnetic resonance imaging (MRI) once an initial assessment is done.

4. **Notify the neurosurgical team or specialized spinal unit, if available.**

Direct trauma to the spinal cord can produce a myelopathy, but it is the secondary effects from bleeding, dislocation, or osseous or articular instability that can be devastating; these secondary effects are preventable if properly identified and addressed.

Inform RN

"Will arrive at the bedside in . . . minutes."

Spinal cord compression is a medical emergency. Delay may cause irreversible neurologic dysfunction.

■ ELEVATOR THOUGHTS (DIFFERENTIAL DIAGNOSIS OF SPINAL CORD COMPRESSION)

Physical examination and often radiographic evaluation are needed to confirm a compressive myelopathy. You should be thinking first of the three categories of disease that are the most likely to cause spinal cord compression: trauma, infection, and neoplasm. Four other categories complete the differential diagnosis list.

1. **Trauma**

    This is the most acute form of spinal cord compression. A history of a motor vehicle accident or sports-related accident is commonly elicited. Flexion, extension, compression, or rotation injuries in addition to direct blunt or penetrating trauma may produce a compressive myelopathy. Cervical disks tend to herniate centrally, producing an anterior cord syndrome.

2. **Infection**

    Infections of the spine most often occur in the thoracic or lumbar spine. Infections can take the following forms:

    - Epidural abscesses. Seen commonly in intravenous (IV) drug users, these are most often bacterial (e.g., *Staphylococcus aureus, Escherichia coli*).
    - Spinal tuberculosis (Pott's disease). This occurs in debilitated or immunocompromised patients or in those known to have pulmonary tuberculosis.
    - Vertebral osteomyelitis. *Staphylococcus* species, *Streptococcus* species, *E. coli,* or *Brucella* species may cause pathologic fractures or produce epidural abscesses.

3. **Neoplasm**

    Metastases are the most common neoplasm seen in bony disease of the spine (Fig. 8–2). The thoracic spine is most often affected because of venous drainage of visceral organs through spinal extradural venous plexuses. Meningiomas may appear as extradural tumors, with a predominance in the thoracic region. The female/male ratio is 9:1. Neurofibromas or schwannomas may arise on spinal roots and cause cord compression as they expand. Ependymomas are intrin-

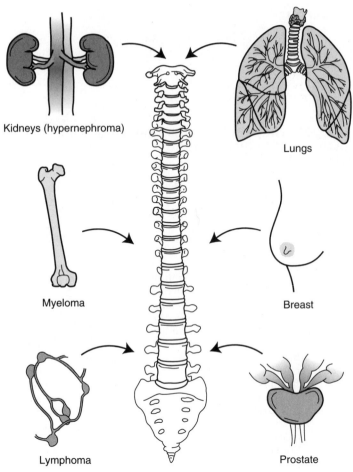

Figure 8–2 □ Neoplasms that commonly metastasize to the spine: carcinoma of the lung, breast, colon, and prostate; hypernephroma; myeloma; and lymphoma.

sic cord tumors that could mimic extra-axial compressive lesions.

4. **Degenerative disease**

Cervical disks herniate centrally, in contrast to lumbar disks, which herniate laterally and cause radicular symptoms. Thoracic disk protrusions are rare. An acute cauda equina syndrome may be produced by herniation at L1–L2.

5. **Congenital disease**

Arnold-Chiari malformation, with or without syringomyelia, may produce cervical myelopathy. Congenital defects of the atlantoaxial joint may predispose to subluxation or dislocation. A tethered cord produces a spastic diplegia of the legs. Relatively minor trauma may bring an occult malformation to clinical prominence.

6. **Inflammatory disease**

Rheumatoid arthritis is the most common disease affecting the stability of the upper cervical spine and may allow atlantoaxial translocations.

7. **Vascular disease**

Epidural and subdural hematomas of the spine are very rare. They may be seen in patients taking anticoagulant medication. Arteriovenous malformations of the spine are rare.

■ MAJOR THREAT TO LIFE

- **Respiratory compromise** (cervical lesions) may require immediate intubation. Diaphragm weakness may result in hypoventilation and respiratory acidosis.
- **Autonomic dysregulation may produce hypotension** that does not respond to volume challenge. This phenomenon may be part of spinal shock. The hypotension may respond to pressors (e.g., dopamine).

■ BEDSIDE

Quick Look Test

What is the general condition of the patient?

Respiratory distress may necessitate immediate intubation. Look for retraction of the supraclavicular muscles as a sign of accessory respiratory muscle use because of diaphragmatic weakness.

Does the patient look cachectic or ill, suggesting cancer or general debilitation?

Is there urinary or bowel incontinence, suggesting sacral cord involvement?

Is there flushing or diaphoresis, suggesting autonomic dysregulation?

Management

If, after a quick look, the patient appears unstable, notify the surgical team, the anesthesiology service, and/or the neurosurgery service and address cardiopulmonary dysfunction. Stability of the neck should be ensured.

1. **Anti-inflammatory treatment**
   a. **Trauma**
      For **acute traumatic spinal cord injury,** the following protocol for methylprednisolone administration should be initiated:
      (1) **Methylprednisolone 30 mg/kg IV bolus over 15 minutes**
      (2) 45-minute pause
      (3) **Methylprednisolone 5.4 mg/kg/hr continuous IV infusion over the next 23 hours**
   b. **Tumor**
      For known or suspected **spinal neoplasm,** administer **dexamethasone 100 mg IV bolus** immediately.

2. **Blood tests**
   In any patient with suspected spinal cord compression, routine blood tests should be performed in preparation for possible surgical decompression: complete blood count (CBC), chemistry panel, coagulation profile, and blood type and hold.

3. **Imaging**
   If the patient is hemodynamically stable and not in respiratory distress, notify the appropriate radiologic personnel. Your patient will require a CT scan or an MRI scan as soon as your examination can provide anatomic localization and a working differential diagnosis. Myelography in combination with CT is still used at some centers at which high-quality MRI is not readily accessible.

Selective Physical Examination

Do not move the patient with a suspected spine injury until adequate immobilization of the neck or back has been ensured (e.g., with a Philadelphia collar).

The anatomy of the white matter tracts and cell groups in the spinal cord is consistent from patient to patient. Precise localization of the involved level and structure of the cord will, therefore, provide valuable early information about the likely pathogenesis of the injury. An anterior cord syndrome localized to the cervical region, for example, suggests cervical disk herniation. A posterior cord syndrome at the thoracic level suggests bony metastasis. Figure 8–3 shows a representative cross section of the spinal cord. Table 8–1 outlines the features of the main spinal cord syndromes. Note that at each level, lower motor neuron signs result from cell groups exiting the cord at that level, and upper motor neuron signs are present below the level of injury.

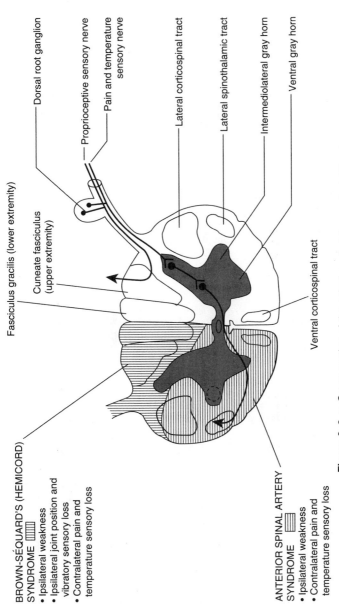

Fasciculus gracilis (lower extremity)

Cuneate fasciculus (upper extremity)

Dorsal root ganglion

Proprioceptive sensory nerve

Pain and temperature sensory nerve

Lateral corticospinal tract

Lateral spinothalamic tract

Intermediolateral gray horn

Ventral gray horn

Ventral corticospinal tract

BROWN-SÉQUARD'S (HEMICORD) SYNDROME
• Ipsilateral weakness
• Ipsilateral joint position and vibratory sensory loss
• Contralateral pain and temperature sensory loss

ANTERIOR SPINAL ARTERY SYNDROME
• Ipsilateral weakness
• Contralateral pain and temperature sensory loss

Figure 8–3 □ Cross section of the spinal cord at the cervical *B* level.

Table 8–1 □ MAJOR SPINAL CORD SYNDROMES

Syndrome	Common Causes	Features
Hemicord syndrome (Brown-Sequard's paralysis)	Penetrating injury Extrinsic compression	Contralateral spinothalamic loss Ipsilateral paresis Ipsilateral dorsal column loss Preserved light touch *Note:* deficits appear 1 to 2 levels below injury
Anterior cord syndrome	Anterior spinal artery infarct "Watershed" (T4–T6) ischemia Acute cervical disk herniation	Bilateral spinothalamic loss Preserved dorsal column sensation Upper motor neuron paralysis below lesion Lower motor neuron paralysis at lesion Sphincter dysfunction
Central cord syndrome	Syringomyelia Hypotensive spinal cord ischemia Spinal trauma (flexion-extension injury) Spinal cord neoplasm	Lower motor neuron weakness in arms Variable leg weakness and spasticity Severe pain and hyperpathia Spinothalamic loss in arms Sphincter dysfunction or urinary retention
Posterior cord syndrome	Trauma Posterior spinal artery infarct	Dorsal column sensory loss Pain and paresthesias in neck, back, or trunk Mild paresis

Vital signs:	Evaluate as described earlier; look for any signs of autonomic instability.
HEENT:	Trauma to the neck should be suspected when there is trauma to the face and body. Battle's sign (ecchymosis over the mastoid process) and raccoon sign (periorbital ecchymosis) suggest basilar skull fracture. Hemotympanum or cerebrospinal fluid (CSF) otorrhea are also signs of skull fracture.
Spine:	Percuss the spine with a fist or lightly with a tendon hammer. Tenderness to percussion suggests bony disease and will help localize the lesion for the rest of the examination and for a focal radiographic evaluation. Remember that the spinal cord comes down only to L1 in adults, unless there is a tethered cord. Tenderness in the lower lumbar or sacral spine may cause radicular symptoms but does not suggest cord compression.
Musculo-skeletal:	Look for signs of rheumatoid arthritis, which can be associated with atlanto-occipital dislocation.

Neurologic examination:

- **Motor**

    Test strength in the legs and the arms. Symmetric loss of lower extremity power with preserved strength in the arms may be the first clue to thoracic cord involvement. If there is bilateral weakness in both the arms and the legs, suggesting cervical involvement, there should be upper motor neuron signs in the legs. Note that if the spinal injury is acute, muscle tone may be decreased below the level of the injury.

- **Sensory**

    Look for a sensory level. Bilateral weakness with a concordant sensory level is pathognomonic for spinal cord injury. Vibratory sense may be the first to go, particularly with a posterior cord syndrome, but the pinprick test (with a previously unused safety pin) is the most precise and reproducible. Remember, pain and temperature sensory neurons entering the cord ascend ipsilaterally for two to three spinal segments before crossing just anterior to the central canal to join the contralateral spinothalamic tract located in the lateral cord. Therefore, loss of pinprick or temperature sensation at a given level may indicate pathology two to three segments above the level detected on examination. A dermatome chart can be found in Appendix A–5.

    Perineal sensory loss (saddle anesthesia) suggests injury to the conus medullaris. Patchy sensory loss in the lower extremities with pain and bilateral weakness may suggest involvement of the cauda equina, rather than of the spinal cord.

Mark the borders of a sensory disturbance with a pen for comparison with future examinations.

- **Reflexes**

    Hyporeflexia is often present at the level of the spinal cord injury, with hyperreflexia below the level of injury. If the injury is acute, the only upper motor neuron sign may be a Babinski's sign. Loss of the "anal wink" (contraction of the anal sphincter in response to pinprick in the perineum) indicates possible conus medullaris involvement.

- **Cranial nerves and mental status examination**

    These may be done briefly to rule out involvement of central nervous system (CNS) structures above the spinal cord. A perisagittal mass lesion, such as a falx meningioma or a CNS lymphoma, may produce bilateral leg weakness and urinary incontinence, mimicking a thoracic cord lesion. Other mental status signs, such as personality change, lethargy, or disinhibition, may be a clue to CNS pathology. Lower brain stem signs may accompany high cervical cord injury, particularly if there is a congenital deformity of the brain or atlantoaxial joint.

Selective History and Chart Review

1. *Reassess the timing, duration, and course of the symptoms.*

    Development over minutes to hours suggests trauma or infarction. Progression over hours to days suggests an infectious etiology. An epidural abscess may be present even in the absence of fever or an elevated white blood cell count. Development of weakness or sensory loss over days to weeks suggests a neoplasm.

2. *Review the presence and character of pain.*

    Radicular pain will help localize and confirm extramedullary spinal involvement. Abrupt onset of radicular or diffuse pain, flaccid weakness, sphincter dysfunction, and a thoracic sensory level suggest spinal cord infarction. Bilateral radicular pain in an unusual distribution (e.g., L2 or L3) may indicate a cauda equina syndrome. Rectal pain may be the first sign of a conus medullaris lesion.

3. *Review the chart for history of illicit drug use* (this predisposes to epidural abscess and osteomyelitis), tuberculosis, or cancer.

4. *Check recent laboratory values* to assess for possible infection or chronic disease.

■ MANAGEMENT II

Imaging

Once the anatomic localization and a working differential diagnosis have been established, the patient must be sent for an appropriate radiologic examination. **In most cases, MRI will be the radiologic modality of choice.** MRI is particularly useful in distinguishing intramedullary from extramedullary tumors. Extramedullary intradural tumors can be identified well with myelography, particularly when this technique is complemented by CT. Likewise, extradural tumors may be detected well with CT and myelography, especially when there is bony involvement. MRI with gadolinium remains the modality of choice, however, because of its noninvasiveness and low risk to the patient. Osteomyelitis, bony metastases, and epidural abscesses can be delineated well by MRI. One situation in which CT is superior to MRI is spinal trauma. Thin cuts through the region of injury can provide high-quality computed reconstructions in any plane. If intrathecal contrast is given prior to the CT scan, cord deformations as well as subtle fractures of the bony elements can be identified.

Surgical Intervention

Fractures, subluxations, and dislocations require reduction into normal alignment. Cervical traction may succeed in reducing a displacement, but it should be performed only by experienced personnel, usually under radiographic guidance. Open reductions may be required for more complex fractures or dislocations.

Neurosurgical decompressive laminectomy is the operation of choice for epidural abscess. Investigations should proceed without delay when an epidural abscess is suspected to avoid its progression to irreversible spinal cord injury. Patients who are paraplegic at the start of the operation rarely regain function. For pyogenic osteomyelitis, direct ventral spinal canal decompression is often necessary. A second, reconstructive operation may be required after the infection is brought under control with appropriate antibiotics. Decompressive laminectomy may also be needed for acute myelopathy or cauda equina syndrome resulting from disk herniation in the lumbar region. An anterior approach may be necessary to remove a herniated cervical disk. Finally, in the rare case of epidural or subdural hematoma, decompressive laminectomy is again the treatment of choice.

For **neoplastic spinal cord compression,** the first step after administration of high-dose steroids and accurate localization by examination and MRI is surgical decompression. Once the pressure has been relieved, further treatment usually requires tissue biopsy. Many tumors may be radiosensitive, but most radiotherapy units require a definite tissue diagnosis. If the surgeons have performed a decompression procedure, open biopsy may be possible. An alternative procedure is CT-guided needle biopsy.

9

DELIRIUM

The term *delirium* is synonymous with the term *acute confusional state*. Delirium is common in hospitalized patients, particularly in the elderly, and refers to an acute, global disorder of thinking and perception, characterized by impaired consciousness and inattention. Restlessness, agitation, and combativeness may be seen, as well as bizarre behavior and delusions. A call to evaluate delirium may therefore be one for "agitation" or "confusion." Delirium may be distinguished from dementia by the fact that with dementia alone, the sensorium remains clear, despite the occurrence of confusion and disorientation. Furthermore, it should be emphasized that although delirium is often defined as a transient condition, it may take days to weeks to clear and, if left untreated, mortality may be as high as 25% in elderly inpatients. As with other mental status alterations discussed in this book, delirium is a symptom, not a disease. Successful management depends on accurate diagnosis of the underlying condition.

■ PHONE CALL

Questions

1. **Is the patient fully awake and alert? In what way is the patient confused? When did the change occur?**
   Clarify the acuteness and nature of the mental status change. It is important to distinguish between acute and chronic changes and also to distinguish delirium from dementia (see Chapter 19) and stupor (see Chapter 6).
2. **What are the vital signs?**
   Fever suggests infection; tachypnea may suggest hypoxia, metabolic acidosis, or hyperglycemia (Kussmaul's respiration); and irregular heart rhythm may suggest cardioembolic stroke.
3. **Was there any head injury?**
4. **What is the patient's underlying medical condition?**
   Diseases that are likely to cause metabolic disarray, such as renal or liver disease, endocrinopathies, diarrheal illnesses, or malignancy, may alter electrolytes. Human immunodeficiency virus (HIV) infection or acquired immune deficiency syndrome (AIDS) opens a wider array of differential diagnoses.

5. **Is the patient diabetic?**
   Both hypoglycemia and hyperglycemia can cause altered mental status.
7. **Is the patient known to be a user of alcohol or other nonprescription drugs?**

Orders

1. Order a finger stick glucose level.
2. If the patient is tachypneic or drowsy, obtain arterial blood gas measurements. A pulse oximeter may be useful for monitoring oxygen saturation.
3. Provide orientation and reassurance to the patient. Make sure the room is well lit. The treatment of the behavioral and emotional manifestations of delirium, to the extent possible, will make the subsequent etiologic evaluation easier.
4. Restrain the patient with a Posey chest restraint if necessary. Significant agitation or combativeness may put the patient or those nearby at risk for physical injury.
5. Do not medicate. Perform the evaluation first. If sedation is given before a good neurologic examination can be obtained, the opportunity for making a diagnosis may be lost.

Inform RN

"Will arrive at the bedside in . . . minutes."

■ ELEVATOR THOUGHTS

What are the causes of delirium?

V (vascular): stroke (infarct or hemorrhage causing a sensory aphasia), subarachnoid hemorrhage, hypertensive encephalopathy, cholesterol emboli syndrome

I (infectious): herpes simplex encephalitis or other viral encephalitis; bacterial, fungal, or rickettsial meningoencephalitis; neurosyphilis; Lyme disease; parasitic abscess (e.g., toxoplasmosis, cysticercosis), bacterial abscess; HIV encephalitis; systemic infection such as urosepsis or pneumonia

T (traumatic): open or closed head trauma, acute or chronic subdural hematoma

A (autoimmune): systemic lupus erythematosus (SLE), multiple sclerosis

M (metabolic/toxic): hypo- or hyperglycemia, hyponatremia, hypercalcemia, hepatic encephalopathy, uremia, porphyria; drug or alcohol ingestion or withdrawal

I (iatrogenic): drug toxicity (particularly in the elderly): psychotropic drugs, steroids, digoxin, cimetidine, anticonvulsants, anticholinergics, dopaminergics (see Table 9–1 for common medications with central nervous system [CNS] side effects); rare: heavy metal poisoning, pellagra, vitamin B_{12} or folate deficiency, Wilson's disease

N (neoplastic): primary brain tumor, metastatic brain disease, paraneoplastic syndrome (limbic encephalitis with small-cell lung cancer)

S (seizure): postictal state, nonconvulsive status epilepticus (rare)

Other (psychiatric): bipolar disorder/mania, psychosis

■ MAJOR THREAT TO LIFE

- **Expanding mass lesion with impending herniation**

    Although it is rare for a mass lesion to progress to impending herniation without focal neurologic signs, the first changes may be confusion or altered state of consciousness. Progression can be rapid if there is an expanding subdural hematoma or edema from subarachnoid hemorrhage.

- **Bacterial meningitis or encephalitis**

    Bacterial meningitis is a major treatable illness that can be fatal if missed. Other meningitides are likely to be less fulminant yet can also be fatal if left untreated. Herpes simplex encephalitis is the most common sporadic encephalitis. Aside from direct brain damage from infection, encephalitides can produce edema and subsequent herniation.

- **Delirium tremens**

    Usually occurring more than 48 hours after cessation of alcohol consumption, the autonomic instability of delirium tremens may produce high fevers, tachycardia, and severe fluctuations in blood pressure (Fig. 9–1). Mortality is about 15%.

■ BEDSIDE

Quick Look Test

Does the patient look ill or well?

Is the patient in respiratory distress?

What are the vital signs?

    If there is a fever, meningitis must be ruled out. An irregular rhythm may suggest atrial fibrillation. Markedly elevated blood pressure, particularly diastolic blood pressure greater than 120 mm Hg, may produce hypertensive encephalopathy, which is characterized by headache, confusion, and irritability, with lethargy developing over hours to days.

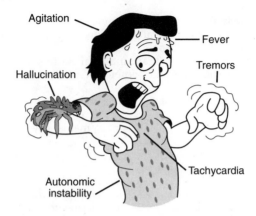

Figure 9–1 □ Delirium tremens.

Selective Physical Examination I

Breath:	The odor of alcohol or fetor hepaticus may suggest the etiology.
HEENT:	Look for external signs of head trauma—scalp lacerations or bruises, Battle's sign, raccoon eyes, papilledema.
Neck:	Nuchal rigidity, Kernig's sign, Brudzinski's sign
Cardiopulmonary:	Tachypnea can indicate hypoxia or metabolic acidosis. Rales or decreased breath sounds may help diagnose a pneumonia. Listen for irregular heart rhythm and for murmurs to suggest valvular heart disease.
Abdomen:	Percuss the liver. Hepatomegaly may be the physical manifestation of hepatic encephalopathy or may direct your management to consideration of alcohol withdrawal. Look for ascites.
Extremities:	Look for clubbing as a sign of chronic pulmonary disease, peripheral edema as a sign of cardiac or renal failure, and splinter hemorrhages as a sign of emboli. **Asterixis** is a sign of metabolic disarray, for example, from renal or hepatic failure.

Neurologic examination:
- **Mental status**:
  1. Assess the patient's **alertness:** Is the patient fully awake and alert? Assess the patient's **attentiveness.** Does the

patient maintain eye contact? Does he or she glance about the room as if having hallucinations? One simple test of sustained attention is to ask the patient to recite the days of the week backward or to ask him or her to count backward from 20 to 1.

2. Listen for **paraphasias** in spontaneous speech to suggest a sensory aphasia. Test **comprehension.** Ask the patient to follow progressively complex commands (e.g., "Show two fingers," "Point to the ceiling and then to the floor," and "Tap each shoulder twice with your eyes closed").

3. Assess **thought content.** Tangential or pressured speech, delusions, flight of ideas, hallucinations, perceptual illusions, and disorientation may all be seen.

- **Cranial nerves**:
  1. **Pupils.** Pinpoint pupils may result from opiate overdose. Widely dilated pupils could be a sign of cholinergic overdose (e.g., organophosphate poisoning). Asymmetric pupils can indicate uncal herniation from intracranial mass effect. Argyll Robertson pupils are seen with CNS syphilis (periaqueductal midbrain lesion (see Chapter 3).
  2. **Facial asymmetry** in the form of a flattened nasolabial fold or a wider palpebral fissure may be a subtle sign of an intraparenchymal mass.
  3. Assess swallowing capacity and gag reflex.
- **Motor**: Depending on how cooperative your patient is, you may be able to test strength by confrontation. An inattentive patient, however, will often show impersistence of sustained power. Observe the movements of the limbs for any asymmetry of use. Any lateralizing weakness should make you suspicious of an intracranial lesion. A tremor should make you suspicious of alcohol withdrawal or intoxication.
- **Sensory**: A detailed sensory examination requires sustained cooperation that an inattentive patient often cannot give. Response to a brief noxious stimulus (e.g., a pinch or pulling hair on the arm) is a quick way to assess gross sensory function. If the limb is paretic, the response may be a facial grimace.
- **Gait**: Ataxia may suggest intoxication.
- **Reflexes**: Babinski's response or reflex asymmetry alone is not enough to make a diagnosis of stroke or intracranial focal lesion; however, reflex changes add weight to other elements on an examination that may suggest intracranial pathology.

Selective History and Chart Review

1. **Review medications.**

    Have any new medications been started recently? Particularly in the elderly, drug toxicity is a common cause of change in mental status. Table 9–1 lists common medications that can cause delirium.

2. **Review medical or psychiatric history.**

Known metabolic disorders such as renal or hepatic disease or past episodes of psychosis would be crucial to make a diagnosis.

■ MANAGEMENT I: CONTROL OF DELIRIUM

1. **Treatment of agitation**

Treatment of delirium depends on the correct identification of the underlying condition. If agitation or combativeness is likely to interfere with the investigation or if there is physical threat to the patient or to the staff, the best medications to use are butyrophenones (e.g., haloperidol), group 3 phenothiazines (e.g., trifluoperazine), or benzodiazepines. **Haldol 2 to 10 mg intramuscularly (IM)** may be expected to reach peak serum levels in 20 to 40 minutes. Repeating

Table 9–1 □ COMMON MEDICATIONS THAT CAN CAUSE DELIRIUM

Anticholinergics
  Trihexyphenidyl HCl (Artane)
  Benztropine mesylate (Cogentin)
Anticonvulsants
  Phenytoin (Dilantin)
  Phenobarbital
  Valproic acid (Depakene/Depakote)
Antihistamines
  Diphenhydramine (Benadryl)
  Dextromethorphan hydrobromide + promethazine (Phenergan)
  Cimetidine (Tagamet)
Benzodiazapines
  Diazepam (Valium)
  Temazepam (Restoril)
  Triazolam (Halcion)
Corticosteroids
  Prednisone
  Dexamethasone (Decadron)
Dopaminergic drugs
  L-dopa (Sinemet)
  Pergolide (Permax)
  Bromocriptine (Parlodel)
Digoxin
Disulfiram
Indomethacin
Lithium
Opiates

the dose up to 20 mg may be necessary in severe cases. For mild agitation or in the elderly, an initial dose of 1 to 2 mg may be sufficient. For moderate agitation, use 4 mg initially. For violent, combative patients, 6 to 10 mg can be used as an initial dose. If an acute dystonic reaction occurs with Haldol, **diphenhydramine 25 to 50 mg IM** may be given, even though the anticholinergic effect may worsen the delirium. Haloperidol should be avoided in alcohol withdrawal, benzodiazepine withdrawal, and hepatic encephalopathy. For acute agitation in these settings, a benzodiazepine such as **lorazepam 1 to 2 mg IM** may be given. (Higher doses may be required if tolerance has developed in the setting of chronic alcohol or benzodiazepine abuse.) **Naloxone (Narcan) 1 to 2 ampules, given intravenously (IV), IM, or subcutaneously (SC) every 5 minutes,** should be reserved for the lethargy of suspected opiate intoxication.
2. **The following blood tests should be ordered immediately:**
   - Complete blood count (CBC) with differential
   - Electrolyte panel, including stat glucose
   - Full chemistry panel, including liver function tests
   - Urine toxicology screen (if drug intoxication is suspected)
   - Urine and blood cultures (if fever is present)
   - Arterial blood gas
   - Calcium, phosphate

A **chest x-ray** should be obtained if fever or dyspnea is present. Erythrocyte sedimentation rate may be measured, but its specificity is low.

■ **MANAGEMENT II: TREATMENT OF THE LIFE-THREATENING DISORDERS**

1. **Bacterial meningitis**
   Delirium with fever should be treated as bacterial meningitis until proven otherwise. As a rule, a head computed tomography (CT) scan should be ordered before a lumbar puncture is performed. If there is no papilledema on examination, no coagulopathy, and no focal deficit (including gait ataxia), and a head CT is not readily available, a lumbar puncture may almost always be done without risk of herniation. (See Chapter 4 for a discussion of lumbar puncture.) Cerebrospinal fluid (CSF) should be sent for cell count, protein and glucose determinations, microbial cultures (bacterial, fungal, mycobacterial), and Venereal Disease Research Laboratory (VDRL) test, and for Gram, acid-fast bacillus, and India ink stains. CSF findings in bacterial meningitis are cloudy fluid with 50 to 20,000 white blood cells, predominantly leukocytes, elevated protein level, and decreased glu-

cose level (see Table 23–1.). The causative organism may be identified and antibiotic sensitivity may be obtained in more than 80% of the cases. Empirical treatment of bacterial meningitis prior to definitive identification in adults should be **ampicillin 1 g IV every 6 hours** and a third-generation cephalosporin (e.g., **ceftazidime 1 g IV every 8 hours**). **Decadron 4 mg IV every 4 hours** may be necessary to normalize elevated intracranial pressure from edema in advanced cases. Steroids are used routinely in pediatric cases.

2. **Delirium tremens**

   The autonomic instability of delirium tremens is treated supportively, with acetaminophen (Tylenol) or a cooling blanket for fevers. Continuous cardiac monitoring may be necessary if arrhythmias develop. **Valium 5 to 10 mg IV load**, with **subsequent doses of 2 to 5 mg IV every 30 to 60 minutes,** should be used. Sedation should be titrated to minimize agitation. Tremulousness may be used as a clinical monitor of the effectiveness of the benzodiazepine. An alternative is **chlordiazepoxide 25 to 100 mg every 6 hours by mouth (PO).** The dose should be tapered as the symptoms subside. **Thiamine 100 mg IV, IM, or PO** should be given daily for 3 days to prevent the development of Wernicke's encephalopathy.

3. **Suspected mass lesion**

   If there is papilledema or a focality on examination, an emergent head CT or MRI scan should be obtained. For mass lesions, refer to the appropriate chapter for treatment of acute stroke (Chapter 7), increased intracranial pressure (Chapter 13), or brain tumor (Chapter 24).

Selective History and Chart Review

Once it is clear that the patient does not have a mass lesion, bacterial meningitis, or delirium tremens, you have time to make a more complete assessment of the situation. If family members are available, try to sort out the acuteness of the change. A chronic or fluctuating course in an elderly person may suggest that the apparent delirium is really a component of dementia. Alzheimer's disease and vascular dementia are the most common causes (see Chapter 19). A subacute course over days, with intermittent fevers, suggests a subacute or chronic encephalomeningitis, such as herpes simplex encephalitis, tubercular meningitis, or cryptococcal meningitis.

Review the chart. What are the patient's medical conditions? What medications is he or she on? Were any medications recently added that are known to have CNS effects? (see Table 9–1). The offending agent should be stopped or substituted. Do the most recent laboratory values suggest metabolic abnormalities? Renal

---

Box 9–1. HEPATIC ENCEPHALOPATHY

Hepatic encephalopathy usually appears in a patient with liver function already compromised from alcoholic cirrhosis, chronic hepatitis, or malignancy. An increased protein load, such as from a gastrointestinal bleed, causes ammonia to accumulate in the brain. Whether the high level of ammonia itself or the increase in concentration of its metabolites produces the alterations in consciousness is not known. Examination may reveal abdominal ascites, an enlarged (or shrunken) liver, and asterixis, in addition to changes in mental status, namely inattention, disorientation, and confusion. In the later stages, focal signs such as hemiparesis or dysconjugate gaze may appear. Management is directed at reducing the protein load with dietary protein restrictions and **neomycin 2 to 4 g per day PO**, which reduces the population of ammonia-producing bacteria in the bowel. **Lactulose 15 to 45 ml two to four times per day** to induce diarrhea may also help reduce intestinal bacteria. Ammonia levels should be followed as an indication of the effectiveness of therapy. If acute agitation requires treatment, use benzodiazepines such as **diazepam 5 to 10 mg every 8 hours. Haloperidol should be avoided.** When hepatic encephalopathy is suspected, be sure to obtain a stool guaiac test and a hematocrit.

---

and hepatic failure are the most common sources of metabolic encephalopathy (Box 9–1). The laboratory tests that you sent off will suggest whether there are acute changes in progress. Is the patient HIV positive? Acute HIV infection may cause a meningoencephalitis. Immunocompromised patients are at risk for a variety of opportunistic infections that can cause encephalopathy, particularly cryptococcal and tuberculous meningitis, toxoplasmosis, and CNS syphilis. Malignancy, most notably small-cell lung carcinoma, can cause a paraneoplastic "limbic encephalitis," in addition to altering electrolytes with syndrome of inappropriate antidiuretic hormone (SIADH).

■ MANAGEMENT III: TREATMENT OF OTHER DISORDERS

1. **Hypoglycemia and hyperglycemia**

Hypoglycemia may be rapidly corrected with a bolus of **50 ml D50W IV by direct injection.** Do not forget that thiamine **(100 mg PO or IM)** must be given first to prevent possible induction of Wernicke's encephalopathy. Maintenance with D5W may be necessary if the hypoglycemia is prolonged. Hyperglycemia (diabetic ketoacidosis) requires administration of insulin, repletion of intravascular volume, and often, management of acidosis and potassium. The level of monitoring required is best handled in an intensive care unit (ICU).

2. **Hyponatremia and hypernatremia**

   Management of hypo- and hypernatremia usually involves treating the underlying cause (e.g., renal disease, vomiting and diarrhea, hypothalamic or adrenal dysfunction, or SIADH from malignancy or medications). Treatment with IV fluids and electrolytes differs depending on volume status. Too rapid a correction of hyponatremia may precipitate central pontine myelinolysis, an acute demyelinating syndrome occurring mostly in patients with poor nutritional status, causing quadriplegia, dysarthria, and pseudobulbar palsy.

3. **Hypocalcemia**

   Severe hypocalcemia (<7.0 ml/dl) may be treated with **10 to 20 ml (1 to 2 g) of 10% calcium gluconate IV in 100 ml D5W over 30 minutes.** If the patient is hyperphosphatemic, correction with glucose and insulin is required before giving calcium IV. Patients on digoxin should have continuous cardiac monitoring, as calcium potentiates digoxin's action.

4. **Uremia with renal failure**

   Symptomatic uremia with renal failure causing delirium may necessitate urgent hemodialysis.

5. **Sepsis**

   Delirium caused by sepsis should clear spontaneously with appropriate treatment of the infection.

6. **Psychiatric causes**

   Psychiatric causes of delirium may generally be treated acutely with **haloperidol 1 to 5 mg PO or IM.** Psychiatric consultation should be obtained for definitive treatment.

7. **Seizures.**

   Delirium from a **postictal state** should clear progressively over minutes to hours. An EEG should be ordered within the next few days. **Nonconvulsive status epilepticus** is a neurologic emergency that requires EEG for definitive diagnosis. (See Chapter 5 for further discussion of seizure management.)

10

HEAD INJURY

The initial assessment of head injury in the emergency room can be frantic, with resuscitation measures, history taking, and examination occurring simultaneously. An organized approach is essential to ensure that vital components of the evaluation are not omitted. **The immediate goal is to judge the severity of the injury as mild, moderate, or severe.** This can be quickly assessed at the time of arrival.

■ PHONE CALL

Questions

1. **What are the vital signs?**
   If the patient is in respiratory distress, the spine should be immobilized (this should have been done already) and nasotracheal intubation should be performed.
2. **What were the circumstances and the mode of injury?**
   The force and location of head impact should be determined as precisely as possible.
3. **Did the patient experience loss of consciousness?**
   Concussion refers to temporary loss of consciousness that occurs at the time of impact. Because patients are amnestic following concussion, only an eyewitness can accurately gauge the duration of loss of consciousness.
4. **Has the patient's neurologic status deteriorated since the time of impact?**
   Progressive decline in level of consciousness after an injury suggests an expanding *subdural or epidural hematoma*.
5. **What is the patient's level of consciousness now?**
   This should be assessed using the Glasgow Coma scale (see Table 6–2).
6. **Has the patient recently ingested drugs or alcohol?**
   Intoxication can confound assessments of mental status and may lead to withdrawal symptoms.
7. **Is there significant extracranial trauma?**
   The patient should be quickly examined for external signs of trauma to the neck, chest, abdomen, and limbs.

Determination of the Severity of Injury

At this juncture, you should have enough information to classify the injury as **mild, moderate,** or **severe.** Subsequent diagnostic testing and management will proceed according to the perceived severity of injury:

1. **Mild head injury** (low-risk group)
   - Glasgow Coma scale score of 15 (alert, attentive, and oriented)
   - No loss of consciousness (e.g., concussion)
   - No drug or alcohol intoxication
   - Patient may complain of headache and dizziness
   - Patient may have scalp abrasion, laceration, or hematoma
   - Absence of moderate or severe injury criteria
2. **Moderate head injury** (intermediate-risk group)
   - Glasgow Coma scale score of 9 to 14 (confused, lethargic, or stuporous)
   - Concussion
   - Posttraumatic amnesia
   - Vomiting
   - Signs of possible skull fracture (Battle's sign, raccoon eyes, hemotympanum, cerebrospinal fluid [CSF] drainage from nose or ear)
   - Seizure
3. **Severe head injury** (high-risk group)
   - Glasgow Coma scale score of 3 to 8 (comatose)
   - Progressive decline in level of consciousness
   - Focal neurologic signs
   - Penetrating skull injury or palpably depressed skull fracture

Orders

1. **For *all patients*, order cervical spine x-rays (anteroposterior, lateral, and odontoid views).**
   All patients with traumatic injury above the level of the clavicles should have cervical spine films to rule out a fracture. Before a cervical collar can be removed, the cervical spine must be cleared completely from C1 to C7.
2. **For all patients with *moderate or severe injury*, give the following orders:**
   a. **Start an intravenous (IV) line with normal (0.9%) saline or lactated Ringer's solution.**
      Isotonic fluids replace intravascular volume more effectively than do hypotonic fluids, and they do not aggravate cerebral edema.
   b. **Perform diagnostic blood tests.**
      (1) Spun hematocrit
      (2) Complete blood count (CBC) and platelets
      (3) Serum chemistries (glucose, electrolytes, blood urea nitrogen [BUN], creatinine)

    (4) prothrombin time (PT)/partial thromboplastin time (PTT)
    (5) Toxicology screen and serum alcohol level
    (6) Type and hold
  c. Obtain a head CT scan with bone windows.
      Skull x-rays are not neccessary if a head CT is performed, because CT is more sensitive for detecting fractures. The chances of detecting intracranial hemorrhage on CT in patients with mild, moderate, or severe head injury are shown in Table 10–1. CT scans should be assessed for the following (Fig. 10–1):
    (1) Epidural and subdural hematoma
    (2) Subarachnoid and intraventricular blood
    (3) Parenchymal contusions and hemorrhages
    (4) Cerebral edema
    (5) Effacement of perimesencephalic cisterns
    (6) Midline shift
    (7) Skull fractures, sinus opacification (air fluid levels), and pneumocephalus
3. **For** *comatose patients* **(Glasgow Coma scale score ≤8) or in patients with signs of herniation, give the following orders:**
  a. **Elevate head of bed 30 degrees.**
  b. **Hyperventilate the patient.**

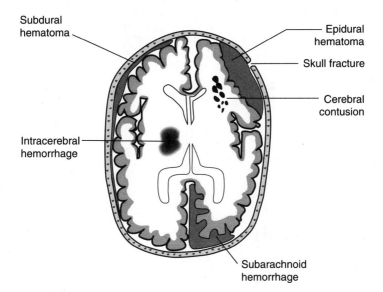

Figure 10–1 □ Schematic diagram of important CT scan abnormalities in patients with head injury.

Table 10–1 □ RISK OF MAJOR INTRACRANIAL HEMORRHAGE ACCORDING TO CLINICAL SEVERITY OF HEAD INJURY

Severity of Injury*	Glasgow Coma Scale Score on Arrival	Percentage of Emergency Room Visits	Intracranial Hemorrhage Risk		Overall Mortality
			No Skull Fracture	Skull Fracture	
Minor	15	95%	1:10,000	1:100	<1%
Moderate	9–14	4%	1:380	1:15	5%
Severe	3–8	1%	1:50	1:8	35%

Adapted from Teasdale GM: Head injury. J Neurol Neurosurg Psychiatry 1995; 58:526–539.
*See text for definitions.

Intubate the patient. Use intermittent mandatory ventilation (IMV) at a rate of 16 to 20 beats per minute with tidal volumes set at 10 to 12 ml/kg. Adjust settings for a partial pressure of carbon dioxide (PCO_2) of 28 to 32 mm Hg. Severe hypocapnia (<25 mm Hg) may lead to excessive vasoconstriction and cerebral ischemia and should be avoided.

c. **Administer mannitol 20% 1 g/kg IV.**

Mannitol should be given "wide open." The patient should be re-examined 30 minutes after mannitol is given to assess for signs of improvement. Additional doses should be guided by an intracranial pressure (ICP) monitor (see Chapter 13).

d. **Insert a Foley catheter.**

e. **Obtain a neurosurgical consultation.**

■ ELEVATOR THOUGHTS

What are the most important sequelae of traumatic head injury?

1. **Concussion**

Concussion refers to temporary loss of consciousness that occurs at the time of impact. It is usually associated with a short period of amnesia. The majority of patients with concussion have normal CT or MRI scans, reflecting the fact that concussion results from physiologic (rather than structural) injury to the brain. *Approximately 5% of patients who have sustained concussion will have an intracranial hemorrhage.*

2. **Epidural hematoma**

Epidural bleeding usually results from a tear in the middle meningeal artery. Approximately 75% of such cases are associated with a skull fracture. The classic clinical course (seen in only one third of patients) proceeds from immediate loss of consciousness (concussion) to a lucid interval, which is followed by a secondary depression of consciousness as the epidural hematoma expands. Epidural blood takes on a bulging convex pattern on the CT scan (see Fig. 10–1) because the collection is limited by firm attachments of the dura to the cranial sutures. Progression to herniation and death can occur rapidly because the bleeding is from an artery.

3. **Subdural hematoma**

Subdural bleeding usually arises from a venous source, with blood filling the potential space between the dural and arachnoid membranes. CT usually reveals a crescentic collection of blood across the entire hemispheric convexity (see Fig. 10–1). *Elderly and alcoholic patients are particularly prone to subdural bleeding;* in these patients, large hematomas can result from trivial impact or from acceleration/deceleration injuries (e.g., whiplash injury).

4. **Parenchymal contusion and hematoma**

Cerebral contusions result from "scraping" and "bruising" of the brain as it moves across the inner surface of the skull. The inferior frontal and temporal lobes are the common sites of traumatic contusion (see Fig. 10–1). With lateral forces, contusions can occur just deep to the site of impact (coup lesions) or at the opposite pole as the brain impacts on the inner table of the skull (contrecoup lesions). Contusions frequently evolve into larger lesions over 12 to 24 hours, and in rare instances, contusions can develop de novo 1 or more days after injury ("spät hematoma").

5. **Axonal shearing injury**

Persistent coma occurs frequently in patients with severe head injury with normal CT scans and normal intracranial pressure. In these cases, coma results from widespread stretching, shearing, and disruption of axons as a result of rotational forces. Bilateral motor posturing and hyperreflexia are common and result from injury to the corticospinal tracts in the brain stem. Diffuse axonal injury is thought to be the single most important cause of persistent disability in patients with traumatic brain damage.

6. **Skull fracture**

Skull fractures are important markers of potentially serious intracranial injury, but they rarely cause symptoms themselves. If the scalp is lacerated over the fracture, it is considered an open, or compound, fracture. *Linear fractures* account for 80% of all skull fractures and can usually be managed conservatively. *Basilar skull fractures* occur with more serious trauma and are frequently missed on routine skull x-ray films. These may be associated with cranial nerve injury or CSF leakage from the nose or ear. *Comminuted and depressed fractures* are often associated with contusions of the underlying brain and usually require surgical débridement.

■ MAJOR THREAT TO LIFE

- Epidural hematoma
- Subdural hematoma
- Increased intracranial pressure

■ BEDSIDE

Quick Look Test

What is the level of consciousness?

Almost all patients with potentially life-threatening lesions will have depressed level of consciousness (lethargy, stupor, or coma).

Airway and Vital Signs

Is the airway protected? What is the respiratory rate?
Indications for intubation include depressed level of consciousness, respiratory distress (rapid, shallow breathing), or respiratory depression.

What is the heart rate and blood pressure?
If the patient is hypotensive, bleeding into the abdomen, thorax, retroperitoneal space, or tissues surrounding a long-bone fracture should be excluded. *Spinal shock* can occur with cord injury and results from acute loss of sympathetic outflow. Hypertension associated with a wide pulse pressure and bradycardia (Cushing's reflex) may reflect increased ICP.

Selective Physical Examination

Head:
: The skull should be palpated for fractures, hematomas, and lacerations. *Battle's sign* (ecchymosis over the mastoid process) and *raccoon sign* (periorbital ecchymosis) suggest, but do not confirm, basilar skull fracture.

Ear, nose, and throat:
: *CSF otorrhea* and *CSF rhinorrhea* result from skull fracture with disruption of the dura. CSF can be differentiated from mucus by its high glucose content on dipstick testing; bloody CSF can be differentiated from frank blood by a positive *halo test* (a "halo" of CSF forms around the blood when CSF is dropped on a cloth sheet). *Hemotympanum* is also highly suggestive of skull fracture. *Tongue biting* suggests an unwitnessed seizure.

Neck:
: Do not manipulate the neck until a cervical fracture has been ruled out.

Chest, abdomen, back, pelvis, and extremities:
: It is essential to rule out important coexisting injuries in patients with head injury. The patient should be thoroughly examined, and x-rays, diagnostic peritoneal lavage, and other interventions should be performed prior to CT scanning as clinically indicated.

Neurologic examination:

Rapid neurologic examination of the patient with head injury should focus on the following:

- **Mental status**
  1. **Level of consciousness**

     Level of consciousness is best documented by using the Glasgow Coma scale (see Table 6–2) and by describing specific stimuli and responses (i.e., "answers with brief confused responses to repeated questioning" or "moans and localizes in response to sternal rub").
  2. **Attention and concentration**

     Ask the patient to count from 20 to 1 or recite the months in reverse.
  3. **Orientation**

     Check for orientation to time, place, and situation.
  4. **Memory**

     Document *retrograde amnesia* by asking the patient to recall the last thing he or she remembers prior to the injury. Check for *anterograde amnesia* by asking about the first thing remembered after the injury. Check recall for three objects at 5 minutes.
- **Cranial nerves**
  1. **Pupils**
  2. **Extraocular movements**

     Nystagmus may be found in alert patients with dizziness or vertigo following concussion. An *exodeviated eye with a large pupil* suggests CN 3 compression from uncal herniation.
  3. **Facial nerve**

     The facial nerve is the most commonly injured cranial nerve in patients with closed head injury.
- **Motor**
  1. **Spontaneous movements**

     Preferential movement of the limbs on one side indicates paresis of the unused limbs. If the patient is unresponsive, check for a lateralized localizing response to sternal rub.
  2. **Limb tone**

     Increased tone may reflect an early stage of decortication (flexor posturing) or decerebration (extensor posturing).
  3. **Arm (pronator) drift**

     If the patient is unable to follow commands, passively elevate both arms and check to see whether one falls preferentially.
  4. **Power**

     Check strength against active resistance at the shoulders, wrists, hips, and ankles.

   5. **Reflexes**
- **Gait**
   1. **Normal gait**
   2. **Tandem (heel-to-toe) gait**
       It is particularly important to check gait in patients with "mild injury" who are treated and released without a CT scan.

■ MANAGEMENT

Mild Head Injury

   Patients with mild injury (who meet the criteria described previously) can generally be discharged from the emergency room **without a head CT scan** as long as the following criteria are met:
- Neurologic examination (especially mental status and gait) is normal
- Cervical spine x-ray is cleared
- A responsible person is available to observe the patient over 24 hours, with instructions to return the patient to the emergency room if late symptoms (listed on a head injury warning card) develop

Moderate Head Injury

   Among patients who have suffered concussion, a Glasgow Coma scale score of 15 (alert, fully oriented, and follows commands) and normal CT scan eliminate the need for hospital admission. These patients can be discharged home for observation, even in the presence of headache, nausea, vomiting, dizziness, or amnesia, because the risk of development of a significant intracranial lesion thereafter is minimal. Criteria for hospital admission after head injury are shown in Box 10–1.

Box 10–1. CRITERIA FOR HOSPITAL ADMISSION FOLLOWING HEAD INJURY

- Intracranial blood or fracture identified on head CT scan
- Confusion, agitation, or depressed level of consciousness
- Focal neurologic signs or symptoms
- Alcohol or drug intoxication
- Significant comorbid medical illness
- Lack of a reliable environment for subsequent observation

Severe Head Injury

Following initial assessment and stabilization, the immediate consideration in the patient with severe head injury is whether there is an indication for emergent neurosurgical intervention. If the decision is made to operate, surgery should proceed immediately, because delays can only increase the likelihood of further brain damage during the waiting period.

The medical management of patients with severe injury should be carried out in an intensive care unit (ICU). Although little can be done about brain damage that occurs on impact, ICU care can play a major role in reducing secondary brain injury from hypoxia, hypotension, or increased ICP.

Checklist for Management of Severe Head Injury in the Intensive Care Unit

1. **Reassess airway and ventilation**
   In general, patients in stupor or coma (those unable to follow commands because of a depressed level of consciousness) should be intubated for airway protection. If there is no evidence of increased ICP, ventilatory parameters should be set to maintain PCO_2 at 40 mm Hg and PO_2 at 90 to 100 mm Hg.

2. **Monitor blood pressure**
   If the patient shows signs of hemodynamic instability (hypo- or hypertension), monitoring is best accomplished with an arterial catheter. Because autoregulation is frequently impaired with acute head injury, mean BP must be carefully maintained to avoid hypotension (mean BP<70 mm Hg), which can lead to cerebral ischemia, or hypertension (mean BP >130 mm Hg), which can exacerbate cerebral edema.

3. **Consult neurosurgery to insert an ICP monitor in patients with a Glasgow Coma scale score of 8 or less**
   Because severe ICP elevations (Lundberg A waves or plateau waves) occur suddenly and without warning, a monitor should be inserted even if the patient does not currently show signs of increased ICP. Ventricular catheters are advisable if significant intraventricular hemorrhage with hydrocephalus is present. Otherwise, a parenchymal or epidural monitor should be used, because the associated risk of infection is significantly lower (see Chapter 13).

4. **Fluid management**
   Only isotonic fluids (normal saline or lactated Ringer's solution) should be administered to patients with head injury because the extra free water in half-normal saline or D5W can exacerbate cerebral edema.

5. **Nutrition**

    Severe head injury leads to a generalized hypermetabolic and catabolic response, with caloric requirements that are 50 to 100% higher than normal. Enteral feedings via a nasogastric or a nasoduodenal tube should be instituted as soon as possible (usually by hospital day 2).

6. **Temperature management**

    Fever (temperature >101°F) exacerbates cerebral injury and should be aggressively treated with acetaminophen or cooling blankets.

7. **Anticonvulsants**

    Fosphenytoin (15 to 20 mg/kg IV loading dose, then 300 mg/day IV) reduces the frequency of early (i.e., first week) posttraumatic seizures from 14% to 4% in patients with intracranial hemorrhage but does not prevent later seizures. If the patient has not experienced a seizure, phenytoin should be discontinued after 7 to 10 days. Levels should be monitored closely, because subtherapeutic levels frequently result from hypermetabolism of phenytoin.

8. **Steroids**

    Steroids have not been shown to favorably alter outcome in patients with head injury and may lead to increased risk of infection, hyperglycemia, and other complications. For this reason, we use steroids only as a treatment of last resort for acute brain herniation **(dexamethasone 10 mg IV every 4 to 6 hours over 48 to 72 hours).**

9. **Prophylaxis for deep vein thrombosis (DVT)**

    Pneumatic compression boots are routinely used in immobilized patients to protect against lower-extremity DVT and the associated risk of pulmonary thromboembolism. **Heparin 5000 U subcutaneously (SC) every 12 hours** may be started 72 hours after injury in patients with prolonged immobilization, even in the presence of intracranial hemorrhage.

10. **Prophylaxis for gastric ulcer**

    Patients on mechanical ventilation or with coagulopathy are at increased risk of gastric stress ulceration and should receive **ranitidine 50 mg IV every 8 hours** or **sucralfate 1 g by mouth (PO) every 6 hours.**

11. **Antibiotics**

    The routine use of prophylactic antibiotics in patients with open skull injuries is controversial. Penicillin may reduce the risk of pneumococcal meningitis in patients with CSF otorrhea, rhinorrhea, or intracranial air but may increase the risk of infection with more virulent organisms.

12. **Follow-up CT scan**

    In general, a follow-up head CT scan should be obtained 24 hours after the initial injury in patients with intracranial hemorrhage to assess for delayed or progressive bleeding.

Selected Complications of Severe Head Injury

1. **CSF leaks**

   CSF leaks result from disruption of the leptomeninges and occur in 2 to 6% of patients with closed head injury. CSF leakage ceases spontaneously with head elevation alone after a few days in 85% of patients; a lumbar drain may speed this process in persistent cases. Although patients with CSF leaks are at increased risk for meningitis (usually from pneumococci), administration of prophylactic antibiotics is controversial. Persistent CSF otorrhea or rhinorrhea or recurrent meningitis is an indication for operative repair.

2. **Carotid cavernous fistulae**

   Carotid cavernous fistulae, characterized by the triad of pulsating exophthalmos, chemosis, and orbital bruit, may develop immediately or several days after injury. Angiography is required to confirm the diagnosis. Endovascular balloon occlusion is the most effective means of repair and can prevent permanent visual loss.

3. **Diabetes insipidus**

   Diabetes insipidus may result from traumatic damage to the pituitary stalk, resulting in cessation of antidiuretic hormone secretion. Patients excrete large volumes of dilute urine, resulting in hypernatremia and volume depletion. **Arginine vasopressin (Pitressin) 5 to 10 U IV, intramuscularly (IM), or SC every 4 to 6 hours or desmopressin acetate (DDAVP) SC or IV 2 to 4 μg every 12 hours** is given to maintain urine output to less than 200 ml/hour, and volume is replaced with hypotonic fluids (0.25% or 0.45% saline) depending on the severity of hypernatremia.

4. **Posttraumatic seizures**

   Posttraumatic seizures may be **immediate** (occurring within 24 hours), **early** (occurring within the first week), or **late** (occurring after the first week). Immediate seizures do not predispose to later seizures; early seizures, however, indicate an increased risk of late seizures, and these patients should be maintained on anticonvulsants. The overall incidence of late posttraumatic epilepsy (recurrent, unprovoked seizures) after closed head injury is 5%; the risk is approximately 20% in patients with intracranial hemorrhage or depressed skull fractures.

■ PROGNOSIS

The outcome after head injury is often a matter of great concern, particularly in patients with serious injuries. The admission

Glasgow Coma scale score has substantial prognostic value: patients scoring 3 or 4 have an 85% chance of dying or remaining in a vegetative state, whereas these outcomes occur in only 5 to 10% of patients with a score of 12 or higher. The *postconcussional syndrome* refers to a chronic syndrome of headache, fatigue, dizziness, inability to concentrate, irritability, and personality changes that develops in many patients following head injury. Often, there is overlap with symptoms of depression.

11

ATAXIA AND GAIT FAILURE

True ataxia implies a decomposition of coordinated posture and movement that is normally integrated by the cerebellum. Because almost every component of the nervous system contributes to maintenance of normal movement, gait, and posture, a call for a patient with gait failure requires consideration of a broad differential diagnosis. Successful evaluation begins with assessing the acuteness of the syndrome. Associated signs on examination will help with anatomic localization. Your management may range from emergent neurosurgical decompression of a cerebellar hematoma to a thorough laboratory evaluation to seek a cause for a chronic degenerative disease.

■ PHONE CALL

Questions

1. **When did the patient last walk normally?**
    This is the key question from which your route of investigation and management will spring. **If the patient was known to have been walking normally within the past 24 hours, you must rule out spinal cord compression** (see Chapter 8) **or a mass lesion in the posterior fossa.** These are medical emergencies. A subacute course (days to weeks) suggests an infectious, inflammatory, or neoplastic process. If the gait deterioration has occurred over weeks to months, your differential diagnosis will be weighted toward degenerative processes, either inherited or acquired.
2. **Has there been any trauma to the head, neck, or back?**
    Although the cerebellum coordinates normal posture and gait, a traumatic subdural hematoma or injury to the spinal cord or peripheral nerves may alter gait.
3. **What is the patient's level of consciousness?**
    Is the patient alert and awake, agitated, or confused? If a patient has an abnormal mental status in combination with ataxia or gait failure, acute intoxication or significant brain injury is likely.
4. **What are the vital signs?**
    Your ability to carry out appropriate diagnostic testing requires knowledge of, if not treatment of, the patient's cardiopulmonary status. Irregular heart rhythm may suggest cardioembolic stroke; fever may suggest an infectious process.

Orders

1. Maintain the patient at bed rest.
2. Use a chest restraint, if necessary, to prevent the patient from injuring himself or herself.
3. If there has been trauma to the head or neck, stabilize the cervical spine with a cervical collar (see Chapter 8).

■ ELEVATOR THOUGHTS (DIAGNOSING GAIT FAILURE)

Gait failure may occur as a result of damage to almost any part of the neural axis. Your initial examination of the patient will help establish whether you are dealing with disturbance of motor, sensory, or cerebellar function. Table 11–1 is an outline of the categories of diseases that cause gait dysfunction and the characteristic features of the gait disturbance. Table 11–2 provides a more detailed differential diagnosis of ataxia.

■ MAJOR THREAT TO LIFE

- **Cerebellar hemorrhage or infarction**
  Hematoma or infarction in the posterior fossa may progress to herniation and death if the lesion is large. It may require emergent neurosurgical evacuation.
- **Acute intoxication**
  Intoxication with sedatives such as barbiturate or alcohol may present initially as ataxia and may lead to respiratory failure.

■ BEDSIDE

Quick Look Test

Is the patient awake and alert?
A decreased level of consciousness in the presence of ataxia means you will need to move swiftly to evaluate for a posterior fossa mass lesion that may be causing herniation.

Is there any evidence of head or neck trauma?
Head trauma rarely presents as ataxia alone but may require more immediate management. Vertebral artery dissection may result from trauma to the neck.

Has the patient been vomiting?
Nausea, vertigo, and vomiting are common symptoms that accompany posterior fossa disease.

Table 11–1 □ CLINICAL FEATURES OF GAIT DISTURBANCES

Disease Category	Features of Gait Failure
Focal brain injury (hemiparesis)	Spastically extended leg Spastically flexed arm Circumduction of paretic foot
Spinal cord injury (paraparesis)	Stiff, effortful movements at knees and hips Bilateral circumduction Toe-walking or scissoring gait
Peripheral or central deafferentation (sensory ataxia)	Wide-based stance and gait High-stepping gait Positive Romberg's sign
Cerebellar disease	Titubation (unsteady, oscillating posture) on sitting or standing Wide-based stance and gait Ataxia: staggering or lurching may be unilateral or bilateral
Normal-pressure hydrocephalus	"Magnetic," shuffling gait Many steps taken to turn 180 degrees
Lower motor neuron disease	Distal weakness (e.g., footdrop) High-stepping gait
Myopathy	Proximal leg weakness Difficulty arising from seated position Difficulty climbing stairs
Parkinsonism	Stooped posture Shuffling gait Retropulsion Difficulty initiating and terminating ambulation
Congenital/perinatal injury (cerebral palsy)	Spastically extended legs Spastically flexed arms Scissoring gait Adventitial movements (abnormal posturing or movements of one or more limbs)
Movement disorders (chorea, athetosis, or dystonia)	Adventitial movements may be present at rest Lurching gait

Selective History and Chart Review

The diagnosis for the etiology of gait failure can often be made on the history alone. If the patient is awake and alert, ask him or her to recount the circumstances of being unable to walk. If the patient is unable to give a history, get the history from a relative,

Table 11–2 □ **DIFFERENTIAL DIAGNOSIS OF ATAXIA BY MODE OF ONSET**

Mode of Onset	Disease Process
Acute (minutes to hours)	Cerebellar hemorrhage Cerebellar infarction Acute intoxication Head trauma Basilar migraine (mostly in children) Dominant periodic ataxia (in children)
Subacute (hours to days)	Posterior fossa tumor Posterior fossa abscess Multiple sclerosis Toxins/intoxications Hydrocephalus Miller-Fisher variant of Guillain-Barré syndrome Viral cerebellitis (mostly in children)
Chronic (days to weeks)	Alcoholic cerebellar degeneration Paraneoplastic cerebellar syndrome Foramen magnum compression Chronic infection (e.g., Jakob-Creutzfeldt disease, rubella, panencephalitis) Hydrocephalus Vitamin E deficiency Hypothyroidism Inherited ataxias (autosomal recessive or dominant) Idiopathic degenerative ataxias
Episodic	Recurrent intoxications Multiple sclerosis Transient ischemic attacks Dominant periodic ataxia (children)

Modified from Harding AE: Ataxic disorders. *In* Bradley WG, Daroff RB, Fenichel GM, Marsden CD (eds): Neurology in Clinical Practice. Boston, Butterworth-Heinemann, 1991.

nurse, or other witness. In the absence of a witness, review the chart.

1. **When did the gait disturbance begin?**
2. **Was the onset sudden or gradual?**
3. **Why was the patient unable to walk? Was it because of weakness, imbalance, pain, or numbness?**
4. **Were there any accompanying symptoms?**
   Diplopia, dysarthria, vertigo, or nausea suggests posterior fossa involvement. Unilateral weakness or numbness implies focal hemispheric brain injury (e.g., stroke). Urinary or fecal incontinence suggests spinal cord involvement. Pain radiating into the legs implies nerve root disease.
5. **Is the patient taking any medications that might cause ataxia?**

Table 11–3 □ **MEDICATIONS KNOWN TO CAUSE ATAXIA**

Anticonvulsants	Immunosuppressants
Phenytoin	Cyclosporine A
Carbamazepine	Cytosine arabinoside
Primidone	Fluorouracil
Ethosuximide	Other medications (rarely cause ataxia)
Methosuximide	Phenothiazines
Sedatives	Monoamine oxidase inhibitors
Barbiturates	Reserpine
Benzodiazepines	Thiothixene
Chloral hydrate	Lithium salts
Paraldehyde	Nitrofurantoin

Most of the effects of medications are dose dependent (Table 11–3).

Selective Physical Examination I

Vital signs:	Fever may suggest an infectious etiology, such as **abscess, viral cerebellitis, or fungal infection.** Fever may also occur in some of the inherited metabolic ataxias (mostly in children). Irregular heart rhythm may suggest cardioembolic stroke.
HEENT:	Look for signs of head trauma. **Subdural or epidural hematoma** may produce hemiparesis
Abdomen:	Look for signs of **chronic alcohol use,** such as hepatomegaly, caput medusae, or ascites. Hepatosplenomegaly may also appear in **Wilson's disease** and in some **inherited metabolic ataxias.**

Neurologic examination:
- **Mental status:** Establish level of alertness and attentiveness by asking the patient to count backward from 20 to 1 or to recite the months of the year backward.
- **Cranial nerves: Gait failure with almost any cranial nerve finding means there is brain stem or cerebellar involvement.**
  1. **Pupils:** Pinpoint pupils may suggest **opiate intoxication;** asymmetric pupils may be a part of Horner's syndrome (miosis, ptosis, and anhidrosis), which, in combination with ataxia and contralateral pain and temperature sensory loss, makes up Wallenberg's (lateral medullary) syndrome. Small, irregular pupils that react to accommodation but not to light (Argyll Robertson pupils) may be a sign of **CNS syphilis, brain stem encephalitis, or mass effect on the midbrain.**
  2. **Extraocular movements: Nystagmus, particularly if verti-**

cal or dysconjugate, is a sign of injury to the brain stem or cerebellum. Vertical (upbeat or downbeat) nystagmus is a reliable indicator of cerebellar or brain stem damage (see Chapter 14 for a more detailed discussion of nystagmus). Horizontal gaze palsies localize disease to a large hemispheric or small pontine lesion. Impaired upgaze, particularly in combination with retraction nystagmus and loss of pupillary accommodation, implies pressure on or damage to the tectum of the midbrain and can be seen in pineal region tumors or in hydrocephalus (Parinaud's phenomenon). CN 6 palsies may be a nonspecific sign of increased intracranial pressure. Oculoparesis, in combination with ataxia and areflexia, makes the diagnosis of the **Miller-Fisher variant of Guillain-Barré syndrome.**

3. **CN 7:** Upper motor neuron facial paresis may be part of a hemiparesis or may indicate brain stem involvement if CN 6 is affected on the same side.

4. **CN 8:** Tinnitus or hearing loss with ataxia suggests a **peripheral vestibular neuropathy or labyrinthitis,** particularly if there is a rotational component to the nystagmus.

5. **CN 9 to CN 12:** Dysphagia, nasal speech, dysarthria, or tongue deviation may suggest a **brain stem stroke or mass lesion at the skull base,** producing spastic paraparesis and gait failure in addition to the lower cranial nerve findings

- **Cerebellar testing:** Rapid, repetitive finger-thumb opposition (rapid alternating movements [RAM]) and finger-nose-finger (FNF) movements are two sensitive screening tests for cerebellar function. Irregular rhythm (dysdiadochokinesis) on finger tapping or ataxia of movements as the finger approaches the target on the FNF test suggests cerebellar dysfunction. The heel-knee-shin (HKS) test is the equivalent of the FNF test for the lower extremities. Figure 11–1 illustrates three common cerebellar tests (the FNF, RAM, and HKS tests). **Unilateral limb ataxia implies ipsilateral cerebellar hemisphere damage** because the cerebellar circuits that coordinate movement cross twice, once while descending in the frontopontocerebellar pathway and a second time while ascending in the dentatothalamic, dentatorubral, and dentatocortical pathways. **Titubation (truncal ataxia) on sitting or standing or gait ataxia in the absence of limb ataxia suggests midline cerebellar damage.**

If the patient is able to stand, the gait evaluation is a crucial part of the examination for anatomic localization and determining the underlying pathophysiology. Table 11–1 reviews the features of gait dysfunction that characterize different disease processes. The gait should be tested with the patient walking normally, walking on the toes, walking on the heels, and doing a tandem walk. Observe for symmetry of balance, stride, and arm swing.

Finger-nose-finger test

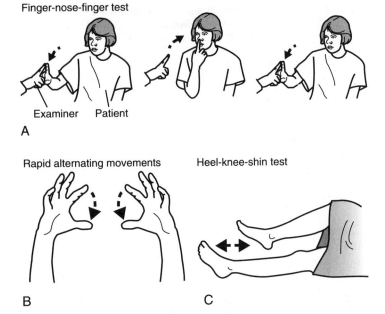

Examiner   Patient

A

Rapid alternating movements   Heel-knee-shin test

B   C

Figure 11–1 □ Cerebellar function tests. *A,* Finger-nose-finger test. Patient touches the finger of the examiner and his or her own nose sequentially. *B,* Rapid alternating movements. Patient taps the forefinger and thumb together as rapidly as possible. *C,* Heel-knee-shin test. Patient runs the heel up and down the opposite shin as accurately and rapidly as possible.

- **Motor:** Test for strength by confrontation and look for pronator drift with the arms extended and palms up. (Pronator drift may be the only sign of a subtle hemiparesis.)
- **Sensory:** Temperature and vibration are the most sensitive parameters for testing sensory loss. Proprioceptive loss may indicate damaged posterior columns, as occurs in **vitamin B$_{12}$ deficiency** (subacute combined degeneration) or **tabes dorsalis** (a now rare, late complication of syphilis).
- **Reflexes:** Unilateral hyperreflexia usually accompanies hemiparesis; bilateral hyperreflexia may indicate myelopathy; and areflexia is seen in peripheral neuropathy and in the **Guillain-Barré syndrome.**

■ MANAGEMENT I

Acute ataxia, particularly with any accompanying signs or symptoms of posterior fossa disease or increased intracranial pressure, must be treated with utmost urgency.

1. **Obtain a noncontrast head computed tomography (CT) or magnetic resonance imaging (MRI) scan.**
   If cerebellar hematoma or infarction is identified, proceed with the next steps.
2. **Admit the patient to an intensive care unit.**
3. **Consult with the neurosurgery service.** If there is hematoma near the brain stem or if the hematoma is large, rapid and irreversible neurologic deterioration may occur. Delayed deterioration may be the result of a rebleed or reactive edema formation. **Surgical evacuation of cerebellar hematoma greater than 3 cm in diameter has been shown to reduce morbidity and mortality.** Consideration for surgical evacuation is warranted particularly if the patient is relatively young and is following a deteriorating course. **It may be necessary to place an intraventricular drain if hydrocephalus develops.**
4. **Cerebellar hematomas smaller than 3 cm may be managed medically with reasonably good results.** Therapy is largely supportive, with blood pressure control to a target maximum systolic blood pressure (SBP) of 160 to 180 mm Hg and control of coagulopathy with fresh frozen plasma if necessary. Hydrocephalus can develop even with smaller hematomas, necessitating neurosurgical placement of an intraventricular drain.
5. **Cerebellar infarction, if large, may produce the same syndrome of rapid progression to coma as does cerebellar hematoma.** As the infarcted territory becomes edematous, compression of the fourth ventricle may produce **obstructive hydrocephalus,** leading to further increase in intracranial pressure. Cerebellar infarction in the posterior inferior cerebellar artery territory carries a worse prognosis than infarction in the anterior inferior cerebellar artery or superior cerebellar artery territories. **Surgical evacuation of a large cerebellar infarction may be lifesaving.** As above, placement of an intraventricular drain may become necessary with cerebellar infarction if hydrocephalus develops.

Other causes of gait failure that require immediate management include cord compression or acute myelopathy (see Chapter 8), **subdural or epidural hematoma from head trauma** (see Chapter 10), **acute cerebral infarction** (see Chapter 7), **and acute intoxication** (see Chapter 6).

■ SELECTIVE PHYSICAL EXAMINATION II

Once posterior fossa lesions have been ruled out by imaging, further examination for systemic signs associated with chronic ataxic disorders should be performed:

Hair: Alopecia may be a sign of **thallium poisoning, hypothyroidism, or adrenoleukomyeloneuropathy.**

Skin: Telangiectases, particularly in the conjunctivae, nose, and ears, or flexures, may be seen in **ataxia-telangiectasia.** Pigmentation may be seen in adrenoleukomyeloneuropathy.

HEENT: Kayser-Fleischer rings appear as a brown border at the edge of the iris in **Wilson's disease.** Retinal angiomas seen on fundoscopic examination may be a part of **von Hippel-Lindau disease** that also includes cerebellar hemangioblastomas. Deafness in combination with short stature is often a sign of **mitochondrial encephalopathy.**

Heart: Cardiomegaly, murmurs, arrhythmias, and heart failure may accompany **Friedreich's ataxia.** Conduction defects on electrocardiogram (ECG) may be present in mitochondrial encephalopathy.

Musculoskeletal: Short stature is characteristic of mitochondrial encephalopathy and ataxia-telangiectasia. Other skeletal deformities may be a part of hereditary ataxias and **hereditary motor and sensory neuropathy.**

■ MANAGEMENT II

Diagnostic Testing

Laboratory Investigation

Laboratory investigation should begin with an attempt to diagnose treatable or reversible causes of ataxia or gait failure. Laboratory tests to be performed include the following blood tests:

1. Chemistry panel, including electrolytes, glucose, and liver function tests
2. Urine and serum toxicology screen
3. Vitamin B_{12} and folate levels
4. Venereal Disease Research Laboratory (VDRL) test
5. Thyroid function tests
6. Anticonvulsant levels if the patient is taking anticonvulsants
7. Lithium level if the patient is taking lithium
8. Anti-Yo serum antibodies to investigate paraneoplastic cerebellar degeneration from ovarian, lung, or breast carcinoma, or Hodgkin's lymphoma (see Chapter 24)
9. Ceruloplasmin levels (Wilson's disease)

Other Diagnostic Tests

1. **Chest x-ray.** A chest x-ray may disclose occult neoplasm, raising the possibility of metastatic disease or a paraneoplastic cerebellar degeneration.

2. **Transcranial Doppler ultrasonogram or MR angiogram.** Vertebrobasilar transient ischemic attacks (TIAs) or vertebrobasilar insufficiency may be suggested if there is stenosis of the basilar or vertebral arteries.
3. **Visual evoked responses.** Delayed P100 suggests multiple sclerosis.
4. **Lumbar puncture.** Oligoclonal bands are present in multiple sclerosis. Abnormal cerebrospinal fluid (CSF) cell count, protein, or glucose may point to an infectious or neoplastic process. Cytology may be performed if a CNS- or meninges-based tumor is suspected.
5. **Electromyography (EMG)/nerve conduction studies (NCS).** The Miller-Fisher variant of the Guillain-Barré syndrome includes ataxia, oculoparesis, and areflexia. A typical demyelination pattern of slowed conduction velocities and prolonged F waves supports this diagnosis. Gait failure on the basis of neuropathy can also be diagnosed with EMG/NCS.

Treatment of Some of the Reversible Causes of Ataxia

1. **Acute sedative intoxication:** Administer **naloxone (Narcan) 0.4 to 0.8 mg IV** for opiate overdose; **flumazenil (Romazicon) 0.5 mg IV** for benzodiazepine overdose; admit for observation and supportive therapy.
2. **Anticonvulsant overdose:** Stop administering the anticonvulsant, admit for observation and cardiovascular monitoring, and follow anticonvulsant levels.
3. **Hypothyroidism:** Administer **Synthroid 0.05 to 0.15 mg every day.**
4. **Lithium toxicity:** Admit patient for cardiac monitoring, adjust dose, and follow lithium and electrolyte levels.
5. **Paraneoplastic disorder:** Treating the underlying malignancy may reverse the symptoms in some patients. Immunosuppressive therapy and plasmapheresis have not been proven effective.
6. **Vertebrobasilar TIAs:** Admit patient for workup for etiology of TIAs. Anticoagulation may be required (see Chapter 25).
7. **Multiple sclerosis:** Treat with IV methylprednisolone and interferon beta (see Chapter 22).
8. **CNS infections:** Treat with appropriate antimicrobial agents (see Chapter 23).
9. **Miller-Fisher variant of Guillain-Barré syndrome:** A several-day course of plasmapheresis or intravenous immune globulin (IVIG) early in the disease may be effective in halting progression and speeding recovery (see Chapter 16).

12

ACUTE VISUAL DISTURBANCES

No symptom may be as disturbing or dramatic to a patient as acute visual loss. Although acute ocular diseases such as glaucoma, uveitis, and retinal detachment may require urgent evaluation by an ophthalmologist, a high percentage of visual disturbances fall within the province of the neurologist. Neurologic visual symptoms may be reported as blurriness, focal obscurations, or positive visual phenomena. Because the visual pathway from the retina to the calcarine cortex is constant from individual to individual, anatomic localization can be made with a high degree of accuracy on physical examination. The progression, associated symptoms and signs, and clinical setting will help you make the correct diagnosis and suggest the proper acute management.

■ PHONE CALL

Questions

The following questions will need to be repeated during the selective history and physical examination of the patient. Nonetheless, these questions, asked prior to your arrival at the bedside, will form the starting point for your diagnostic and management algorithm.

1. Is the visual loss in one or both eyes?

This is the first point for anatomic localization. Visual disturbances affecting one eye indicate pathology between the retina and the optic chiasm. Binocular disturbances suggest lesions in the visual pathway between the chiasm and the calcarine cortex.

2. What is the nature of the visual disturbance?

This is an elaboration of question one. Vision can be altered in one of the following ways: monocular visual loss (temporary or permanent), bilateral blindness, a hemifield cut, diplopia, scotomata, or positive phenomena (e.g., flashes or lines). The first description of the disturbance will allow the visual problem to be categorized into specific disease entities.

3. How old is the patient?

Certain disorders, such as ischemic optic neuropathy or transient monocular blindness (TMB), are rare in patients under 45 years of age, whereas a first presentation of multiple sclerosis, pseudotumor cerebri, or migraine is much more common in a younger patient.

4. **Is the patient still experiencing the visual symptom?**
   Although persistent acute visual loss may require immediate, specific therapy, transient visual loss may be no less ominous as a warning sign for further visual, cerebrovascular, or inflammatory events.

5. **When did the visual disturbance begin?**
   This important question is the first step in understanding the pathology of the condition. **Acute monocular blindness is a neuro-ophthalmologic emergency.** Ischemia in the retina resulting from a central retinal artery occlusion may be irreversible after 105 minutes. Furthermore, even if the patient presents many hours after the onset of visual loss, efficient and accurate diagnosis may prevent contralateral visual loss or stroke.

6. **Was there any trauma or injury to the eyes?**
   Eye injury will nearly always require ophthalmologic evaluation. Because a dilated fundoscopic examination by an ophthalmologist will interfere with your ability to get an accurate assessment of pupillary reactivity, you should try to perform your assessment first.

Orders

If there has been eye trauma or if there is a pre-existing ophthalmologic condition such as glaucoma, call the ophthalmology service for consultation.

Inform RN

"Will arrive at the bedside in . . . minutes."

■ ELEVATOR THOUGHTS (DIFFERENTIAL DIAGNOSIS OF ACUTE VISUAL DISTURBANCE)

The differential diagnosis of acute visual disturbance can be divided into processes affecting one eye or both eyes.

1. **Monocular visual loss**
   - **Retinal ischemia (central [or branch] retinal artery occlusion [CRAO])**
     This is usually caused by an embolus from the ipsilateral internal carotid artery or from the heart or aortic arch. If the symptoms are transient (TMB or amaurosis fugax), the mechanism may be hemodynamic rather than embolic. Hemodynamic TMB may be caused by perfusion failure in

the retinal artery from high-grade carotid stenosis. Patients with vascular causes for retinal ischemia usually have risk factors for cerebrovascular disease, such as hypertension, diabetes, or a history of smoking.

- **Optic nerve head ischemia (anterior ischemic optic neuropathy [AION])**

    Although its pathophysiology is uncertain, this entity is often associated with arteritis. Patients in their 50s or 60s may have systemic lupus erythematosus, polyarteritis nodosa, sickle cell trait, or polycythemia. In patients over 60 years of age, the most common associated arteritis is giant cell (temporal) arteritis, which must be treated emergently.

- **Inflammatory/demyelinating optic neuritis**

    The most common cause for optic neuritis in a patient under 40 years of age is multiple sclerosis, but idiopathic forms and sarcoidosis can be present in older individuals.

- **Retrobulbar mass lesion**

    The lesion may be a **tumor such as optic glioma, neurofibroma, meningioma, or metastasis, or a giant aneurysm in the cavernous segment of the carotid. Pseudotumor cerebri** (benign intracranial hypertension) can mimic a mass lesion, causing papilledema and visual loss in young women who are often obese and dysmenorrheic. Visual loss may begin unilaterally.

2. **Binocular visual loss**

    Binocular involvement with visual field defects implies pathology at or behind the optic chiasm. Acute binocular visual loss affecting the chiasm, the optic tracts, the thalamus (lateral geniculate body), the optic radiations, or the calcarine cortex is nearly always due to an anatomic lesion such as a **tumor, abscess, or stroke. Migraine** is a notable exception, in which "spreading depression" (a wave of depolarization) is thought to produce neuronal deactivation that moves slowly across the cortex and produces scotomata in one visual field. **Pituitary adenomas** often produce bitemporal visual field defects as pressure from the mass disrupts midline-crossing fibers from both nasal retinae (Fig. 12–1). The farther back along the visual pathway the lesion is located, the more congruous is the visual field defect.

3. **Diplopia**

    Double vision implies some form of oculoparesis. If diplopia persists when one eye is covered, the etiology is either factitious or an ophthalmologic condition such as retinal detachment, dislocated lens, or keratoconus. For true binocular diplopia, the lesion is almost always in the brain stem or involves CN 3, CN 4, or CN 6. The most common conditions affecting the brain stem are **stroke** and **multiple sclerosis,** although **brain stem tumors** and **progressive multifocal**

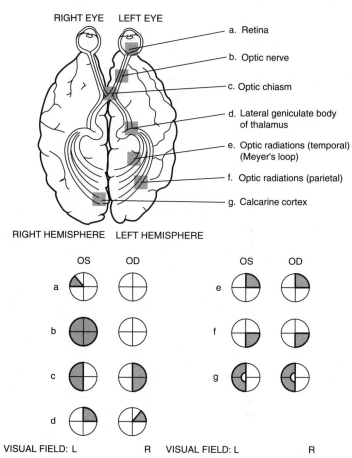

Figure 12–1 □ Visual field cuts produced by lesions at different points along the visual pathway. a. Monocular segmentanopia produced by a retinal artery branch occlusion in the left eye. b. Monocular blindness produced by a lesion in the left optic nerve. c. Bitemporal hemianopia produced by a mass lesion at the optic chiasm. d. Right segmentanopia produced by a lesion in the lateral geniculate body of the left thalamus. e. Right upper quadrantanopia produced by a lesion in the left temporal optic radiation (Meyer's loop). f. Right lower quadrantanopia produced by a lesion in the left parietal optic radiation. g. Left homonomous hemianopia produced by a lesion in the calcarine cortex of the right occipital lobe. Note that macular vision is sometimes spared because of middle cerebral artery collateral blood flow to the occipital pole. OS, Oculus sinister; OD, oculus dexter.

leukoencephalopathy (PML) may rarely present with diplopia. The most common systemic condition that affects the ocular cranial nerves is **diabetes mellitus.** A **berry aneurysm** of the posterior communicating artery may also produce diplopia by stretching CN 3 as it passes over the artery on its way forward toward the cavernous sinus. Invasive or metastatic **tumor in the cavernous sinus region** or late **chronic meningitis** may cause oculomotor disturbances. Unilateral or bilateral CN 6 palsies can be a "false localizing" sign of **increased intracranial pressure** (see Chapter 13). **Hyperthyroidism** may cause diplopia by mechanical limitation of infiltrated, fibrotic ocular muscles. Finally, weakness of the extraocular muscles because of **myasthenia gravis** must be considered in the differential diagnosis of diplopia, particularly if the symptoms fluctuate or appear with fatigue.

Diagnoses for which immediate, specific therapy may arrest or restore vision loss are the following:
- Central retinal artery occlusion
- Ischemic optic neuropathy from temporal arteritis
- Pseudotumor cerebri
- Acute glaucoma

Diagnoses for which urgent management may prevent further vision loss or stroke are the following:
- Transient monocular blindness with carotid stenosis
- Retrobulbar mass lesion (aneurysm or tumor)

■ MAJOR THREAT TO LIFE

Acute visual loss in the absence of other neurologic signs is rarely life threatening.

■ BEDSIDE

Quick Look Test

Are there any signs of trauma?

Is the patient in any pain or discomfort?

Is one eye affected or are both?

Selective History and Chart Review

Some of the questions asked in the initial telephone interview should be discussed with the patient.

1. **Was one eye affected or were both?**

   It may be difficult for a patient to distinguish between a visual field loss and monocular blindness. A patient will often refer to "the left eye" as being defective when in fact the left hemifield was affected. Ask if the symptoms improve if "the bad eye" is covered.

2. **When and how did the visual disturbance begin?**

   Ask the patient to describe the onset of the symptoms, with particular reference to the location and pattern of the visual disturbance. An obscuration that moves across the visual field "like a shade coming down" is a common description of an arterial occlusion. An altitudinal defect is common with ischemic optic neuropathy. An expanding blind spot may suggest worsening papilledema. Slowly marching lights, particularly the jagged-edged "fortification scotomata," is a common description of migraine, whether or not it is followed by headache. Sudden loss of vision over seconds to minutes suggests a vascular cause. Progression over hours to days may suggest ischemic optic neuropathy, demyelination, mass lesion, or pseudotumor cerebri.

3. **Was there pain?**

   Headache is common in temporal arteritis, pseudotumor cerebri, and migraine. Masticatory claudication and other myalgias may be a tip-off for arteritis. Pain with eye movement is the rule for the inflammatory optic neuritis of multiple sclerosis, but pain is usually absent with retinal embolism and ischemic optic neuropathy. The exception is in carotid artery dissection, which may cause pain in the side of the head or jaw, with radiation into the orbit.

4. **Were there any associated neurologic symptoms?**

   Dysarthria, vertigo, nausea, vomiting, and ataxia suggest stroke or mass lesion in the posterior fossa. Urinary incontinence, ataxia, diplopia, and patchy weakness or sensory loss are other presenting symptoms of multiple sclerosis.

Selective Physical Examination

Vital signs:	Fever may be a feature of temporal arteritis. Cardiac arrhythmia and hypertension are risk factors for cerebrovascular disease.
HEENT:	▪ **Palpate the temporal arteries** just anterior and superior to the ear and along the side of the head (Fig. 12–2). Exquisite tenderness strongly suggests temporal arteritis. Listen for **carotid bruits.**
	▪ **Eye examination.** Check for **proptosis** by viewing the orbits from above. A retrobulbar mass lesion may cause the eye to protrude. Gentle palpation of the globe may disclose more resistance to posterior motion. The high pressure of glaucoma may also be detected, if present.

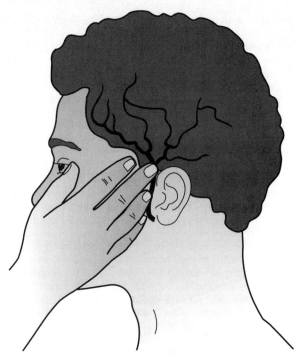

Figure 12–2 □ Palpation of the temporal artery just anterior to the superior insertion of the auricle.

Neurologic examination:

- **Mental status**

    Aphasia or hemineglect may rarely accompany a disruption of optic radiations through the parietal lobe.

- **Cranial nerves**

    Check **ocular motility** with the following steps:

    1. **Pupillary reactivity.** Examine each pupil's direct and consensual response to light. Use low ambient light and a bright flashlight for the stimulus. A relative or absolute **afferent pupillary defect (APD)** may be detected by swinging the flashlight from one eye to the other. If the pupil enlarges when the flashlight swings to that eye **(Marcus Gunn pupil)**, there is pathology in the retina or optic nerve.

    2. **Visual fields.** Test for visual fields by having the patient visually fix on your nose and by holding your hands in two of the four visual quadrants, an arm's length from the patient. Move a finger or briefly display a number of fingers on one or both hands. Test all four quadrants.

More subtle visual field loss may be tested by comparing the brightness of a red button or hatpin. Red desaturation may occur without frank blindness. Be sure to check macular vision in the central 6 degrees of vision. Figure 12–1 illustrates the visual field defects expected with lesions at various points along the visual pathway.

3. **Fundoscopic examination.** This can reveal a specific pathology, although an examination adequate to make a definitive diagnosis may require pharmacologic dilation of the pupil. Table 12–1 lists the fundoscopic features of the most important diagnoses of monocular blindness.

4. Have the patient follow your finger through horizontal and vertical range of motion. Note oculoparesis if it occurs. Simple observation of the eye movements may be sufficient to diagnose a CN 3 or CN 6 lesion.

5. A latent or subtle nonconjugate gaze may be revealed by the cover-uncover test. Ask the patient to fix on one point such as your finger. Cover one eye, then uncover it. Repeat with the other eye. If the eyes shift when the eyes are uncovered, there is a nonconjugate gaze. Although a positive cover-uncover test may suggest brain stem or cranial nerve pathology, benign, latent phorias in patients with normal vision may cause a positive test.

6. If there is pre-existing amblyopia or if the patient is suppressing one eye's image, it may be difficult to identify diplopia without isolating the images from the two

Table 12–1 □ **FUNDOSCOPIC FEATURES OF SOME NEURO-OPHTHALMOLOGIC ENTITIES**

Diagnosis	Fundoscopic Appearance
Central retinal artery occlusion	White, ground-glass retina "Boxcar segmentation" (clumped red blood cells) in retinal veins (<1 hour) Macular cherry-red spot (hours to days)
Branch retinal artery occlusion	Embolic material (bright calcium flecks or lipid yellow Hollenhorst plaques) at arterial branch points Arcuate band of retinal infarction
Ischemic optic neuropathy	Disk head pallor, often in the superior or inferior half only Papilledema Superficial flame hemorrhages Optic disk cupping (late)
Optic neuritis	Disk pallor
Pseudotumor cerebri	Papilledema

eyes. Isolation may be accomplished with a **Maddox rod.** Correct use of the Maddox rod takes practice, but it can be invaluable in identifying subtle oculoparesis. To check for horizontal diplopia, have the patient cover one eye with the Maddox rod, with the slats oriented vertically, and then have the patient fix on a point light source. Two images should be seen: the point of light will be seen by the uncovered eye and a vertical red line will be seen by the covered eye. If gaze is conjugate, light should bisect the red line. As you move the light laterally, the light and line will move farther apart if there is a paresis of lateral gaze in one eye. This occurs as the image is projected onto the retina, away from the macula in the affected eye. The rules are as follows: (1) the "false" image is always the one on the outside, and (2) the false image always comes from the affected eye. Figure 12–3 diagrams the use of the Maddox rod. The same procedure can be used to check for a vertical nonconjugate gaze by orienting the slats of the Maddox rod horizontally and moving the light up or down. Again, the image that is on the outside (farther up on upgaze or farther down on downgaze) comes from the affected eye. Impairment of abduction indicates CN 6 or lateral rectus palsy. Impairment of adduction indicates CN 3 or medial rectus palsy. If adduction palsy is accompanied by abduction nystagmus in the opposite eye, this is likely an **internuclear ophthalmoplegia,** suggesting multiple sclerosis in a younger patient or a paramedian midbrain infarct in an older person.

- **Coordination and gait**
  Ataxia or dysdiadochokinesis may be a sign of multiple sclerosis or may suggest posterior circulation infarction affecting the cerebellum and the occipital cortex.
- **Sensation**
  Unilateral sensory loss may accompany visual field cuts produced by lesions in the thalamus or parietal lobe.
- **Reflexes**
  Asymmetry may be a subtle sign of brain injury.

■ MANAGEMENT

Order the following blood tests:
1. Erythrocyte sedimentation rate (ESR)
2. Complete blood count (CBC) with platelet count
3. Prothrombin time (PT) or International Normalized Ratio (INR)/partial thromboplastin time (PTT)
4. Chemistry panel including glucose and cholesterol levels

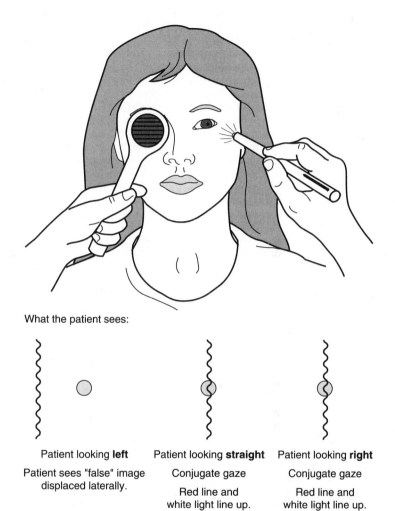

What the patient sees:

Patient looking **left**

Patient sees "false" image displaced laterally.

Patient looking **straight**

Conjugate gaze

Red line and white light line up.

Patient looking **right**

Conjugate gaze

Red line and white light line up.

Figure 12–3 □ Use of the Maddox rod in a patient with a right CN 3 palsy. Patient sees the red line to the left of the white light on left gaze. This occurs because the red line projects farther laterally onto the retina of the abnormal eye, giving a "false" image that appears displaced laterally. The gaze is conjugate on primary gaze and on rightward gaze. Right CN 3 palsy would be confirmed by holding the Maddox rod so that the red line is oriented horizontally and asking the patient to look upward. The red line would then appear above the white light.

If there is monocular blindness or any suspicion of injury to the eye, have someone call for an ophthalmologic consultation to follow your assessment.

1. Central retinal artery occlusion

Restoration of vision is usually possible only within the first 90 to 120 minutes after the occlusive event, although rare instances of reversal of blindness have been reported up to 12 hours after embolus. Treatment between 12 and 24 hours would be considered heroic. Treatment in the hyperacute phase is aimed at dislodging the embolic particle and lowering the intraocular pressure. This is accomplished by laying the patient flat and applying firm **ocular massage.** If segmentation can still be seen in the retinal veins, you should consult an ophthalmologist to perform an anterior oculocentesis. The presence of a cherry-red spot suggests that the retina has been infarcted.

Apart from treating the eye itself, CRAO requires a search for an embolic source. **Duplex Doppler ultrasonography** of the carotid arteries and echocardiography seeking a cardioembolic source should be performed urgently. **Intravenous (IV) heparin at 800 U/hour (no bolus), aiming for a PTT of 1.5–2.0 times the control value,** is recommended while the search for an embolic source is underway, provided there are no contraindications to anticoagulation therapy. **Patients with ipsilateral carotid stenosis greater than 70% should be referred for carotid endarterectomy** to reduce the risk of stroke. Long-term anticoagulation with coumadin is probably indicated if a cardioembolic source is identified.

2. Arteritic ischemic optic neuropathy

Identifying temporal arteritis is of utmost importance. Because the prognosis for recovery of vision is less than 15% for the first eye, and because contralateral blindness may occur in up to 40% of patients, early recognition is important. Realistically, if visual loss is the presenting symptom, therapy is aimed at preventing involvement of the contralateral eye. Anorexia, fever, myalgias, and jaw claudication accompanying visual loss and headache in a patient over 65 years of age firmly establishes the diagnosis clinically. Less typical presentations are possible. Sedimentation rate and fibrinogen levels are usually markedly elevated. **Prednisone 100 mg by mouth (PO)** once a day should be started immediately, then tapered slowly after several weeks. **IV methylprednisolone 1 g/day** may also be used. Temporal artery biopsy should be arranged within a week. Corticosteroids generally have to be continued for 1 to 2 years. The ESR can be used as a marker of disease activity.

3. Transient monocular blindness

Patients with painless transient monocular visual loss, particularly those with risk factors for cerebrovascular disease, should be evaluated for risk of stroke. TMB is a classic warning sign for high-grade carotid stenosis. As in CRAO, the patient should be referred for duplex Doppler ultrasonography, echocardiography, and usually magnetic resonance (MR) angiography. Maintaining the patient on an antithrombotic agent, either **acetylsalicylic acid (aspirin) 325 mg once a day** or **IV heparin at 800 U/hour** if he or she is awaiting imminent endarterectomy, will reduce the risk of stroke or recurrent TIA (see Chapter 25).

4. **Retrobulbar mass lesion**

In a patient with a suspected retro-orbital mass, high-quality imaging is the key to accurate diagnosis. **MRI with gadolinium contrast enhancement** will help define soft-tissue masses. **Computed tomography (CT) with thin cuts through the orbits** can help define any bony erosion. Appropriate **surgical referral** to an ophthalmologist or neurosurgeon should be made.

5. **Inflammatory optic neuritis**

Optic neuritis is the presenting symptom for multiple sclerosis in about 15% of patients. Optic neuritis occurs at some point in the course of the disease in about 50% of patients with multiple sclerosis. As with treatment of other flares of multiple sclerosis (see Chapter 22), treatment of optic neuritis is **IV methylprednisolone 1 g for 7 to 10 days,** followed by a tapering dose of oral prednisone. Oral prednisone as a first line of treatment for acute optic neuritis has been shown to be ineffective. Patients older than 45 years of age may have idiopathic optic neuritis that is steroid responsive.

6. **Pseudotumor cerebri**

Visual loss is the most significant and dreaded complication of pseudotumor cerebri. Papilledema may occur with or without decreased acuity, but once visual loss begins, urgent therapy is imperative to prevent progression to blindness. Visual disturbance usually begins with an expanding blind spot or with constriction of the peripheral fields. Formal visual field testing may help evaluate the extent of loss. For mild visual loss, give **acetazolamide 500 mg PO two times a day.** This treatment is aimed at relieving increased intracranial pressure. For severe visual loss, the addition of **methylprednisolone 250 mg IV four times a day** (with an appropriate gastrointestinal protective medication such as ranitidine) may be vision saving. For patients whose visual loss is unresponsive to medical therapy, consult an ophthalmologist for **optic nerve sheath fenestration.** Periodic lumbar punctures or lumboperitoneal shunting has been advocated by some physicians, but the results of these treatments are inconsistent (see also Chapter 15).

13

INCREASED INTRACRANIAL PRESSURE

Increased intracranial pressure (ICP) is not a symptom. Rather, increased ICP is a pathologic state common to a variety of serious neurologic illnesses (Table 13–1). All conditions that result in increased ICP are characterized by an increase in intracranial volume. Accordingly, all therapies for ICP (hyperventilation, mannitol, etc.) are directed toward reducing intracranial volume.

Normal ICP is less than 200 mm H_2O, or 15 mm Hg. Because elevations beyond these levels can rapidly lead to brain damage and death, prompt recognition and treatment are essential. This chapter will be most useful in cases in which the pathology is known, and increased ICP is the suspected cause of clinical deterioration.

■ PHONE CALL

Questions

1. **What is the patient's underlying neurologic problem?**
2. **Why is increased ICP suspected?**
3. **What is the patient's current level of consciousness?**

■ BEDSIDE

Quick Look Test

Does the patient have clinical signs of increased ICP?
Increased ICP should be suspected in patients with known or suspected intracranial pathology (e.g., stroke, trauma, or neoplasm) who exhibit the following symptoms and signs:
Signs that are almost always present:
- Depressed level of consciousness (lethargy, stupor, coma)
- Hypertension, with or without bradycardia

Symptoms and signs that are sometimes present:
- Headache
- Vomiting
- Papilledema
- CN 6 palsies

Table 13–1 □ **CONDITIONS ASSOCIATED WITH INCREASED ICP**

Intracranial mass lesions
   Subdural hematoma
   Epidural hematoma
   Intracerebral hemorrhage
   Brain tumor
   Cerebral abscess
Increased CSF volume (or resistance to outflow)
   Hydrocephalus
   Benign intracranial hypertension (pseudotumor cerebri)
Increased brain volume (cytotoxic cerebral edema)
   Cerebral infarction
   Global hypoxia-ischemia
   Reye's syndrome
   Acute hyponatremia
Increased brain and blood volume (vasogenic cerebral edema)
   Head trauma
   Meningitis
   Encephalitis
   Lead encephalopathy
   Eclampsia
   Hypertensive encephalopathy
   Dural sinus thrombosis

Remember, however, that these signs may be nonspecific. For this reason, *the only way to confirm the diagnosis and properly treat increased ICP is to measure it.*

Does the patient have clinical signs of herniation?

Clinical signs of herniation, listed below, result from *brain stem compression:*

- Loss of pupillary reactivity
- Impairment of eye movements
- Hyperventilation
- Motor posturing (flexion or extension)

When ICP is differentially increased across the tentorium (as is usually the case with hemispheric mass lesions), pressure gradients lead to downward displacement of brain tissue into the posterior fossa. Herniation is often rapidly fatal but can be reversed in some cases by treatments that reduce intracranial volume and ICP.

■ MANAGEMENT I

Emergency Measures for Reduction of ICP

If the clinical signs described under **Bedside** are identified in a comatose patient, the following emergency measures can "buy time" prior to computed tomography (CT) and a definitive neurosurgical procedure (craniotomy, ventriculostomy, or placement of an ICP monitor):

1. Elevate head of bed 30 to 45 degrees.
2. Intubate and hyperventilate (target partial pressure of carbon dioxide (PCO_2) is 25 to 30 mm Hg).
3. Insert a Foley catheter.
4. Administer **mannitol 20% 1 g/kg intravenous (IV) rapid infusion.**
5. Administer **normal saline (0.9%) at 100 ml/hour (avoid hypotonic fluids).**
6. Consult the neurosurgery service.

(The rationale for these measures is elaborated on further in Management II).

Placement of an ICP Monitor

Most clinicians would not treat a patient with suspected high blood pressure (BP) without measuring it. However, empirical therapy for increased ICP (i.e., repeated doses of mannitol) without monitoring is used all the time, to the great disadvantage of the patient. This approach is unsatisfactory because most ICP treatments are effective for a short time only, lose their efficacy with prolonged use, and have side effects. Optimally, therapy should be given when ICP is high and should be withheld when it is normal. Only use of an ICP monitor can make this possible.

Indications for ICP monitoring (all three conditions should be met):

1. The patient is in a coma (patient does not open eyes, speak, or move purposefully to pain; equivalent to a Glasgow Coma scale score of ≤8)
2. Increased ICP is suspected.
3. The prognosis is such that aggressive treatment in the intensive care unit (ICU) is indicated.

ICP Monitors

If the decison has been made to treat the patient for suspected ICP, and surgical reduction of intracranial volume (e.g., craniotomy for removal of hematoma) is not feasible, an ICP monitor should be placed. There are three main types of monitors (Fig. 13–1):

1. **Ventricular catheter**

   Once inserted, a ventricular catheter is connected to both a pressure transducer and an external drainage system via a three-way stopcock. The major advantage to ventricular catheters is that they allow treatment of increased ICP via drainage of cerebrospinal fluid (CSF). The main disadvan-

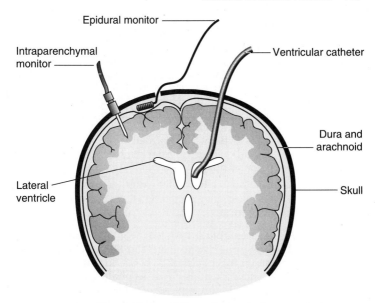

Figure 13–1 □ ICP monitoring devices.

tage is the high infection rate (10 to 20%), which increases dramatically after 5 days.

2. **Intraparenchymal fiberoptic transducer (Camino, Honey-well)**

These devices are very accurate and the infection rate is exceedingly low (approximately 1%). The fiberoptic cable is somewhat inflexible and is prone to breakage.

3. **Epidural transducer (Ladd, Gaeltec)**

These devices are inserted deep to the inner table of the skull and superficial to the dura. They are associated with a minimal infection rate (less than 1%) but have a tendency to malfunction and to have a baseline drift (>5 to 10 mm Hg) after more than a few days of use.

■ ELEVATOR THOUGHTS

What are the physiologic principles of ICP?

If you are caring for a patient with increased ICP, a firm understanding of intracranial physiology is essential.

Intracranial Anatomy

There are three principal components of volume within the cranium of the normal adult: brain (1400 ml), blood (150 ml), and CSF (150 ml). CSF is produced by the choroid plexus within the ventricles at a rate of approximately 20 ml/hour, resulting in the formation of almost 500 ml/day. Normal ICP ranges from 50 to 200 mm H_2O (4 to 15 mm Hg). CSF is reabsorbed across the convexity of the meninges into the venous circulation via arachnoid granulations. These pathways normally offer little resistance to CSF outflow. For this reason, jugular venous pressure is normally the principal determinant of ICP.

Intracranial Compliance

Because the cranial vault is a rigid, fixed container, any increase in intracranial volume can lead to increased ICP. In clinical practice, the most common mechanisms of increased intracranial volume are **extrinsic mass lesions, hydrocephalus, and cerebral edema (brain swelling).** Initially, as volume is added to the intracranial space, minimal increases in pressure occur. This is due to the highly compliant nature of the intracranial contents; as intracranial volume increases, CSF is displaced through the foramen magnum into the paraspinal space, and blood is displaced from compressed brain tissue. When these mechanisms are exhausted, however, intracranial compliance decreases, and further increases in intracranial volume lead to dramatic elevations of ICP (Fig. 13–2).

Cerebral Perfusion Pressure

Cerebral perfusion pressure (CPP) is routinely monitored in conjunction with the ICP because it is an important determinant of cerebral blood flow (CBF). CPP is defined by the equation

$$CPP = MABP \text{ (mean arterial blood pressure)} - ICP$$

When autoregulation is intact, CBF is maintained at a constant level across a wide range of CPPs (50 to 150 mm Hg). However, in injured brain with impaired autoregulation, CBF approximates a straight-line relationship with CPP; that is, reductions of CBF are more severe at any given level of reduced CPP (Fig. 13–3). **CPP must be closely regulated within a relatively narrow range (70 to 120 mm Hg) in patients with increased ICP,** because reductions below this level can lead to secondary hypoxic-ischemic damage, whereas excessive increases can lead to

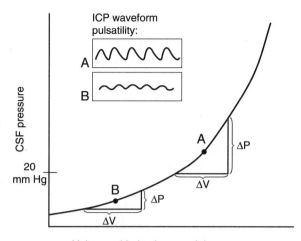

Figure 13–2 □ Intracranial pressure-volume curve. At low pressures (point B) the intracranial compartment is compliant, meaning that large increases in volume (ΔV) lead to small increments in pressure (ΔP). At higher pressures (point A) the intracranial space becomes less compliant. As a result, the amplitude and pulsatility of the arterial reflection in the ICP waveform increases (*inset*).

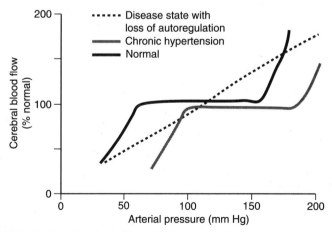

Figure 13–3 □ Cerebral autoregulation curve. In disease states (e.g., vasospasm or ischemia), cerebral blood flow becomes pressure passive *(dotted line)*. With chronic hypertension, the autoregulatory curve shifts to the right.

"breakthrough" hyperperfusion and aggravation of cerebral edema.

ICP Waveforms

The normal ICP waveform (see Fig. 13–2) reflects the effects of systemic arterial and venous pressures on the intracranial contents. Normally, a large initial upward deflection corresponds with the systemic arterial pressure wave. As ICP rises and intracranial compliance decreases, the amplitude of the ICP waveform increases, and superimposed pathologic ICP elevations can occur. Two types of pathologic ICP waves have been described (Fig. 13–4):

1. **Lundberg A waves (plateau waves).** Plateau waves are dangerous elevations of ICP; they can reach levels of 20 to 80 mm Hg and are generally from 5 minutes to 1 hour in duration. When severe, they are associated with reduced CPP (less than 60 mm Hg) and CBF and with global hypoxic-ischemic injury.
2. **Lundberg B waves.** These waves are of lesser amplitude (10 to 20 mm Hg) and duration (1 to 5 minutes) than plateau waves and thus are less dangerous. Clinically, they are a useful marker of abnormal autoregulation and reduced intracranial compliance.

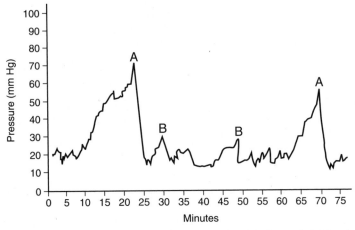

Figure 13–4 □ Pathologic ICP elevations. A = Lundberg A (plateau) waves; B = Lundberg B waves. (Redrawn from Chestnut RM, Marshall LF: Treatment of abnormal intracranial pressure. Neurosurg Clin North Am 1991;2:267–284.)

■ MANAGEMENT II

General Measures for Treating Patients with Increased ICP

1. **Elevate head of bed by 30 to 45 degrees and maintain a straight head position**
   Head elevation reduces ICP by reducing jugular venous pressure and by enhancing venous outflow. Sharp head angulation should be avoided, because it may cause jugular venous compression, increased venous backpressure, and increased ICP.
2. **Prevent seizures**
   Seizures can lead to profound elevations of CBF, intracranial blood volume, and ICP, even in patients who are paralyzed. **Fosphenytoin (10 to 20 mg/kg loading dose; then 3 to 5 mg/kg per day)** is the preferred agent for seizure prophylaxis.
3. **Treat fever aggressively**
   Fever can exacerbate ICP, and it lowers the threshold for neuronal death. Treatment with **acetaminophen (650 mg every 4 hours), indomethacin (25 mg every 6 hours),** or a cooling blanket can be effective.

Steps for Treating an "ICP Crisis" in Intubated, Monitored Patients

Proper treatment of increased ICP requires an organized, stepwise approach (Box 13–1). Brief elevations of ICP (lasting only 1 to 5 minutes) occur frequently with suctioning, coughing, and repositioning and do not require aggressive treatment. **In general,**

Box 13–1. SUMMARY OF STEPWISE TREATMENT FOR ELEVATED ICP *(ICP HIGHER THAN 20 mm Hg FOR MORE THAN 10 MINUTES)*

1. Surgical removal of an intracranial mass lesion or CSF drainage
2. Hyperventilation to P_{CO_2} levels of 25 to 30 mm Hg
3. IV sedation to attain a motionless, quiet state
4. Reduction of blood pressure if CPP remains higher than 120 mm Hg, or pressor infusion if CPP is less than 70 mm Hg.
5. Administration of **mannitol 0.25 to 1.0 g/kg every 4 to 6 hours**
6. Administration of pentobarbital

the following measures should be instituted only when the ICP is elevated above 20 mm Hg for a period of 10 or more minutes.

1. **Removal of intracranial mass or drainage of CSF**

    Remember that reduction of intracranial volume is the only definitive treatment for increased ICP. Consider a repeat CT scan in a patient with increasing ICP. If a ventricular catheter is in place, the system should be opened for drainage, and 5 to 10 ml of CSF should be removed.

2. **Hyperventilation**

    By acutely lowering the P_{CO_2} level to 25 to 30 mm Hg, *hyperventilation can lower ICP within minutes.* The alkylosis caused by hypocarbia leads to cerebral vasoconstriction, reduced cerebral blood volume, and decreased ICP.

    - Hyperventialtion is best accomplished by increasing the ventilatory rate (16 to 20 cycles/minute) in mechanically ventilated patients, or by using a face mask with an Ambu bag in nonintubated patients.

    - *The peak effect of hyperventilation on ICP is generally reached within 30 minutes.* Over the next 1 to 3 hours, the effect gradually diminishes, as compensatory acid-base buffering mechanisms correct the alkylosis.

    - Once ICP is stabilized, hyperventilation should be tapered slowly over 6 to 12 hours, because abrupt cessation can lead to vasodilatation and rebound increases in ICP.

    Note: Beware that prolonged severe hyperventilation (P_{CO_2} less than 25 mm Hg) may actually exacerbate cerebral ischemia by causing excessive vasoconstriction.

3. **Sedation and paralysis**

    In patients with reduced intracranial compliance, physical agitation or resisting mechanical ventilation can lead to significant elevations of ICP because of increases in intrathoracic, jugular venous, and arterial pressures. *Before further measures are instituted, agitated patients with increased ICP should be sedated to the point at which they are motionless and quiet.*

    Note: Intravenous sedatives cause apnea and hypotension and thus require intubation and intravascular blood pressure monitoring. The following agents can be used:

    - **Morphine IV** is an opiate with sedative-hypnotic and analgesic effects. The dose is **2 to 5 mg IVP every hour.**

    - **Fentanyl IV** (supplied as 50 µg/ml) is also an opiate and is 100 times more potent than morphine. For rapid control of agitation, give **25 to 100 µg IVP.** For sustained sedation, give **fentanyl IV infusion 4 mg/250 ml normal saline (NS).** Start at 5 ml/hour (1.33 µg/min); the range is 8 to 23 ml/hour (2 to 6 µg/min).

    - **Propofol IV (10 mg/ml)** is a powerful sedative-hypnotic drug whose effect is more rapidly reversible than that of fentanyl. The typical maintenance dose is **5 to 50 μg/ kg/min (0.3 to 3 mg/kg/hour);** this translates into 2 to 20 ml/hour for a 70-kg person.

4. **Blood pressure management**

If mean arterial blood pressure and ICP remain elevated in a hyperventilated and sedated patient, treatment of arterial hypertension can sometimes lead to further reduction of ICP. If CPP is greater than 120 mm Hg and ICP is greater than 20 mm Hg, hypertension should *definitely* be treated. *However, CPP should not be allowed to fall to less than 70 mm Hg.* Agents for controlling hypertension include the following:

- **Labetalol IV (5 mg/ml)** is a combined alpha-1 and beta-1 blocker. For immediate control of BP, **push 20 to 80 mg every 10 to 20 minutes.** Once the desired BP is attained, start **200 mg/200 ml NS (1 mg/ml) at 2 mg/min (120 ml/hour) and titrate.**

- **Nicardipine IV** is a rapidly titratable calcium channel blocker. Start with **25 mg/250 ml NS at 5 ml/hour (8 μg/ min)** and titrate.

- If CPP is less than 70 mm Hg and ICP is greater than 20 mm Hg, elevation of blood pressure with **dopamine 800 mg/500 ml NS** (start at 13 ml/hour and titrate) can lead to a reflex reduction of ICP by eliminating cerebral vasodilatation that occurs in response to inadequate perfusion.

5. **Mannitol**

Mannitol, an osmotic diuretic, lowers ICP via its cerebral dehydrating effects. The effects of mannitol appear to be biphasic. Rapid infusion immediately creates an osmotic gradient across the blood-brain barrier, resulting in movement of water from brain to the intravascular compartment. The result is decreased brain tissue volume and, hence, reduced ICP. The secondary effect of mannitol results from its action as an osmotic diuretic. As mannitol is cleared by the kidneys, it leads to free water clearance and increased serum osmolality. As a result, even after the mannitol is gone, an intracellular dehydrating effect is maintained as water flows down the osmotic gradient, from the intracellular to the extracellular space.

- **The initial dose of mannitol 20% solution is 1 g/kg, followed every 4 to 6 hours with doses of 0.25–0.5 g/kg as needed.** The effect on ICP is maximal when mannitol is given rapidly (over 10 minutes).

- The effect of mannitol on ICP begins in 10 to 20 minutes, reaches its peak between 20 and 60 minutes, and lasts for 3 to 6 hours.

- Adverse effects of mannitol therapy include exacerbation of congestive heart failure (because of the initial intravascular volume load); volume contraction, hypokalemia, and profound hyperosmolality (after prolonged use); acute tubular necrosis (because of excessive hyperosmolality); and "rebound" increases in ICP.

- Patients treated repeatedly with mannitol require measurements of serum electrolytes and osmolality every 6 hours, and careful measurement of intake and output. Volume lost through urine should be replaced with normal (0.9%) saline to avoid volume depletion.
- Mannitol tends to lose its efficacy once serum osmolality increases to more than 315 mOsm/kg, but exceptions can occur.

6. **Pentobarbital**

High-dose barbiturate therapy, given in doses equivalent to those inducing general anesthesia, can effectively lower ICP in most patients refractory to the steps outlined above. The effect of pentobarbital is multifactorial but most likely stems from coupled decreases in cerebral metabolism, blood flow, and blood volume. In addition, pentobarbital causes profound hypotension and usually requires the use of vasopressors to maintain CPP at or higher than 70 mm Hg.

- **Pentobarbital typically requires a loading dose of 10 to 20 mg/kg, given in repeated 5 mg/kg boluses,** until a state of flaccid coma with preserved pupillary reactivity is attained. Intravenous pressors (dopamine, phenylephrine) should be ready at the bedside to maintain BP.
- **Maintenance doses are usually 1 to 4 mg/kg/hour (order as 250 mg/250 ml NS, starting at 70 ml/hour).** Continuous or intermittent electroencephalogram (EEG) monitoring should be used, with the infusion rate titrated to a burst-suppression pattern.
- If ICP is adequately controlled with pentobarbital, it is generally maintained for 24 to 48 hours. It can then be discontinued abruptly, with a wash-out period lasting from 24 to 72 hours.
- Failure of ICP to respond to pentobarbital is an ominous sign. If ICP remains markedly elevated (higher than 30 mm Hg), discontinuation of all aggressive measures should be considered.

14

DIZZINESS AND VERTIGO

Dizziness and vertigo are among the most common neurologic complaints. The etiology of these conditions may range from benign labyrinthitis to serious cardiac syncope to life-threatening cerebellar hemorrhage. Vertigo may be defined specifically as a sensation of movement—either of the environment or of the patient. A spinning sensation is most commonly described, but feelings of acceleration or other movement may also be reported. Dizziness, on the other hand, may be used to mean vertigo, but it may also mean lightheadedness, fatigue, or a general sense of illness.

■ PHONE CALL

Questions

1. **Does the patient have a normal level of consciousness?**
   Vertigo followed by a decreased level of consciousness may be a sign of impending herniation, a neurologic emergency.
2. **When did the dizziness or vertigo begin?**
   In general, a more acute onset requires a greater urgency in making a diagnosis.
3. **What are the vital signs?**
   Rapid, slowed, or irregular heart rhythm may suggest cardiac syncope or cardioembolic stroke. Fever may suggest infection. Tachypnea may be a sign of heart failure or an anxiety attack.

Orders

1. Obtain a finger stick glucose.
2. Obtain orthostatic blood pressure.
3. Obtain an electrocardiogram (ECG).

Inform RN

"Will arrive at the bedside in . . . minutes."

■ ELEVATOR THOUGHTS (DIFFERENTIAL DIAGNOSIS OF DIZZINESS AND VERTIGO)

The most common causes of dizziness and vertigo are **orthostatic hypotension, medication side effect, benign positional vertigo,** and **labyrinthitis.** A more complete differential diagnosis follows.

> **V (vascular):** brain stem stroke (most often pontine, brachium pontis, or cerebellar), cerebellar hemorrhage, arteriovenous malformation (AVM) (rare), brain stem transient ischemic attacks (TIAs) resulting from vertebrobasilar stenosis ("insufficiency") or embolism, vasodepressor syncope, postural hypotension, cardiac arrhythmia
>
> **I (infectious):** syphilis, viral or bacterial meningitis, otitis media with labyrinthitis, Lyme disease involving the vestibular cranial nerve, viral cerebellitis (mostly in children)
>
> **T (traumatic):** head trauma or postconcussional syndrome
>
> **A (autoimmune):** multiple sclerosis
>
> **M (metabolic/toxic):** diabetes with hypoglycemia, dehydration, drug toxicity (Table 14–1)
>
> **I (idiopathic/iatrogenic):** benign positional vertigo, Meniere's disease
>
> **N (neoplastic):** neurofibroma, schwannoma, or meningioma of the acoustic nerve, brain stem glioma, posterior fossa metastasis
>
> **S (Seizure/pSychiatric)**

■ MAJOR THREAT TO LIFE

- Cerebellar infarction or hemorrhage

■ BEDSIDE

Quick Look Test

Is the patient awake and alert?
Lethargy may indicate a brain stem or cerebellar stroke with potential for herniation or progression to coma.

Selective History and Chart Review

1. **Is the dizziness lightheadedness or true vertigo?**

   Lightheadedness, a swimming sensation, faintness, or other similar symptoms point to a systemic disorder such as cardiac syncope, postural hypotension, or systemic infection. True **vertigo,** on the other hand, suggests neurologic dysfunction. The physical examination will help clarify the differential diagnosis, which will focus on distinguishing a

Table 14–1 □ **COMMON MEDICATIONS THAT CAUSE VERTIGO AND DIZZINESS***

Anticonvulsants: carbamazepine, phenytoin, primidone, ethosuximide, methosuximide
Antidepressants: nortriptyline and other tricyclic antidepressants
Antihypertensives: enalapril
Antihistamines: ranitidine, cimetidine
Antiarrhythmics: flecainide
Antibiotics: streptomycin, tobramycin, gentamycin
Analgesics: propoxyphene (Darvocet), naproxen, indomethacin
Neuroleptics: phenothiazines
Tranquilizers: diazepam, chlordiazepoxide, meprobamate
Aspirin
Digoxin

---

*Many medications have dizziness as a side effect. This is a partial list.

peripheral cause from a central nervous system cause for vertigo.

2. **What is the time course of the symptoms?**

As described earlier, an acute onset of vertigo may indicate posterior fossa stroke or hemorrhage. Rapid onset of light-headedness can occur with cardiac disease. A more gradual onset may suggest medication toxicity, infection, tumor, or demyelinating disease. If this is an episode in a series of recurrences, Meniere's disease or benign positional vertigo may be the cause.

3. **Do the symptoms change with changes in head position?**

Dizziness on standing may indicate orthostatic hypotension; dizziness or vertigo with head turning may be a sign of benign positional vertigo or labyrinthitis.

4. **Has the patient begun any new medications recently?**

Table 14–1 shows common medications that cause vertigo. Dizziness without true vertigo is one of the most common side effects of medication. Refer to the *Physician's Desk Reference* for medications not listed in the table.

5. **Are there any accompanying symptoms?**

Ask about symptoms specific to the brain stem, such as diplopia, dysarthria, and ataxia. Tinnitus may localize the problem to the inner ear. If there is posterior neck or head pain, consider vertebral artery dissection and stroke.

Selective Physical Examination

HEENT: Be sure to look into the external auditory canal for vesicles of herpes zoster. Unilateral hearing loss and tinnitus are reliable signs of injury outside the brain stem.

Abdomen: Hepatomegaly, ascites, and caput medusae are signs of chronic alcohol abuse.

Neurologic examination:

1. Mental status

Ensure that the patient is awake, alert, and attentive. Decreased attentiveness may suggest drug toxicity or metabolic disarray. If there is vertigo with decreased alertness, see Chapter 6 for further management.

2. Cranial nerves

Any cranial nerve abnormality in combination with dizziness or vertigo should be considered a sign of brain injury until it is proven otherwise.

a. Nystagmus

When vestibular input to the brain stem is disrupted, the eyes will drift toward the affected side. Repeated corrective saccades result in nystagmus, with the fast phase away from the lesion. The sensation of movement experienced with vertigo is the illusion of environmental drift as the eyes move through the slow phase of nystagmus in the other direction. Corrective saccades are suppressed by visual tracking systems so that there is a sensation of continued field shift in one direction. Oscillopsia—the illusion of the environment's jumping or oscillating—is actually quite rare. Nystagmus subtypes are listed in Table 14–2. A common and crucial differential diagnosis that arises in almost every case of vertigo is whether the process is peripheral, and often benign, or whether it represents a lesion in the brain stem. Certain characteristics of nystagmus can help identify the site of pathology (Table 14–3).

(1) Look for nystagmus in the primary gaze by having the patient fix on your finger. More subtle nystagmus can be seen by looking for oscillations of the fundus on indirect ophthalmoscopy.

(2) Have the patient follow your finger through the full range of horizontal and vertical gaze. The hand should be kept at a distance of 2 to 3 feet to minimize convergence, which should be tested separately.

(3) Provocative tests may be helpful in distinguishing peripheral from central injury.

(a) Nystagmus should be looked for with the patient in different positions, particularly if the patient notes a positional component to the vertigo. The Bárány maneuver is useful in helping to distinguish the positional vertigo of a benign vestibular disorder from a brain stem lesion (Fig. 14–1). A

Table 14–2 □ SUBTYPES OF NYSTAGMUS

Physiologic nystagmus
  Fine nystagmus at ends of gaze, extinguishes after a few beats
  Significance: none, if symmetric

Asymmetric horizontal nystagmus
  Horizontal or rotational
  Fast phase always in one direction
  Worse with gaze in one direction than in the other
  Often made worse with change in head position
  Significance: most often labyrinthine or vestibular disease (benign
    positional vertigo, labyrinthitis, Meniere's disease)

Vertical nystagmus
  Upbeat or downbeat nystagmus
  May be present with sedative or anticonvulsant medication
  Significance: if no drug toxicity is present, vertical nystagmus almost
    always means brain stem disease at the midbrain or craniocervical
    junction

Dissociated or abduction nystagmus
  Unilateral horizontal fast component in direction of gaze in the
    abducted eye
  Significance: internuclear ophthalmoplegia, e.g., in multiple sclerosis

Convergence-retraction nystagmus
  Part of Parinaud's syndrome of impaired upgaze, impaired pupillary
    reaction, convergence insufficiency
  Fast component is convergence and retraction of both globes
  Significance: mass lesion compression of the tectum of the midbrain,
    for example, by pineal tumor, or a midbrain stroke in the region of
    the aqueduct of Sylvius

Pendular nystagmus
  Usually horizontal
  Sinusoidal waveform (oscillation, equal velocity in either direction)
  Significance: congenital; if acquired, most commonly multiple sclerosis;
    also cerebrovascular disease of the cerebellum or brain stem

Periodic alternating nystagmus
  Horizontal, with fast phase alternating directions in cycles of 1 to 3
    minutes
  May coexist with downbeat nystagmus
  Significance: congenital or acquired lesions at the craniocervical
    junction

Ocular dysmetria
  Overshooting on attempt to refix on an eccentric target (e.g., moving
    from the examiner's nose to a finger held to the side)
  Overshooting may be followed by ever-shortening saccadic corrections
  Significance: cerebellar disease

Table 14–3 □ CHARACTERISTICS OF NYSTAGMUS ARISING FROM PERIPHERAL OR CENTRAL CAUSES

Nystagmus from peripheral causes
    Extinguishes with repetitive provocative maneuvers
    Exhibits latency of several seconds with provocative maneuvers
    Rotational nystagmus
    Hearing loss or tinnitus
    No accompanying brain stem signs
Nystagmus from central causes
    Any vertical nystagmus
    Accompanying brain stem signs
    Does not extinguish with provocative maneuvers
    No latency with provocative maneuvers

        rotational component, a latency of a few seconds in onset of the nystagmus, and a lessening of the magnitude of the response with subsequent trials all suggest peripheral lesions.
    (b) Injecting cold water into the ear on the side of an intact vestibular pathway (see Fig. 6–2) will result in nystagmus, with the fast component beating away from the stimulus. If the peripheral vestibular input is dysfunctional, the response will not occur. Be sure you view an intact tympanic membrane before attempting this test. Also be warned that the stimulus may produce nausea in your patient.
  b. Diplopia, dysarthria, facial motor or sensory asymmetry, decreased gag response, or asymmetry of tongue protrusion
      Any of these should alert you to the possibility of a CNS lesion.
3. **Cerebellar**
    Evaluate for limb ataxia and gait ataxia.

■ MANAGEMENT

  1. **Rule out a posterior fossa mass lesion.**
    Because the consequences of missing a cerebellar hematoma or posterior fossa tumor can be serious, a **noncontrast computed tomography (CT) scan** should be obtained in all cases of first-time vertigo, particularly in the elderly, and certainly if there is any hint of brain stem involvement. CT is poor at identifying smaller lesions and infarcts in the posterior fossa because of the substantial bony artifact. If a

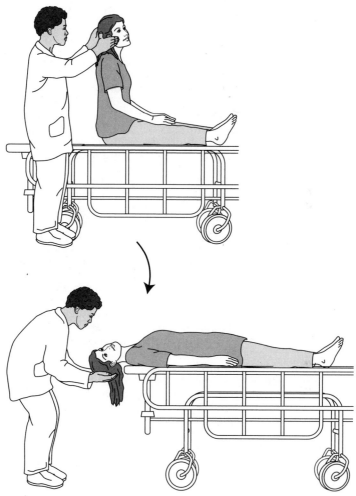

Figure 14–1 □ Bárány maneuver. The physician moves the patient from a sitting to a supine position, with the head rotated to one side and hyperextended 30 degrees. The test is positive if vertigo is re-created. Nystagmus should be seen with the onset of symptomatic vertigo.

brain stem lesion is suspected but not identified on CT, a **magnetic resonance imaging (MRI) scan** should be obtained.

2. **Correct any obvious metabolic disorder,** or discontinue, taper, or substitute any toxic medication. Treat cardiac syncope if present.

3. **Identify a possible peripheral cause.**

    If no posterior fossa lesion and no metabolic abnormality is identified, a peripheral cause for vertigo may be present. Such causes include labyrinthitis (postinfectious congestion or inflammation of the labyrinths), Meniere's disease (recurrent attacks of severe vertigo, nausea and vomiting, tinnitus, and hearing loss) and benign positional vertigo (see below). An **electronystagmogram** may be useful in making a diagnosis of peripheral vestibulopathy. An audiogram may be useful in diagnosing Meniere's disease.

4. **Treat benign positional vertigo empirically.**

    Benign positional vertigo is a type of vertigo that occurs in adults over 50 years of age. This type of vertigo is thought to arise when particulate debris accumulates in the posterior semicircular canal (Fig. 14–2). Particular head positions or head movement may cause the particles to stimulate hair cells and produce the sensation of movement. Benign positional vertigo may respond to **meclizine 25 mg by mouth (PO) three times a day.** Central causes of dizziness generally do not respond to meclizine. Nonmedicational treatment of benign positional vertigo has been successful in many cases. The two approaches are desensitization exercises, in which the patient moves through a series of repetitive head and body positions twice daily, and canalith repositioning procedures, such as the modified Epley maneuver, in which the head is rotated slowly from the bad side to the good side in an effort to move the particles out of the posterior semicircular canal (Fig. 14–3). Following the Epley maneuver, the patient is asked to sleep sitting up for two nights.

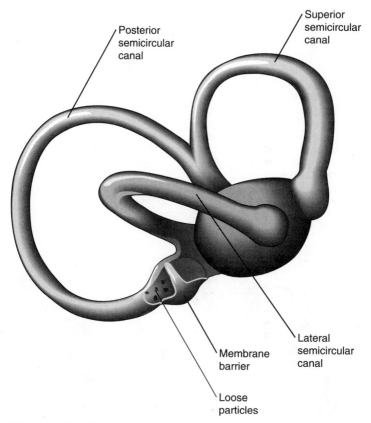

Figure 14–2 □ Particles accumulated in the posterior semicircular canal.

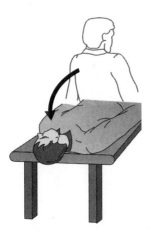

Step 1: Move from sitting to reclining position with the head extended 45 degrees over the end of the table, turned with the "bad" ear down (e.g., left)

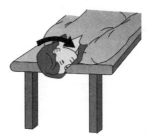

Step 2: Turn the head to the right slowly over 1 minute

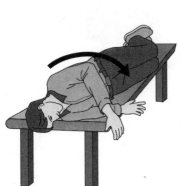

Step 3: Roll over onto the right side, with the head looking down at the floor

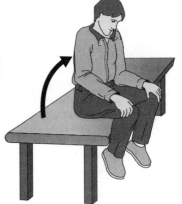

Step 4: Slowly return to sitting position with the chin tilted down

Figure 14–3 □ Four-step canalith repositioning procedure for benign positional vertigo (modified Epley maneuver). The clinician should support and rotate the patient's head in steps 1 and 2.

15

HEADACHE

Headache is one of the most common complaints presented to neurologists. In general, headaches can be grouped into two broad diagnostic categories. One group comprises the **primary headache disorders,** for example, migraine, tension, and cluster headache. The second category comprises **symptomatic headache** resulting from intracranial lesions, systemic diseases, or local diseases of the eye or nasopharynx. The goal in evaluating headache is to establish the diagnosis and initiate effective treatment.

■ **PHONE CALL**

Questions

1. **How severe is the headache?**
2. **Was the onset sudden or gradual?**
   Sudden onset of extremely severe headache is suggestive of subarachnoid hemorrhage or meningitis.
3. **When did the headaches begin?**
   Recent-onset headaches or headaches that have become progressively worse over time suggest a symptomatic etiology such as subdural hematoma or brain tumor.
4. **What are the vital signs?**
5. **Has there been a change in level of consciousness?**
6. **Is the patient experiencing nausea or vomiting?**
   Nausea and vomiting can occur with severe migraine or with conditions associated with increased intracranial pressure (ICP).

Orders

1. Place the patient in a quiet, darkened room.
2. Start **D5NS IV at 80 ml/hour if** nausea and vomiting are severe.
3. Obtain a temperature if this has not already been obtained.
4. Order an erythrocyte sedimentation rate (ESR) if the patient is older than 50 years of age.
5. If you are confident that the headache represents a chronic, previously diagnosed problem, the patient can be treated with an agent that has previously relieved the headache or with **acetaminophen 650 mg.**

■ ELEVATOR THOUGHTS

What causes headache?

Primary Headache Disorders

1. Tension headache
2. Migraine headache
3. Cluster headache
4. Paroxysmal hemicrania
5. Trigeminal neuralgia
6. Occipital neuralgia (cervical osteoarthritis)

Symptomatic Headache Disorders

1. Vascular
   - Subarachnoid hemorrhage
   - Intracerebral hemorrhage
   - Cerebral infarction
2. Infectious
   - Meningitis
   - Sinusitis
3. Posttraumatic (postconcussion) headache
4. Increased intracranial pressure
   - Intracranial mass lesions (brain tumor, hemorrhage, etc.)
   - Malignant hypertension
   - Idiopathic intracranial hypertension (pseudotumor cerebri)
5. Decreased intracranial pressure
   - Spontaneous intracranial hypotension
   - Post–lumbar puncture headache
6. Temporal arteritis
7. Drug exposure or withdrawal
   - Nitrate exposure
   - Caffeine withdrawal

■ MAJOR THREAT TO LIFE

- **Subarachnoid hemorrhage**
  Aneurysmal subarachnoid hemorrhage, if not properly diagnosed, can lead to fatal rebleeding.
- **Bacterial meningitis**
  Bacterial meningitis must be recognized early if antibiotic treatment is to be successful.
- **Herniation from intracranial mass lesions**
  Herniation may occur as a result of a tumor, subdural or epidural hematoma, abscess, or any other mass lesion.

■ BEDSIDE

Quick Look Test

Does the patient look well (comfortable), sick (uncomfortable), or critical (about to die)?
Most patients with chronic headache look well, whereas those with severe migraines, subarachnoid hemorrhage, or meningitis look sick.

Airway and Vital Signs

What is the temperature?
Fever associated with headache suggests meningitis. However, headache can also represent a nonspecific reaction to a systemic febrile illness.

What is the blood pressure (BP)?
Contrary to popular belief, headache is rarely caused by hypertension, unless the hypertension is acute and severe (diastolic pressure greater than 120 mm Hg). Hypertension may also reflect subarachnoid hemorrhage, acute stroke, or increased ICP from an intracranial mass lesion.

Selective History and Chart Review

A detailed, well-focused history is the most important tool in diagnosing the cause of headache. The following questions are important:
1. **What is the quality of the pain?**
   Tension headache is frequently described as tight, aching, and band-like. Migraine often has a throbbing quality.
2. **Where is the pain located?**
   Tension headache is usually generalized and most prominent in the occiput and forehead. Alternating unilateral headaches suggest migraine. Cluster headaches are periorbital.
3. **What time of day do the headaches occur?**
   Tension headaches typically develop in the late morning or the early afternoon and go away with sleep. Cluster headaches frequently strike *after* the patient has gone to sleep and tend to occur at the same time every day.
4. **Do warning symptoms occur before the headaches begin?**
   Migraine is often preceded by prodromal symptoms of hunger, restlessness, or moodiness. Classic migraine is preceded by an aura that is usually visual. Neurologic symptoms that persist once the headache has started are unusual in migraine and suggest a structural lesion (i.e., neoplasm or arteriovenous malformation).

5. **Do any factors precipitate the headaches?**

   Migraine is frequently precipitated by emotional stress, fatigue, foods containing tyramine (e.g., red wine or cheese), or menstruation.

6. **Are any symptoms associated with the headache?**

   Nausea, vomiting, photophobia, and phonophobia are highly characteristic of migraine. Ipsilateral tearing or nasal congestion occur with cluster headache.

7. **Is there a history of chronic or recurring headaches?**

   The longer a headache has lasted in its present form, the more likely it is to be benign. Headaches that are qualitatively different from previous headaches should raise suspicion for a symptomatic etiology.

8. **Do headaches run in the family?**

   Migraine is familial in approximately 50% of cases.

Selective Physical Examination

In most patients with headache, the neurologic and physical examinations are normal. The primary purpose of the initial screening examination is to check for signs of *meningismus, increased intracranial pressure, or neurologic focality.*

HEENT:	Sinus tenderness (sinusitis)
	Temporal artery tenderness (temporal arteritis)
	Conjunctival injection (cluster headache)
	Cranial bruit (arteriovenous malformation)
Neck:	Neck rigidity (subarachnoid hemorrhage, meningitis)
	Neck muscle spasm (tension headache)
	Kernig's and Brudzinski's signs (Fig. 15–1)
Neurologic examination:	Level of consciousness
	Confusion or disorientation
	Pupil symmetry
	Papilledema and spontaneous venous pulsations
	Retinal hemorrhages (flame or subhyaloid)
	Pronator drift
	Deep tendon and plantar reflexes
	Gait

■ DIAGNOSTIC TESTING

Diagnostic testing is not necessary if the patient has a long history of characteristic primary headaches (migraine, tension,

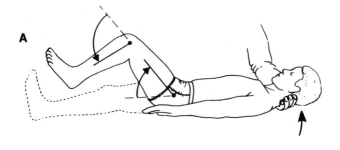

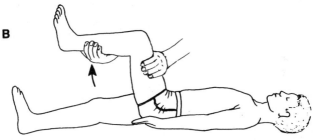

Figure 15–1 □ *A*, Brudzinski's sign. The test result is positive when the patient actively flexes the hips and knees in response to passive neck flexion by the examiner. *B*, Kernig's sign. The test result is positive when pain or resistance prevents full extension of the knee from the 90-degree hip/knee flexion position. (From Marshall SA, Ruedy J: On Call: Principles and Protocols, 2nd ed. Philadelphia, WB Saunders Co, 1993.)

or cluster), a normal neurologic examination, and no fever or meningismus.

1. **Obtain a CT scan in patients with the following:**
   - Acute, extremely severe headache ("thunderclap headache")
   - Headache with progressive onset over days to weeks that is not similar to previous headaches
   - Altered mental status (even if intoxicated)
   - Focal neurologic signs
   - Papilledema

2. **If subarachnoid hemorrhage is suspected and the CT scan is negative, a follow-up lumbar puncture (LP) is mandatory.**

   Fifteen percent of patients with aneurysmal subarachnoid hemorrhage have a negative CT scan. In these instances, the diagnosis can be made only by cerebrospinal fluid (CSF) examination (increased numbers of red blood cells and xanthochromia are present).

3. **Test for bacterial meningitis**

   If bacterial meningitis is suspected, obtaining a CT scan prior to LP is a good idea in most patients, as long as administration of antibiotics is not delayed. *CT scanning prior to LP is mandatory in patients with depressed level of consciousness, neurologic focality, papilledema, or acquired immune deficiency syndrome (AIDS), because of the high likelihood of detecting a mass lesion in these patients.* As long as the patient does not look terribly ill, it is reasonable to withhold antibiotics until after the LP, as long as both the CT and LP can be performed **within 1 hour.** Otherwise, treat first, keeping in mind that the CSF culture results may be negative. **Empirical treatment of suspected meningitis consists of ceftriaxone 1 g intravenously (IV) every 12 hours and ampicillin IV 2 g every 6 hours.**

■ MANAGEMENT: SPECIFIC DISORDERS AND THEIR TREATMENT

Migraine Headache

The term "migraine" is often used to describe any severe headache. However, migraine is a specific clinical syndrome with a distinct pathophysiology. *The diagnosis of migraine is based not on the quality of the pain (i.e., throbbing) but on the characteristic symptoms associated with the headache.*

Common Migraine (Migraine Without Aura). This is defined by the following criteria.

1. Recurrent headaches of 4 to 72 hours' duration with *at least two* of the following characteristics:
   - Unilateral location
   - Pulsating quality
   - Severe enough in intensity to limit daily activity
   - Aggravated by light physical activity (e.g., walking)
2. In addition, *at least one* of the following characteristics must be present:
   - Nausea or vomiting
   - Photophobia and phonophobia

Classic Migraine (Migraine with Aura). This resembles common migraine except that it is preceded by an aura—a fully reversible symptom indicative of focal cerebral dysfunction. Common types of aura include the following:
- Homonymous visual disturbance
- Unilateral paresthesias or numbness

- Unilateral weakness
- Aphasia or other speech disorder

In the typical patient with classic migraine, a visual aura precedes the headache by 10 to 20 minutes. The aura is usually characterized by scintillations (shimmering, geometric patterns known as fortification spectra), migrating scotomata, or waving and blurring of vision. In some patients, aura may occur without the subsequent headache.

Complicated Migraine. This refers to a migraine headache with particularly severe or persistent sensorimotor deficits, suggestive of cerebral infarction. In these patients, vasoconstrictors such as ergotamine should be avoided because of the risk of precipitating cerebral infarction.

Treatment

Start with **identifying and eliminating inciting factors.** Many women experience fewer migraines after discontinuing oral contraceptives. Mild migraine headaches may respond to symptomatic treatment with nonsteroidal anti-inflammatory drugs (NSAIDs) such as ibuprofen or naproxen. Many patients, however, require **abortive therapy** with an *ergot-containing agent* or *sumatriptan*, which is taken as soon as possible after the start of the headache in an attempt to cut it short. Agents used for abortive therapy in migraine are listed in Table 15–1.

Patients with frequent disabling attacks of migraine (more than one per week) who fail to respond to abortive therapy alone should be considered for **preventive therapy.** Agents used for migraine prevention are listed in Table 15–2. *Beta blockers or tricyclic antidepressants* are the usual first-line agents.

A protocol for the **emergency room treatment of severe migraine** is shown in Table 15–3. Intravenous hydration is important for patients with intractable vomiting. If sumatriptan is unsuccessful, "cocktail" treatment with *prochlorperazine, dihydroergotamine,* and *dexamethasone* can break the cycle of intractable migraine in most patients. In severe cases, the migraine headache can last for days (**status migranosus**).

Tension Headache

Tension headaches are also known as "muscle contraction headaches," although muscle contraction has little to do with the pathogenesis. Because most people experience tension headaches to some degree, those who present for medical evaluation (less than 5% of the population) either have unusually frequent or severe symptoms or are depressed. Headache that never goes away or that grows worse as the day progresses is suggestive of tension headache. The pain is usually bilateral, most prominent

Table 15–1 □ **DRUGS USED FOR ABORTIVE THERAPY OF MIGRAINE HEADACHE**

Acetaminophen/butalbital/caffeine (Fioricet)	1 to 2 tablets every 4 hours as needed, maximum 6 tablets per day
Acetaminophen (Tylenol)	325 to 650 mg every 4 hours as needed
Aspirin	325 to 650 mg every 4 hours as needed
Aspirin/butalbital/caffeine (Fiorinal)	1 to 2 tablets every 4 hours as needed, maximum 6 tablets per day
Ergotamine 1 mg (Gynergen)	1 to 2 mg at onset, repeat to maximum of 5 per attack or 10 per week
Ergotamine 2 mg *sublingual* tablets (Ergomar, Ergostat)	1 to 2 mg SL, repeat every 30 minutes as needed, maximum of 3 tablets per day
Ergotamine 1 mg/caffeine 100 mg (Cafergot Wigraine)	1 to 2 tablets at onset, repeat to maximum of 5 per attack or 10 per week
Ergotamine/caffeine *suppositories* (Cafergot)	1 PR at onset, repeat in 1 hour as needed, maximum 2 per day, 5 per week
Ibuprofen (Motrin, Advil)	400 to 800 mg every 4 hours as needed
Indomethacin (Indocin)	25 to 50 mg every 4 hours as needed
Isometheptene/acetaminophen/ dichloralphenazone (Midrin)	2 capsules at onset, repeat 1 every hour as needed, maximum of 5 per day, 10 per week
Ketorolac (Toradol)	10 mg every 6 hours as needed
Naproxen (Naprosyn, Anaprox)	500 to 750 mg at onset, 250 to 375 mg every 4 hours as needed
Sumatriptan (Imitrex)	6 mg SC, maximum 6 doses per month; 25 mg PO, repeat every 2 hours as needed

Table 15–2 □ DRUGS USED FOR PREVENTIVE THERAPY OF MIGRAINE

Beta blockers
    Propranolol (Inderal)   10 to 40 mg four times a day
    Atenolol (Tenormin)   25 to 100 mg once a day
    Metoprolol (Lopressor)   50 to 200 mg two times a day
Tricyclic antidepressants
    Amitriptyline (Elavil)   50 to 200 mg every night
    Nortriptyline (Pamelor)   25 to 150 mg per day at nighttime
Calcium channel blockers
    Verapamil (Calan)   40 to 120 mg three times a day
Ergots
    Ergotamine (Gynergen)   1 mg two times a day (must skip 2 days/week)
    Methylergonovine maleate (Methergine)   0.2 to 0.4 mg three times a day
    Ergotamine/belladonna/ phenobarbital (Bellergal)   1 to 2 tablets two times a day
Serotonin antagonists
    Methysergide (Sansert)   2 mg once to three times a day
    Cyproheptadine (Periactin)   4 to 8 mg three times a day
Anticonvulsants
    Phenytoin (Dilantin)   200 to 400 mg per day
    Valproic acid (Depakote)   250 to 500 mg four times a day
NSAIDs/anti-inflammatory drugs
    Indomethacin (Indocin)   25 to 50 mg three times a day
    Naproxen (Naprosyn, Anaprox)   250 to 375 mg three times a day
    Aspirin   325 to 650 mg per day
Serotonin reuptake inhibitor
    Fluoxetine (Prozac)   20 mg per day

Table 15–3 □ PROTOCOL FOR THE EMERGENCY ROOM TREATMENT OF MIGRAINE

Mild to moderate migraine
    Administer sumatriptan 6 mg SC

Severe or refractory migraine
1. Insert IV line or heplock.
2. Premedicate with **promethazine (Phenergan) 50 mg** or **prochlorperazine (Compazine) 10 mg IV.**
3. Administer **dihydroergotamine (D.H.E. 45 1 mg IV push over 2 minutes).**
4. Follow with **dexamethasone (Decadron) 4 to 12 mg IV.**
5. Repeat 1 mg D.H.E. 45 every 1 to 2 hours as needed (maximum 3 mg/day).

in the occiput and frontal regions, and is described as tight, pressing, or band-like. Associated eye strain or neck and scalp muscle tightness is common. **Chronic daily headache** refers to tension headaches associated with overuse of NSAIDs or other analgesic agents, in which medication withdrawal contributes significantly to the pathogenesis.

Treatment

Most patients respond to **relaxation techniques** and **NSAIDs** such as ibuprofen or naproxen (see Table 15–1). If the patient is depressed, an antidepressant may be helpful. If the patient has chronic daily headache, it may be necessary to taper the analgesics.

Cluster Headache

Cluster headache is characterized by excruciating unilateral head pain, often localized to the orbit, associated with ipsilateral tearing, conjunctival injection, and nasal congestion. The pain is described as sharp, boring, and piercing and occurs in brief episodes (15 minutes to 2 hours) without prodrome. The headaches are distributed into "clusters," occurring daily for 3 weeks to 3 months, then remitting for months or years. Cluster headaches are most common early in the morning or late at night, and they frequently occur with regularity at a particular time of day. Men are affected five times more often than are women. Ipsilateral facial flushing, Horner's syndrome, and exacerbation of symptoms by alcohol are seen in some patients.

Treatment

Any abortive treatment for migraine can be used to abort a cluster headache, but the following agents are particularly effective:

1. **Ergotamine 1 to 2 mg PO**
2. **Sumatriptan 6 mg SC**
3. **Oxygen 100% at 7 to 10 L/min**
4. **Dihydroergotamine (D.H.E.) 1 mg IV**
5. **Lidocaine 4% 1 ml intranasally**

In some patients, the cluster headache can be managed with purely abortive treatment. In many cases, however, daily prophylactic medication must be given. Commonly used preventive agents include the following:

1. **Prednisone 20 to 40 mg per day**
2. **Methysergide 2 mg four times a day (limit to 6 months)**
3. **Cyproheptadine 2 to 4 mg four times a day**
4. **Verapamil 80 mg three times a day**
5. **Lithium 300 mg three to four times a day**
6. **Ergotamine 1 mg two times a day**
7. **Valproate 200 to 500 mg every 6 hours**

Postconcussion Headache

After concussion, patients may complain of headache, dizziness, poor concentration, and irritability (postconcussional syndrome). Brain imaging is normal, as is the neurologic examination, except for the occasional finding of nystagmus. In many cases, there is coexisting depression, anxiety, or potential for secondary gain, such as a disability claim or litigation.

Treatment

Begin with **NSAIDs** (see Table 15–1) and provide reassurance; in most cases, the symptoms remit over a period of weeks to months. In protracted cases with depressive symptoms, a tricyclic agent may be helpful.

Idiopathic Intracranial Hypertension (Pseudotumor Cerebri)

Also known as benign intracranial hypertension, this illness is characterized by the triad of *headache, papilledema, and increased ICP* in the absence of an intracranial mass lesion or hydrocephalus. The disease occurs almost exclusively in obese young women. The key to establishing the diagnosis is excluding other causes of increased ICP. These include dural sinus thrombosis, chronic meningitis, hypervitaminosis A, and tetracycline or steroid exposure. Depressed level of consciousness and focal neurologic deficits do not occur, except for occasional CN 6 palsies.

The main hazard in idiopathic intracranial hypertension is **visual loss** that results from optic nerve damage, which can be permanent. If this diagnosis is suspected, MRI with magnetic resonance venography should be performed to rule out a mass lesion, hydrocephalus, or dural sinus thrombosis. If the MRI is normal, LP establishes the diagnosis by the finding of normal CSF under increased pressure (greater than 200 mm H_2O).

Treatment

About one third of patients have spontaneous remission of headache after the first LP. Many patients will respond to repeated lumbar taps and removal of CSF, performed every few days to every few weeks. If the patient does not respond to serial LPs, start **acetazolamide 250 to 500 mg three times a day. Prednisone 40 to 60 mg PO per day** or **methylprednisolone 250 mg IV every 6 hours** may be added with additional benefit. All patients should have baseline **visual field and acuity testing.** If visual loss progresses despite medical therapy, a lumboperitoneal shunt or optic nerve sheath decompression may be necessary.

Temporal (Giant Cell) Arteritis

Temporal arteritis, a sytemic illness of elderly patients, is characterized by inflammatory infiltrates of lymphocytes and giant cells in cranial arteries. It occurs almost exclusively in patients older than 50. Most patients have systemic symptoms of low-grade fever, diffuse myalgias, weight loss, weakness, and malaise (*polymyalgia rheumatica*). The ESR is elevated in all patients, usually to high levels (60 to 120 mm/hour). Jaw claudication is an uncommon, but useful, diagnostic clue.

Treatment

The main hazard in temporal arteritis is *visual loss* (ischemic optic neuropathy; see Chapter 12), which occurs in 10 to 30% of untreated patients because of involvement of the ophthalmic artery. If the diagnosis is suspected, start **prednisone 100 mg every day** immediately and schedule the patient for a **temporal artery biopsy.** Because false-negative biopsy results are common, biopsy should be repeated on the opposite side if the initial biopsy result is negative. In most patients, prednisone will abolish all symptoms and normalize the ESR in 2 to 4 weeks. Because the illness is self-limited, steroids (10 to 20 mg per day) can usually be discontinued within 6 months to 2 years.

Trigeminal Neuralgia

Also known as tic douloureux, this illness is characterized by brief, sharp, lancinating paroxysms of pain in the distribution of the trigeminal nerve. The maxillary (V2) and mandibular (V3) divisions are most frequently affected, and specific trigger points can often be found on the face. For this reason, the pain is often related to activities such as toothbrushing, shaving, or eating. More than 90% of patients present after age 40, and women are more often affected than men. If trigeminal neuralgia is associated with trigeminal sensory loss, other cranial nerve deficits, or onset before age 40, MRI should be performed to rule out neoplasm, multiple sclerosis, or vascular compression of the trigeminal nerve. **Glossopharyngeal neuralgia,** a rare disorder similar to trigeminal neuralgia, is characterized by lancinating pains in the oropharynx that radiate to the ear. The pain is triggered by swallowing, yawning, sneezing, or coughing. Treatment is the same as for trigeminal neuralgia.

Treatment

The most effective treatment is **carbamazepine, 400 to 1200 mg/day given four times a day.** The initial dose of **200 mg two times a day** is gradually increased to the minimal effective dosage. **Phenytoin (100 to 200 mg two times a day)** may also be effective in some patients. **Baclofen (5 to 10 mg three times a day)** may be used as adjunctive treatment to either carbamazepine or phenytoin. In refractory cases, radiofrequency surgical ablation or microsurgical vascular decompression of the trigeminal ganglion may be required.

Spontaneous Intracranial Hypotension

This unusual disorder, which resembles **post-LP headache,** is characterized by headache that worsens after standing. Associated symptoms include nausea, vomiting, tinnitus, and vertigo. The pathogenesis is related to spontaneous leakage of CSF along the craniospinal axis. By definition, CSF pressure is low (less than 60 mm H_2O), and the diagnosis is confirmed by meningeal enhancement on MRI (because of traction) and demonstration of CSF leakage by CT myelography.

Treatment

If prolonged bed rest fails to relieve the symptoms, most patients will respond to autologous epidural blood patch at the level of CSF leakage.

16

NEUROMUSCULAR
RESPIRATORY FAILURE

Generalized weakness is the primary problem in patients with severe neuromuscular disease. Weakness of the bulbar or respiratory muscles leads to life-threatening respiratory compromise by two mechanisms: (1) lack of upper airway protection and (2) hypoventilation because of respiratory muscle weakness. The most common diseases presenting as acute paralysis and ventilatory failure are **myasthenia gravis** and **Guillain-Barré syndrome** (acute inflammatory polyneuropathy). Your management should be directed toward stabilizing the patient, assessing the need to intubate and ventilate, and establishing a diagnosis. Because patients with neuromuscular disease can deteriorate rapidly, close observation and meticulous airway and ventilatory management in the early stages are critical.

■ PHONE CALL

Questions

1. **What are the vital signs?**
2. **Is the patient in respiratory distress?**
   Rapid, shallow breathing is a danger sign of impending ventilatory failure. Patients with acute weakness who are in obvious respiratory distress should be intubated immediately.
3. **Over what time period has the weakness developed?**
   Fluctuating weakness that has been present for weeks or months is characteristic of myasthenia gravis. Progressive ascending paralysis over hours to days is suggestive of Guillain-Barré syndrome.
4. **Has the patient had difficulty swallowing?**
   Dysphagia (coughing or choking after swallowing) is a symptom of bulbar muscle weakness. Affected patients are at risk for aspiration and should be made nothing by mouth (NPO).

Orders

1. **Administer oxygen.**
   For mild to moderate respiratory distress, order 40% oxygen via face mask and reassess oxygen requirements on arrival at the bedside.

2. **Perform bedside pulmonary function tests.**
   - *Vital capacity* is the maximal exhaled volume after full inspiration and is normally 60 ml/kg (approximately 4 L in a 70-kg person). Patients generally require intubation when vital capacity falls below 15 ml/kg (approximately 1 L).
   - *Peak inspiratory pressure* (normally greater than 50 cm H_2O) measures the force of inhalation generated by contraction of the diaphragm and is an index of the ability to maintain lung expansion and avoid atelectasis.
   - *Peak expiratory pressure* (normally greater than 60 cm H_2O) correlates with the strength of cough and the ability to clear secretions from the airway.
3. **Measure arterial blood gas levels on room air.**
   Hypercarbia (partial pressure of carbon dioxide [PCO_2] greater than 45 mm Hg) results from alveolar hypoventilation.

   Hypoxia (partial pressure of oxygen [PO_2] less than 75 mm Hg) is indicative of impaired ventilation-perfusion matching and is usually related to atelectasis or pneumonia.
4. **Obtain a chest x-ray.**
5. **Keep the patient NPO.**
6. **Insert an intravenous line.**
   IV access should be established in the event of an acute deterioration.

■ **ELEVATOR THOUGHTS**

What can cause generalized weakness leading to respiratory failure?
   An anatomic approach is the most useful way to classify causes of generalized weakness. Further discussion of many of the entities listed below can be found later in this chapter.
1. **Spinal cord lesion**
   - Cervical cord compression
   - Transverse myelitis
2. **Motor neuron lesion**
   - Amyotrophic lateral sclerosis
   - Polio
3. **Peripheral nerve lesion**
   - Guillain-Barré syndrome (acute inflammatory polyneuropathy)
   - Chronic inflammatory demyelinating polyneuropathy
   - Diphtheritic polyneuropathy
   - Carcinomatous meningitis
   - Acquired immunodeficiency syndrome (AIDS)–related demyelinating polyneuropathy

- Toxic neuropathy (lead, arsenic, hexacarbons, dapsone, nitrofurantoin)
- Lyme disease
- Tick paralysis
- Critical illness polyneuropathy
- Acute intermittent porphyria
4. **Neuromuscular junction lesion**
   - Myasthenia gravis
   - Lambert-Eaton syndrome
   - Botulism
   - Organophosphate poisoning
5. **Muscle lesion**
   - Polymyositis or dermatomyositis
   - Critical illness myopathy
   - Hyperthyroid myopathy
   - Mitochondrial myopathy
   - Acid maltase deficiency (Pompe's disease)
   - Periodic paralysis (hyperkalemic or hypokalemic)
   - Hypophosphatemia
   - Congenital myopathy (muscular dystrophy)

■ MAJOR THREAT TO LIFE

- Hypoxia
  Inadequate oxygenation is the most worrisome end result of any process leading to shortness of breath. Hence, your initial assessment should be directed toward ascertaining whether significant hypoxia is present.

■ BEDSIDE

Quick Look Test

Does the patient look well (comfortable), sick (uncomfortable), or critical (about to die)?

This simple observation will help determine the necessity of immediate intubation or admission to an intensive care unit (ICU) for observation.

Airway and Vital Signs

Is the upper airway clear?
- Weakness of the tongue and oropharyngeal muscles can lead to upper airway obstruction, which increases resistance to airflow and the work of breathing. *Stridor* is indicative of potentially life-threatening upper airway obstruction.

- Weakness of the laryngeal and glottic muscles can lead to impaired swallowing and aspiration of secretions. A *wet, gurgled voice* and *pooled oropharyngeal secretions* are the best clinical signs of significant dysphagia.

What is the respiratory rate?

Check for *paradoxical respirations* (Fig. 16–1), inward movement of the abdomen on inspiration, which is indicative of diaphragmatic paralysis.

What is the heart rate?

Sinus tachycardia is expected in patients in respiratory distress, but it can be particularly severe in patients with Guillain-Barré syndrome with dysautonomia.

What is the blood pressure (BP)?

Hypertension or BP lability can result from dysautonomia in Guillain-Barré syndrome. Hypotension can occur with acute cervical spine injury (spinal shock) but otherwise demands a complete investigation to rule out other causes (i.e., myocardial infarction, hypovolemia, or sepsis).

What is the temperature?

Fever should raise suspicion for aspiration pneumonia.

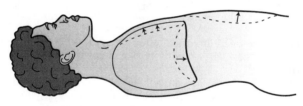

Normal inspiration

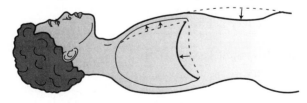

Paradoxical respiration

Figure 16–1 □ Paradoxical respirations. With normal inspiration *(top)*, contraction and downward movement of the diaphragm cause the abdomen to move outward. With paradoxical respiration *(bottom)*, outward expansion of the chest leads to passive upward movement of the diaphragm and inward movement of the abdomen.

Selective History

To make the diagnosis, it is important to establish the time course and distribution of weakness. Key questions to keep in mind when obtaining a history in patients with generalized weakness include the following: (1) Is a spinal cord lesion a possibility? (2) Is the process purely motor or is sensation involved? (3) Is the patient at risk for sudden respiratory failure?

1. **When did the weakness develop?**
   Early symptoms of weakness can be subtle. Ask about difficulty arising from a chair, climbing stairs, lifting packages, combing or brushing hair, or turning keys or doorknobs.

2. **Was there an antecedent illness?**
   Approximately 70% of cases of Guillain-Barré syndrome are triggered by an antecedent viral illness or *Campylobacter jejuni* gastroenteritis. Respiratory crisis in myasthenia gravis is triggered by infection in approximately 40% of patients.

3. **Does the weakness fluctuate?**
   Fluctuating weakness (on an hourly basis) is almost pathognomonic for myasthenia gravis.

4. **Has there been any blurred or double vision?**
   Blurred vision occurs with botulism.

5. **Has there been any neck or back pain?**
   Neck pain should raise suspicion for a cervical cord lesion. Low backache occurs frequently with Guillain-Barré syndrome.

6. **Has there been any numbness or tingling?**
   Distal paresthesias are common in Guillain-Barré syndrome.

7. **Have there been any muscle aches, cramps, or tenderness?**
   Aching and tenderness generally occur with myopathy. Cramps can occur with motor neuron disease or with severe electrolyte derangements.

8. **Has there been any exposure to toxins or insecticides?**
   Organophosphate is the most common toxin that can lead to respiratory failure.

Selective Physical Examination

Once the patient has been stabilized, the goal is to identify signs of airway or respiratory compromise and to search for clues to the diagnosis.

HEENT:
- Oropharynx: Check for *pooled secretions*, which are diagnostic of impaired swallowing and ability to handle secretions. *Exudative pharyngitis* occurs with diphtheria.

- **Swallow test:** Give the patient a small amount (3 oz) of water to drink. Coughing after swallowing is diagnostic of aspiration.
- **Speech:** Check for *dysphonia*. A nasal voice results from palatal paralysis. A soft, strangulated voice results from vocal cord paralysis. Evaluate *dysarthria* by checking the buccal (ma, ma), lingual (la, la), and pharyngeal (ga, ga) components of articulation.

Respiratory:
- **Lungs:** Auscultate for wheezes, rales, rhonchi, or consolidation.
- **Diaphragm:** Palpate for normal, outward abdominal movement during inspiration.
- **Cough:** Check the strength of the patient's cough.
- **Ventilatory reserve:** Ask the patient to inhale fully and count from 1 to 25. A patient with adequate ventilatory reserve should be able to do this in a single breath.

Skin:
- **Rashes:** Check for a rash (Lyme disease, dermatomyositis).

Neurologic examination:
- **Pupils:** Pupillary reactivity may be lost with botulism or in the Miller-Fisher variant of Guillain-Barré syndrome (triad of ophthalmoplegia, ataxia, and areflexia).
- **Extraocular muscles:** *Ptosis and ocular muscle weakness* is characteristic of myasthenia gravis but can occur with the Miller-Fisher variant of Guillain-Barré syndrome, botulism, diphtheria, polymyositis, Graves' disease, mitochondrial myopathy, or critical illness myopathy.
- **Face, palate, tongue, and neck strength**
- **Limb strength**
- **Fasciculations:** Fasciculations are seen with motor neuron disease or organophosphate poisoning.
- **Reflexes:** *Areflexia* is **always** seen with Guillain-Barré syndrome.
- **Coordination:** Ataxia occurs with the Miller-Fisher variant of Guillain-Barré syndrome.
- **Sensation:** A cervical or upper thoracic *sensory level* associated with quaraparesis suggests a cervical cord lesion. Mild sensory loss in the distal extremities is common in Guillain-Barré syndrome.

■ MANAGEMENT

Airway Management and Mechanical Ventilation

Criteria for Intubation

A number of factors must be considered when deciding when to intubate and ventilate. The most important factor, perhaps, is the overall comfort level of the patient. Decisions must be individualized, but the following criteria may be helpful:

- *Reduction of vital capacity to 15 ml/kg (approximately 1 L in a 70-kg person)*
- *PO_2 less than 70 mm Hg on room air*
- *PCO_2 greater than 50 mm Hg associated with acidosis (pH less than 7.35)*
- *Severe oropharyngeal paresis with inability to protect the airway*

Remember that conservative, early intubation and institution of positive pressure ventilation can minimize the development of atelectasis and pneumonia and may lead to earlier extubation.

Initial Ventilator Management

The initial goals of ventilator management immediately after intubation are (1) to provide rest and (2) to promote lung expansion. These goals are best accomplished using *synchronized intermittent mandatory ventilation (SIMV)* at a rate of 6 to 8 breaths per minute, using tidal volumes of 10 to 15 ml/kg. Adjust these parameters to maintain normal minute ventilation (6 to 10 L/min) and PCO_2 (approximately 40 mm Hg) values.

Patients with long-standing weakness and CO_2 retention should be intentionally hypoventilated (PCO_2 at or higher than 45 mm Hg). Overventilating to normal or reduced PCO_2 levels will result in alkalosis and renal serum bicarbonate wasting, which in turn will make it more difficult to successfully wean the patient.

In general, we advocate using larger tidal volumes in combination with lower ventilatory rates. *Positive end-expiratory pressure (PEEP)* aids in the expansion of collapsed alveoli and should be used in all patients at levels of 5 to 15 cm H_2O.

Bronchoscopy

Fiberoptic bronchoscopy for pulmonary toilet should be performed aggressively in patients with hypoxia, severe atelectasis, or lobar collapse because of mucus plugging.

Tracheostomy

After the patient has been on mechanical ventilation for approximately 2 weeks, tracheostomy should be performed. Compared to prolonged (more than 2 weeks) endotracheal intubation, tracheostomy (1) is more comfortable, (2) poses less risk of permanent laryngeal or tracheal injury, (3) facilitates weaning from mechanical ventilation by reducing dead space and airway resistance, and (4) makes it easier to clear airway secretions by cough or suctioning.

Weaning to Extubation

The criteria to be met before weaning is initiated are listed in Box 16–1.

Continuous positive airway pressure (CPAP) with pressure support is the preferred initial mode for weaning patients with respiratory muscle weakness. Each time the patient inhales, "pressure support" delivers additional inspiratory volume until a preset level of pressure is reached. The amount of inspiratory pressure support given (range, 5 to 15 cm H_2O) should be initially adjusted to attain tidal volumes of approximately 500 ml in an adult. We advocate daytime weaning trials and "resting" the patient on SIMV overnight (Box 16–2).

Extubation can be performed once the patient has demonstrated the ability to tolerate long periods (e.g., overnight) on CPAP with pressure support equal to 5 cm H_2O without fatigue. Fluctuating pulmonary function tests, excessive secretions, or concurrent medical problems (i.e., infection or cardiovascular instability) are relative contraindications to extubation. Extubation should always be performed early in the day.

General Care of the Patient with Neuromuscular Respiratory Failure

1. **Elevate the head of the bed**
   With diaphragmatic weakness, lung volumes become diminished and work of breathing increases in the supine position.

Box 16–1. CRITERIA FOR WEANING TO EXTUBATION

1. Vital capacity greater than 15 ml/kg
2. Peak inspiratory pressure greater than 25 cm H_2O
3. Po_2 greater than 80 mm Hg on 40% oxygen
4. No adverse medical conditions: infection, fever, hypotension, anemia, gastric distention, volume overload, or cardiac arrhythmias

---

Box 16–2. WEANING TRIAL PROTOCOL

1. Begin the weaning trial by switching the ventilator mode from SIMV to CPAP with pressure support.
2. After 15 to 30 minutes, record the respiratory rate and mean tidal volume.
3. Every 2 to 4 hours, the level of pressure support may be decreased by 1 to 2 cm H_2O if the patient remains comfortable.
4. In general, the weaning trial should be continued up to 12 hours or until signs of respiratory fatigue occur. *An increasing respiratory rate combined with falling tidal volumes is the most reliable indicator of respiratory fatigue.* Associated signs may include agitation, restlessness, tachycardia, and diaphoresis. At this point, an arterial blood gas measurement may be desirable.
5. When the weaning trial is over, return to SIMV mode overnight.

---

2. **Chest physical therapy**
   Chest percussion and airway suctioning are essential for preventing mucus plugs and aiding in the clearing of secretions. Prescribe *incentive spirometry* every 6 hours if the patient is not intubated.
3. **Serial measurements of vital capacity**
   Vital capacity should be checked every 4 to 6 hours in nonintubated patients and every 12 to 24 hours in intubated patients.
4. **Prophylaxis for deep vein thrombosis (DVT)**
   Order **heparin 5000 U SQ every 12 hours.**
5. **Nutrition**
   Patients with bulbar weakness should be made NPO and fed via a *small-bore nasoduodenal tube.* When attempting to wean a CO_2 retainer, use a nutritional supplement with a high ratio of carbohydrate to lipid (e.g., Pulmocare) to minimize CO_2 production.
6. **Fluids and electrolytes**
   Hypokalemia and *hypophosphatemia* can exacerbate muscle weakness and should be periodically checked for and treated.
7. **Bowel and bladder care**
   Paralysis predisposes to constipation and can be prevented with **docusate sodium (Colace) 100 mg three times a day and milk of magnesia 30 cc every night.** Intermittent

straight catheterization carries a lower risk of infection than an indwelling Foley catheter.

■ SPECIFIC DISORDERS

Guillain-Barré Syndrome

Guillain-Barré syndrome is a monophasic, acute inflammatory demyelinating polyneuropathy. The etiology is related to an auto-immune attack directed against surface antigens on peripheral nerves, resulting in focal segmental demyelination.

Onset

In approximately 70% of cases, the syndrome follows a respiratory or gastrointestinal infection by 5 days to 3 weeks. Viral upper respiratory infection and *Campylobacter jejuni* gastroenteritis are the most common precipitating infections. Other causes include human immunodeficiency virus (HIV) infection, immunization, pregnancy, Hodgkin's disease, and surgery.

Clinical Features

The syndrome usually begins with rapidly progressive ascending paralysis, associated with cranial nerve and respiratory muscle weakness, loss of deep tendon reflexes, and distal paresthesias and sensory loss. Unlike other neuropathies, proximal muscles are often affected more than distal muscles. The weakness progresses over 7 to 21 days; the median duration from onset to maximal weakness is 12 days. Respiratory failure requiring intubation occurs in 20% of patients. Papilledema, autonomic disturbances (e.g., hypertension, hypotension, urinary retention, sinus tachycardia, cardiac arrhythmias), and syndrome of inappropriate antidiuretic hormone (SIADH) are seen in some patients.

Laboratory Data

The cerebrospinal fluid (CSF) classically shows dissociation between albumin levels and cytologic findings, with elevated protein levels and normal white blood cell counts (5 cells/μl or fewer). The elevation in the protein level can sometimes take up to 2 weeks to develop. A mild lymphocytic or monocytic pleocytosis is sometimes seen (10 to 100 cells/mm^3) and should raise suspicion for an infectious polyradiculopathy (e.g., HIV, cytomegalovirus [CMV], or Lyme disease) or polio. Nerve conduction studies show loss of F waves and reduced conduction velocities. Reduced motor fiber amplitudes reflect secondary axonal damage and imply a worse prognosis for recovery.

Treatment (Box 16–3)

Patients with signs of respiratory muscle weakness should be admitted to an ICU for observation until it is clear that the illness has stabilized. **Plasmapheresis,** when initiated within 10 days of the onset of symptoms, can speed the onset of recovery. A total of five treatments is performed every 1 to 2 days, with a total of 2 to 4 L of plasma exchanged for 5% albumin during each treatment. High-dose **intravenous immune globulin (IVIG), 0.4 g/kg per day for 5 consecutive days,** has been shown to be as effective as plasmapheresis and may be slightly superior. "Rebound" deterioration after completing a course of IVIG can sometimes occur.

Prognosis

Features shown to have a poor prognosis in Guillain-Barré syndrome include (1) advanced age, (2) very low distal motor amplitudes, (3) rapidly progressive weakness occurring over the first week, and (4) respiratory failure requiring intubation.

Myasthenia Gravis

Myasthenia gravis is caused by an antibody-mediated attack on nicotinic acetylcholine receptors, resulting in a defect in neuromuscular transmission. This phenomenon manifests clinically as *fluctuating weakness* and *muscle fatigability,* the hallmarks of myasthenia gravis.

Box 16–3. CHECKLIST FOR THE MANAGEMENT OF GUILLAIN-BARRÉ SYNDROME

1. *Diagnostic work-up:* Lumbar puncture, electromyography/ nerve conduction studies, hepatitis and Lyme disease serologies, CMV, Epstein-Barr virus (EBV), herpes simplex virus (HSV), and HIV titers, urine porphyrin levels, urine heavy metal screen, stool analysis for *Campylobacter.*
2. *Pain management:* Pain can be severe and may result from meningeal inflammation or neuropathic mechanisms. Nonsteroidal anti-inflammatory drugs **(NSAIDs) (ketorolac 30 mg IM every 6 hours)** and **narcotics (morphine 10 mg every 2 to 4 hours as needed)** are most effective.
3. *Dysautonomia:* The most frequent cardiovascular manifestation of dysautonomia is sustained hypertension and tachycardia. Treatment with beta-blockers **(propranolol PO 10 to 40 mg every 6 hours** or **labetolol infusion)** is effective and may be required in older patients with coronary artery disease.

Clinical Features

Fluctuating weakness is the hallmark of myasthenia gravis; it tends to involve the eyes (in 90% of patients), face, neck, and oropharynx (in 80% of patients), and limbs (in 60% of patients). The age distribution at onset is bimodal, with an early peak between ages 20 and 40 (primarily in women) and a later peak between ages 50 and 80 (in both sexes). The limbs are almost never affected in isolation. Sensation is always normal, and reflexes are preserved unless the muscle is plegic. Most patients reach the maximum severity of their disease within the first 1 to 2 years; thereafter, spontaneous remission is common (in approximately 30% of patients), and the disease process tends to become less severe. *Malignant thymoma* is present in approximately 15% of patients with myasthenia and is associated with more severe disease.

Myasthenic crisis is defined by respiratory failure requiring intubation and mechanical ventilation. Crisis is most often provoked by infection (in 40% of patients) but can also occur spontaneously (in 30% of patients) or result from aspiration, surgery, pregnancy, medications, or emotional upset. Approximately 25% of patients can be extubated within 1 week, 50% within 2 weeks, and 75% within 1 month. One third of patients intubated for crisis will proceed to experience a second crisis. Although a crisis is by definition life-threatening, with modern ICU management, mortality (approximately 5%) results only from overwhelming medical complications (e.g., myocardial infarction, sepsis).

Laboratory Data

The diagnosis of myasthenia gravis can be established with the following tests:

1. *Edrophonium (Tensilon) testing* reveals transient improvement in patients with ocular and facial weakness. **Edrophonium 10 mg** is used in adults; infuse 2 mg initially and observe for severe cholinergic muscarinic effects such as nausea, bradycardia, and hypotension. **Atropine 0.4 mg** should be kept at the bedside and can be used to reverse these symptoms. If there are no severe effects, inject the remaining 8 mg and observe for improvement, which generally occurs within 2 to 10 minutes.

2. *Repetitive nerve stimulation* at 2 to 3 Hz characteristically produces a greater than 10% decrement in amplitude between the first and fifth compound muscle action potential. Sensitivity and specificity are 90% when weak, proximal muscles are tested; however, sensitivity falls to less than 50% in myasthenic patients without limb weakness.

3. *Single-fiber EMG* reveals "jitter," variation in the time interval between firing of muscle fibers in the same motor unit.

Single-fiber EMG is highly sensitive (sensitivity greater than 95%) for myasthenia gravis but is not specific.

4. *Acetylcholine receptor antibodies* are present in 80 to 90% of patients with generalized myasthenia but in only 50% of patients with ocular myasthenia. Titers do not correlate with the severity of illness.

Treatment (Box 16–4)

Therapeutic options for treating myasthenia gravis can be divided into three categories: *symptomatic therapy* (with acetylcholinesterase inhibitors), *short-term disease suppression* (with plasmapheresis and IVIG), and *long-term immunosuppression* (with thymectomy, steroids, or chemotherapy).

Symptomatic Therapy. Acetylcholinesterase inhibitors (Table 16–2) improve myasthenic weakness by allowing acetylcholine to accumulate at the neuromuscular junction. **Pyridostigmine (Mestinon) is started at 30 mg PO three times a day, increased to 60 to 120 mg every 4 to 6 hours as a maintenance dose, and increased to 120 mg every 3 hours as a maximal dose.** A long-acting 180-mg tablet (Mestinon Timespan) can be given at bedtime for patients with nocturnal or morning weakness. Excessive muscarinic side effects (e.g., pulmonary secretions, diarrhea) can be controlled by concurrently giving an antimuscarinic agent such as **glycopyrrolate (Robinul) 1 to 2 mg PO three times a day** or **propantheline bromide (Pro-Banthine) 15 mg PO four times a day.**

Box 16–4. CHECKLIST FOR THE MANAGEMENT OF MYASTHENIC CRISIS

1. Eliminate and avoid all contraindicated medications (see Table 16–2).
2. *Diagnostic work-up:* Edrophonium test, acetylcholine receptor antibody level, repetitive nerve stimulation, single-fiber EMG, thyroid function tests, chest computed tomography (CT) scan.
3. *Treatment:* Anticholinesterase medications should be *discontinued* while patients are mechanically ventilated because they lead to excessive stimulation of secretions. We restart anticholinesterase therapy at half the baseline dose 1 day before extubation is anticipated. A course of plasmapheresis or IVIG is indicated in all patients.

Table 16–1 □ **DRUGS THAT CAN EXACERBATE WEAKNESS IN MYASTHENIA GRAVIS**

Antibiotics
    Aminoglycosides (gentamycin, streptomycin, others)
    Peptide antibodies (polymyxin B, colistin)
    Tetracyclines (tetracycline, doxycycline, others)
    Erythromycin
    Clindamycin
    Ciprofloxacin
    Ampicillin
Antiarrhythmics
    Quinidine
    Procainamide
    Lidocaine
Neuromuscular junction blockers (vecuronium, pancuronium, others)
Quinine
Steroids
Thyroid hormones (thyroxine, levothyroxine, others)
Beta blockers (propranolol, timolol, others)
Phenytoin

Short-term Disease Suppression. This is indicated to hasten clinical improvement in hospitalized patients. **Plasmapheresis (five exchanges of 2 to 4 L every 1 to 2 days)** can lead to improvement within days, but the effect is short-lived, lasting only 2 to 4 weeks. Similar benefits have been reported in 70% of patients treated with **IVIG (0.4 g/kg daily for 5 days),** but experience with this therapy remains limited.

Long-term Immunosuppression. This treatment is indicated when weakness is inadequately controlled with anticholinesterase medications. **Prednisone** is most commonly prescribed; to use the lowest dose possible, start with **15 to 20 mg per day** and gradually increase to **40 to 100 mg per day over 4 to 8 weeks** until an adequate response is achieved. Temporary worsening of symptoms within the first 2 weeks of starting steroids can be expected in up to 40% of patients. **Azathioprine 100 to 250 mg per day** can also be used for long-term immunosuppression in patients who cannot tolerate the side effects of steroids. **Thymectomy** leads to disease remission in 40% of patients and clinical improvement in another 40%, but these benefits can take months or years to occur. Thymectomy is indicated in any patient between the ages of 15 and 60 with thymoma or with generalized myasthenia.

Uncommon Causes of Paralysis and Respiratory Failure
Botulism
Botulism is caused by an exotoxin produced by *Clostridium botulinum,* an anaerobic, gram-positive, spore-forming rod that

Table 16-2 □ ANTICHOLINESTERASE DRUGS USED FOR MYASTHENIA GRAVIS

	Route	Equivalent Dosage	Onset	Maximal Response	Dosage Range
Pyridostigmine bromide (Mestinon)	PO*	60 mg	30 to 60 minutes	1 to 2 hours	30 to 120 mg every 3 to 8 hours
	IM, IV†	2 mg	5 to 10 minutes	20 to 30 minutes	—
Pyridostigmine long-acting (Mestinon Timespan)	PO	—	1 to 2 hours	3 to 5 hours	180 mg per day at nighttime
Neostigmine bromide (Prostigmin)	PO	15 mg	30 minutes	1 hour	15 to 30 mg every 2 to 3 hours
Neostigmine methylsulfate (Prostigmin injectable)	IV†	0.5 mg	1 to 2 minutes	20 minutes	0.5 to 1 mg every 2 hours
	IM	1.5 mg	30 minutes	1 hour	1.5 to 3 mg every 2 to 3 hours

*Can be given as a tablet or as a liquid.
†Equivalent IV dose of pyridostigmine or neostigmine is one thirtieth of the oral dose.

contaminates food. Weakness occurs because the toxin is a potent inhibitor of presynaptic acetylcholine release. Clinical symptoms begin within 12 to 24 hours of ingestion and are characterized by gastrointestinal complaints, dilated and nonreactive pupils, blurred vision, and weakness that begins with the extraocular and oropharyngeal muscles before becoming generalized. Urinary retention, dry mouth, and anhidrosis may also occur. **Botulism trivalent antitoxin (one vial IV and one vial IM every 2 to 4 hours)** should be given as soon as possible. **Guanidine hydrochloride (40 mg PO every 4 hours)** is an acetylcholine agonist that can counteract the presynaptic blockade caused by the toxin.

Poliomyelitis

Poliovirus is an enterovirus that can cause selective destruction of motor neurons in the spinal cord and brain stem, resulting in flaccid, areflexic paralysis. Modern vaccination has made the disease a clinical rarity. Acute paralysis from polio is differentiated from that caused by Guillain-Barré syndrome by the presence of headache, high fever, mental status changes, asymmetric weakness, and neutrophils in the CSF.

Tetanus

Tetanus results from an exotoxin produced by *Clostridium tetani*, an anaerobic gram-positive coccus that can infect soft-tissue wounds. The toxin results in neuronal hyperexcitability; the result is seizures, autonomic instability, and sustained "tetanic" muscle contractions involving the jaw ("lockjaw"), neck, back, and respiratory muscles. Treatment is directed toward (1) assisting ventilation, which may require intubation and administration of neuromuscular blocking agents; (2) neutralizing the toxin with **tetanus immune globulin 250 units IM (single dose);** and (3) eradicating the soft-tissue infection with **procaine penicillin 1.2 million units every 6 hours for 10 days.**

17

SYNCOPE

Syncope is a brief loss of consciousness caused by sudden reduction of cerebral blood flow. *Presyncope* refers to the situation in which there is reduction of cerebral blood flow and a sensation of impending loss of consciousness, although the patient does not actually pass out. Presyncope and syncope represent degrees of the same disorder and should be addressed as manifestations of the same underlying problem. Your task is to discover the cause of the syncopal attack.

■ PHONE CALL

Questions

1. **Did the patient actually lose consciousness?**
2. **Is the patient still unconscious?**
3. **What are the vital signs?**
4. **Was the patient standing, sitting, or lying down when the attack occurred?**
   Syncope in the recumbent position is almost always cardiac in origin. Syncope that occurs immediately after standing up suggests orthostatic hypotension.
5. **Was any seizure-like activity witnessed?**
6. **Did the patient sustain any injury from the fall?**

Orders

If the patient is still **unconscious,** give the following orders:
1. Administer IV D5W to keep the vein open (KVO) if IV is not already in place.
2. Turn the patient onto the left side (this maneuver minimizes the risk of upper airway obstruction and aspiration).
3. Order a stat 12-lead electrocardiogram (ECG) and rhythm strip.
4. Obtain a finger stick glucose level.

If the patient has **regained consciousness,** if there is no evidence of head or neck injury, and if the vital signs are stable, do the following:
1. Instruct the RN to keep the patient supine for at least 10 to 15 minutes, until the patient feels comfortable. To return the patient to bed, slowly raise the patient to the sitting position, and then to a standing position.
2. Have the RN check orthostatic vital signs (blood pressure

[BP] and heart rate with the patient lying down and standing).
3. Order an ECG and rhythm strip.
4. Have vital signs taken every 15 minutes until you arrive at the bedside. Instruct the RN to call you back immediately if the patient become unstable before you are able to perform your assessment.

Inform RN

"Will arrive at the bedside in . . . minutes."

■ ELEVATOR THOUGHTS

What causes syncope?
A comprehensive list of the differential diagnoses for syncope and the approximate relative frequency of each of the main categories in an emergency room (ER) population is given below. **Note that neurologic and psychiatric causes are at the bottom of the list and in combination account for only 5% of all patients presenting with syncope.** In the majority of patients (90%), syncope results from a transient drop in systemic BP and can be explained on the basis of reflex vasodilation, cardiac disease, orthostatic hypotension, or medications. *Accordingly, your initial evaluation should focus on excluding these conditions before a neurologic diagnosis is seriously considered.*

1. **Reflex vasodilatation (in 60% of ER patients)**
   a. Vasodepressor (vasovagal, neurocardiogenic) syncope
   b. Carotid sinus syncope
   c. Situational syncope
      (1) Micturition syncope
      (2) Defecation syncope
      (3) Cough syncope
2. **Cardiac causes (in 25% of ER patients)**
   a. Arrhythmias
      (1) Tachycardias
         (a) Ventricular tachycardia/fibrillation
         (b) Supraventricular tachycardia
      (2) Bradycardias
         (a) Sick sinus syndrome
         (b) Second- and third-degree heart block
         (c) Pacemaker malfunction
   b. Flow failure
      (1) Obstruction to left ventricular outflow
         (a) Aortic or mitral stenosis
         (b) Hypertrophic obstructive cardiomyopathy

    (c) Aortic dissection
   (2) Obstruction to pulmonary outflow
    (a) Pulmonic stenosis
    (b) Pulmonary embolism
   (3) Pump failure
    (a) Myocardial infarction
    (b) Cardiac tamponade
3. **Orthostatic (postural) hypotension (in 10% of ER patients)**
  a. Volume depletion (anemia, dehydration)
  b. Drug induced (Table 17–1)
  c. Autonomic dysfunction
   (1) Central: Shy-Drager syndrome
   (2) Peripheral: autonomic neuropathy
4. **Neurologic causes (in 5% of ER patients)**
  a. Seizure (technically not syncope but mimics syncope)
   (1) Unwitnessed tonic-clonic seizure
   (2) Atonic seizure (drop attack)
  b. Transient ischemic attack (TIA)
   (1) Brain stem ischemia
    (a) Vertebrobasilar stenosis/occlusion
    (b) Subclavian steal syndrome
   (2) Bilateral hemispheric ischemia from carotid artery stenosis or occlusion

Table 17–1 □ DRUGS AND MEDICATIONS THAT CAN CAUSE SYNCOPE

Antihypertensive agents
 Nitrates
 Calcium channel blockers
 Diuretics
 Angiotensin converting enzyme inhibitors
 Beta blockers
 Others (hydralazine, prazosin)
Antiarrhythmic agents (prolonged QT interval syndrome, torsades de pointes)
 Quinidine
 Procainamide
 Disopyramide
 Sotalol
 Amiodarone
Tricyclic antidepressants
Monoamine oxidase inhibitors
Phenothiazines
Levodopa
Digoxin
Ethanol
Marijuana

    c. Increased intracranial pressure (ICP)
      (1) Subarachnoid hemorrhage (SAH)
      (2) Space-occupying lesion (e.g., brain tumor)
5. **Psychiatric causes (in less than 1% of ER patients)**
    a. Hyperventilation
    b. Conversion disorder (technically not syncope but mimics syncope)

■ MAJOR THREAT TO LIFE

- *Aspiration* is the main threat if the patient is still unconscious.
  Remember that syncope generally lasts only a few minutes. If the patient remains persistently unconscious (longer than 15 minutes), the diagnosis is coma, and your evaluation should proceed as outlined in Chapter 6.
- *Fatal cardiac arrhythmia* is the main hazard once the patient has regained consciousness.
  If a cardiac rhythm disturbance is suspected, the patient should be attached to an ECG monitor, and consideration should be given to observing the patient in an intensive care unit (ICU). Other potentially life-threatening illnesses that can present with syncope include subarachnoid hemorrhage, gastrointestinal bleeding, pulmonary embolism, aortic dissection, and myocardial infarction.

■ BEDSIDE

Quick Look Test

Does the patient look well (comfortable), sick (uncomfortable), or critical (about to die)?

Most cases of syncope are brief (loss of consciousness less than 5 minutes), and many patients look well shortly after regaining consciousness. Others may appear nauseated, pallid, and diaphoretic—these signs represent the systemic autonomic response to hypotension and should resolve rapidly.

Are there any external signs of head or neck trauma?

Significant head injury is unusual after syncope but should be checked for. In most cases, a period of presyncope warns the patient that something is amiss and allows him or her to avoid a hard fall. Cardiac syncope often occurs without warning and is more likely to lead to traumatic injury.

Airway and Vital Signs

Abnormal vital signs can help make your diagnosis of the specific cause of syncope much easier.

Is the airway clear?
If the patient is still unconscious, ensure that he or she is lying on the left side and that respirations are adequate.

What is the heart rate?
Supraventricular or ventricular tachycardia should be documented on ECG tracings. If the patient is hypotensive, call for a cardiac arrest team and treat immediately with electrical cardioversion.

Sinus bradycardia implicates vagally mediated vasodepressor syncope. In this case, both the heart rate and the BP should normalize quickly as the patient remains supine.

What is the BP?
Persistently low BP or significant orthostatic hypotension combined with normal sinus rhythm or sinus tachycardia implicates volume depletion. Begin IV volume resuscitation with D5NS and order a stat hematocrit. Rule out gastrointestinal (GI) bleeding and ruptured aortic aneurysm, which rarely present with syncope.

Hypertension, if found in association with headache, stiff neck, or altered level of consciousness, may indicate subarachnoid hemorrhage.

What is the temperature?
Patients with syncope are rarely febrile. If *fever* is present, it is usually due to a concomitant illness not related to the syncopal attack. If the syncopal attack was unwitnessed, be careful to exclude meningitis or encephalitis associated with a seizure.

Selective History

History should be obtained from the patient as well as from witnesses, if available. Focus on events immediately preceding and following the attack.

1. **Has this ever happened before?**
   If it has, ask the patient if a diagnosis was made after the previous attack.
2. **What do the patient or witnesses recall from the period immediately before the syncope?**
   - Syncope occurring while changing from the supine or the sitting position to the standing position suggests *orthostatic hypotension.*
   - Palpitations or the complete absence of prodromal symptoms suggest *cardiac arrhythmia.*
   - A prodrome of dizziness, lightheadedness, pallor, diaphoresis, and dimming of vision (i.e., presyncope) is highly characteristic of *reflex vasodepressor syncope.*

- Syncope after turning the head to one side, especially if the patient is wearing a tight collar, may represent *carotid sinus syncope.*
- Syncope during or immediately following Valsalva's maneuver (coughing, micturition, defecation) can result from mechanical disruption of venous return and is termed *situational syncope.*
- One or more episodes of vertigo, diplopia, dysarthria, numbness, weakness, or ataxia preceding the attack, alone or in combination, are suggestive of *vertebrobasilar insufficiency.*
- An aura (unusual smell or taste, abdominal sensations, visual or sensory hallucinations) may point to a *seizure* as the cause of an unwitnessed attack.

3. **How does the patient feel upon waking from the syncopal attack?**
   - Headache suggests *subarachnoid hemorrhage.*

   Persistent lethargy and confusion are atypical for true syncope and suggest an unwitnessed *seizure* or *subarachnoid hemorrhage.*

4. **Were any shaking movements observed?**

   Loss of consciousness associated with simultaneous generalized tonic-clonic activity is diagnostic of seizure. *Caution:* Be aware that minor twitching, myoclonic activity, or a single convulsion that **follows** loss of consciousness is common and reflects *secondary* consequences of cerebral hypoxia-ischemia.

5. **Was the patient incontinent of stool or urine?**

   If the attack was unwitnessed, incontinence is highly suggestive of seizure. Be aware that incontinence can also occur with true syncope.

6. **Is there any history of cardiac disease, seizure, stroke, or TIA?**

   These may point to an obvious cause of syncope.

7. **Has the patient been feeling ill recently?**

   Ask about symptoms of infection, diarrhea, peptic ulcer, chest pain, palpitations, or neurologic dysfunction, which may point to a predisposing illness.

8. **What are the medications?**

   Refer to Table 17–1 for a list of medications that can cause syncope.

Selective Physical Examination

Your physical examination is directed toward finding a cause for the syncope. However, a search for evidence of injuries sustained by a fall is equally important at this time.

Vital signs:	- Repeat now, including *orthostatic* tests if not performed yet

HEENT:	▪ Fundoscopy: look for subhyaloid hemorrhages (SAH)
	▪ Tongue lacerations, especially at lateral borders (seizure)
	▪ Ecchymoses, abrasions, lacerations
Neck:	▪ Neck stiffness (SAH)
Cardiac:	▪ Heart murmur (mitral, pulmonic, or aortic stenosis)
	▪ Pericardial rub (cardiac tamponade)
GU:	▪ Urinary incontinence (seizure)
Rectal:	▪ Heme-positive stool (GI bleeding)
Extremities:	▪ Palpate for evidence of fracture

Neurologic examination:
- Lethargy, confusion, or disorientation (seizure, SAH)
- Hemianopia or aphasia (stroke, CNS mass lesion)
- Diplopia, nystagmus, facial weakness or numbness, dysarthria or dysphonia (vertebrobasilar ischemia)
- Hemiparesis/pronator drift (Todd's paralysis, stroke, CNS mass lesion)
- Cogwheel rigidity (Shy-Drager syndrome)
- Stocking-glove sensory loss and areflexia (peripheral and autonomic neuropathy)
- Appendicular or gait ataxia (vertebrobasilar ischemia)

■ DIAGNOSTIC TESTING

Apart from an ECG, there are no laboratory tests that are routinely indicated for the evaluation of syncope. In approximately 50% of cases, a careful history, examination (including orthostatic BP), and ECG are all that are needed to establish a diagnosis (for instance, a clear-cut case of vasovagal syncope in a patient having blood drawn). Initial laboratory tests useful for identifying other nonneurologic causes of syncope have been listed previously in this chapter.

If the cause of syncope is unexplained and the history and examination are not suggestive of a neurologic cause, further work-up should be directed toward ruling out a cardiac cause of syncope. The reason for this is that cardiac causes of syncope carry a substantially higher risk of subsequent sudden death than do noncardiac causes (approximately 30% compared to 10% over 12 months) and thus are important to rule out. Tests to rule out a cardiac cause of syncope may include the following:
- Echocardiography
- Cardiac telemetry
- Holter monitoring
- Head-up tilt table testing

- Signal-averaged electrocardiography (SAECG)
- Electrophysiologic (EP) studies
- Cardiac stress testing
- Coronary angiography

If a neurologic cause of syncope is suggested by history or examination, specific testing may include the following (refer to the next section on specific neurologic causes of syncope to guide your selection):

- 3-minute trial of hyperventilation
- Electroencephalogram (EEG) (with and without sleep)
- Head CT or MRI
- Transcranial Doppler ultrasonography (intracranial vertebral and basilar arteries)
- Duplex Doppler ultrasonography (extracranial carotid and vertebral arteries)
- Magnetic resonance angiography
- Cerebral angiography
- Electromyography (EMG)/nerve conduction studies (NCS)

■ MANAGEMENT

Approach to Syncope: A Neurologist's Perspective

Step 1: Rule out medical causes of syncope

As stated previously, neurologic causes of syncope are unusual. When called in consultation to evaluate for a possible neurologic etiology, the first step is to verify that the more common and easy-to-identify medical causes have been excluded. Important tests to rule out a medical cause of syncope in the ER include the following:

- Orthostatic BP
- ECG
- Cardiac auscultation
- Hematocrit
- Arterial blood gas measurement (rule out pulmonary embolism)
- Review of medications (Table 17–1 lists medications that can cause syncope)
- Toxicology screen and serum ethanol level

Step 2: Know what you are looking for

Syncope results from temporary reduction of cerebral blood flow, and in the majority of cases, the cause is a drop in systemic BP. True neurologic causes of syncope follow the same principle and result from only two basic mechanisms:

1. **Transient focal reduction of cerebral blood flow related to stenosis or embolism of a cerebral artery (i.e., TIA).** With

rare exceptions, the only brain region in which transient focal ischemia can lead to loss of consciousness is the brain stem. Hence, *vertebrobasilar TIA* is the main consideration.

2. **Reduction of cerebral blood flow caused by a transient elevation of ICP.** *Subarachnoid hemorrhage* and an ICP wave associated with a *pre-existing mass lesion* are the main considerations.

Seizures are not a cause of syncope. However, generalized seizures lead to sudden, temporary loss of consciousness and thus can be confused with syncope. As the consulting neurologist, you may be asked to corroborate or rule out the diagnosis.

■ SELECTED DISORDERS THAT CAN CAUSE OR MIMIC SYNCOPE

Nonneurologic Causes

Vasovagal (Vasodepressor, Neurocardiogenic) Syncope

Also known as "the common faint," vasodepressor syncope is apt to occur in the setting of a strong emotional or painful stimulus. A prodrome of presyncope (dizziness, pallor) is the rule. Bradycardia may be identified shortly after the episode, and recovery is usually rapid. If the clinical picture is unclear, *head-up tilt table testing* can be used to provoke vasovagal syncope and establish the diagnosis, with a sensitivity and specificity of approximately 80%. Sudden head-up tilting produces an increase in myocardial contractility, which in turn leads to excessive stimulation of left ventricular mechanoreceptors (C fibers) and an exaggerated reflex vagal response in patients with vasovagal syncope. Isolated episodes require no specific intervention, and the prognosis is excellent. Eighty percent of patients with recurrent vasovagal syncope respond to treatment with a **beta blocker (propranolol 10 to 60 mg four times a day** or **pindolol 5 to 20 mg three times a day)** that blunts the cardiac inotropic response to a fall in BP and thus prevents the overly sensitive reflex vagal response.

Carotid Sinus Syncope

This unusual disorder is seen almost exclusively in older individuals and results from hypersensitivity of baroreceptors in the carotid sinus. External pressure of the neck (e.g., turning the head while wearing a tight collar) results in an exaggerated vagal response and fall in BP. *Carotid massage* with ECG monitoring can be used to establish the diagnosis, but this should be performed with caution.

Neurologic Causes

Transient Ischemic Attack

As stated previously, **vertebrobasilar stenosis or occlusion** is a rare cause of syncope. The diagnosis is suggested by symptoms or signs of focal brain stem ischemia (diplopia, vertigo, ataxia, nystagmus, dysarthria, facial numbness, unilateral or bilateral weakness, or sensory loss) either before or after the event. Deficits referable to the posterior cerebral artery, particularly hemianopia, may also occur. Syncope following prolonged head extension ("beauty parlor syncope") in patients with atherosclerotic vertebrobasilar disease has been described. *Transcranial and duplex Doppler ultrasonography, magnetic resonance angiography,* or *conventional angiography* is required to establish the diagnosis. Management is discussed in Chapter 25.

Subclavian steal syndrome is an unusual cause of vertebrobasilar insufficiency. It results from occlusion of one of the subclavian arteries proximal to the origin of the vertebral artery. The distal subclavian artery is hence supplied by retrograde flow from the ipsilateral vertebral artery, which "steals" flow from the basilar and contralateral vertebral arteries, resulting in intermittent hemodynamic flow failure in the posterior circulation.

Unilateral **carotid stenosis or occlusion** does not cause syncope. However, in very rare instances, syncope may result from severe bilateral disease, particularly with superimposed reduction of blood pressure.

Seizures

Generalized tonic-clonic seizures always result in loss of consciousness and can easily be mistaken for syncope if the event is unwitnessed. **Atonic (akinetic) seizures** manifest as sudden loss of consciousness and muscle tone and thus are clinically indistinguishable from true syncope. They represent an unusual form of generalized-onset seizure and occur most often in children with severe epilepsy, in combination with other seizure types. Atonic seizures are exceedingly rare in adults. If seizures are suspected, identification of interictal epileptiform activity on *EEG* can establish the diagnosis. Refer to Chapter 5 for information regarding the management of seizures.

Subarachnoid Hemorrhage

This frequently presents with sudden loss of consciousness due to a brief surge in ICP. However, in most cases, severe headache and nuchal rigidity are the predominant symptoms once the patient awakens, and these complaints easily point to the diagnosis. *Head CT and LP* are required to establish the diagnosis. Management is discussed in Chapter 25.

Intracranial Mass Lesions

In rare instances, syncope can result from an ICP wave in a patient harboring an unsuspected intracranial mass lesion or in a patient with obstruction to cerebral venous outflow resulting from dural sinus thrombosis. The diagnosis should be evident by the presence of abnormalities on the neurologic examination and can be confirmed with *neuroimaging studies (CT or MRI)*.

Autonomic Dysfunction

Syncope or near-syncope due to autonomic impairment is *always* associated with orthostatic hypotension. **Peripheral neuropathy** from diabetes, amyloidosis, paraneoplastic disease, and other causes can involve the sympathetic nerves, which normally mediate a compensatory pressor response when BP declines upon standing. **Shy-Drager syndrome** is a multiple-system atrophy (MSA) characterized by parkinsonism (tremor, rigidity, bradykinesia, postural instability) and central autonomic failure that manifests primarily as orthostatic hypotension. Idiopathic isolated central and peripheral autonomic failure have also been described but are rare. Autonomic failure leading to orthostatic hypotension can be treated with **support stockings** and **fludrocortisone (Florinef) 0.1 mg one to three times a day,** a pure mineralocorticoid that induces sodium retention and intravascular volume expansion. The alpha-agonist **midodrine 5 to 10 mg three times a day** can be used as an alternative to fludrocortisone.

Conversion Disorder

"Hysterical faints" generally occur as a dramatic loss of consciousness in the presence of other people, without changes in BP or pulse. Patients may betray their state by having complete or partial memory of the spell. The diagnosis should be suspected when pre-existing psychiatric disease (anxiety or personality disorder) is present and the work-up is negative. *Caution:* Many psychiatric medications can cause true syncope.

Hyperventilation

Hypocapnia resulting from hyperventilation leads to syncope or presyncope by decreasing cerebral blood flow because of cerebral vasoconstriction. Acute lowering of P_{CO_2} to 25 mm Hg is sufficient to produce symptoms. Tetany or carpopedal spasm can result from the associated alkylosis and may or may not precede the event. The diagnosis is established by a *3-minute trial of hyperventilation,* which reproduces the symptoms of presyncope or syncope. Hyperventilation usually results from **anxiety or panic disorder;** further management should be directed toward treatment of these conditions. If the problem is recurrent, acute episodes can be managed by having the patient breathe into a paper bag (CO_2 rebreathing).

18

PAIN SYNDROMES

Pain is the chief complaint in many patients. Although pain may arise from a variety of nonneurologic causes, this chapter will cover the diagnosis and management of six pain syndromes that are uniquely neurologic. Headache is covered in Chapter 15. Treatment of pain, independent of the underlying cause, is usually possible with appropriate therapeutic agents, but rational management decisions can be made only after identification of the site of the pain-producing lesion and recognition of the pathophysiology of the particular pain syndrome. Figure 18–1 outlines the possible sites and mechanisms of pain. This chapter will address the following pain syndromes:

- Sympathetically maintained pain (SMP) (reflex sympathetic dystrophy)
- Facial pain (tic douloureux)
- Postherpetic neuralgia
- Painful peripheral neuropathy
- Cervical or lumbar root compression
- Brachial neuritis

■ PHONE CALL

Questions

Questions to be asked at the time of initial contact depend on the pain syndrome. Localization will determine the subsequent path of questioning, but certain questions are pertinent to all pain syndromes. The first three questions can be asked over the phone to prepare for the history taking and examination.

1. **Where is the pain?**
   Is the pain localized, or does it radiate from one region to another, suggesting an anatomic territory?
2. **When did it begin?**
   Acute pain may respond well to specific analgesics, whereas chronic pain may require a combination of therapies, including strong psychologic support.
3. **Is there a history of injury or underlying neurologic disease?**
   Acute injury from lifting or from a mechanical task is common for radicular pain. Traumatic injury to a limb usually precedes SMP. A variety of underlying medical conditions

215

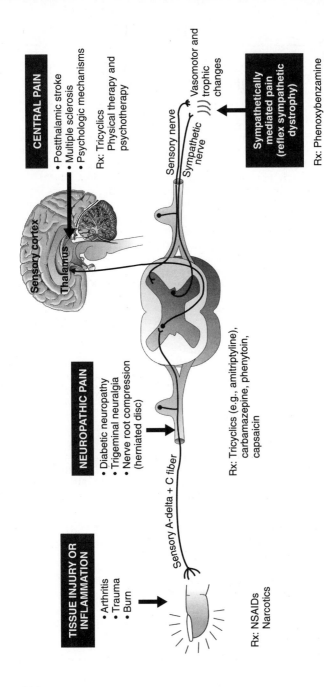

Figure 18–1 □ Sites of origin of pain within the nociceptive pathway.

predispose to painful peripheral neuropathies, including diabetes mellitus, alcoholism, acquired immunodeficiency syndrome (AIDS), and exposures to environmental toxins. Some medications can produce painful neuropathies as well.

Orders

No orders should be given over the phone. Although analgesia may be required in order to obtain an adequate history and perform an adequate physical examination, it is best to evaluate the patient yourself first.

Inform RN

"Will arrive at the bedside as soon as possible."

■ ELEVATOR THOUGHTS (DIFFERENTIAL DIAGNOSIS BASED ON LOCATION OF PAIN)

Face: trigeminal neuralgia (tic douloureux), herpes zoster ophthalmicus (or herpes zoster oticus), temporomandibular joint disease, atypical facial pain, carotid artery dissection

Neck: rheumatoid arthritis, osteoarthritis, meningitis, subarachnoid hemorrhage, vertebral artery dissection, carotid artery dissection, glomus jugulare tumor, tension headache

Low back: herniated nucleus pulposus, epidural abscess, vertebral metastasis, osteomyelitis, osteoarthritis, disk infection, herpes zoster, spinal stenosis, myofasciitis, musculoligamentous strain, ankylosing spondylitis, retroperitoneal disease (referred pain from neoplasm, pancreatitis, ulcer, aortic aneurysm, etc.)

Arms/shoulders: cervical radiculopathy, brachial plexitis, SMP, ischemic heart disease, entrapment syndromes (suprascapular syndrome, radial nerve entrapment, interosseous syndrome, lateral epicondylitis)

Hands/feet (painful peripheral neuropathies): diabetes mellitus, alcoholic neuropathy, AIDS-associated neuropathy, toxin exposure (arsenic, thallium, chloramphenicol, metronidazole), amyloidosis, carpal tunnel syndrome, de Quervain's disease, SMP, paraneoplastic sensory neuropathy, multiple myeloma, inherited neuropathies (Fabry's disease, Tangier disease, dominantly inherited sensory neuropathy)

■ MAJOR THREAT TO LIFE

Neck pain is the only category in which a missed early diagnosis could lead to significant disability or death. Etiology of pain syndromes in this category include carotid artery dissection, meningitis, and subarachnoid hemorrhage.

■ BEDSIDE

Quick Look Test

Does the patient appear acutely ill?
Tachypnea, jaundice, or a decreased level of alertness suggests that the medical illness should be attended to before the pain syndrome is addressed.

How severe does the pain appear to be?
Pain tolerance varies widely from individual to individual. Psychologic factors mediate the response to pain. You should try to get an impression of the relationship between the complaints and the true degree of disability. When you walk into the room, is the patient lying or sitting comfortably in bed or is he or she rolling about, grimacing, moaning, or holding the body in an unmoving posture?

Vital Signs

Fever suggests infection. Tachypnea may mean diabetic ketosis or hyperventilation in response to pain. Tachycardia and elevated blood pressure often accompany acute pain.

Selective History and Chart Review

1. **Define the character of the pain.**
   The questions posed during the phone call should be asked directly (Where is the pain? When did the pain begin?). It is then important to try to determine whether the pain is due to involvement of neural or nonneural tissue.

   Injury to nonneural structures (muscle, bone, or joint) is often abrupt in onset, is continuous or recurrent in specific focal regions, and is usually relieved by rest. Pain caused by injury to neural structures, by contrast, can be delayed or gradual in onset, is often paroxysmal, and is often present at rest. Numbness or tingling between episodes of pain is common. The pain is often described as burning or lancinating. Particularly when the pain is caused by injury to the peripheral nervous system, the pain may be induced by normally innocuous stimuli such as the touch of a shirt or spray from a shower.

2. **What makes the pain better or worse?**
   Dysesthesias from light tactile stimuli suggest injury to peripheral nerves. "Shooting" (radiating) pains induced by

movement of the arm or leg suggest cervical or lumbosacral radiculopathy.

3. **What is the patient's medical history?**

Ask specifically about diabetes, renal disease, and risk for human immunodeficiency virus (HIV) infection when probing for causes of peripheral neuropathy. Any history of trauma may lead to a diagnosis of nerve or root compression or SMP. Malignancy may produce neural pain either by compression from a mass or by neural infiltration. Chemotherapeutic agents such as vincristine can produce a painful neuropathy. A previous stroke, particularly in the thalamus, the lateral medulla, or the parietal lobe, may produce a late pain syndrome.

4. **What medications is the patient taking?**

See Table 18–1 for a list of medications that have pain as a potential side effect.

Selective Physical Examination I

Specific points on examination are discussed under the individual pain syndromes. Certain general principles of examination hold for all pain syndromes, however.

Musculoskeletal:	If there is pain in or around a joint, look for signs of inflammation, palpate for tenderness, and test the joint for active and passive range of motion. Be sure to percuss the spine to check for spinal involvement from infection or neoplastic disease.
Skin:	Rash may accompany an infection or a drug reaction. Vesicles of herpes zoster may precede or follow the associated neuralgia.
Abdomen:	Organomegaly may suggest chronic ethanol

Table 18–1 □ COMMON MEDICATIONS THAT CAN CAUSE PAIN OR PARESTHESIA

Antimicrobials	Psychoactive agents
Chloramphenicol	Amitriptyline
Metronidazole	Phenelzine
Streptomycin	Other medications
Nalidixic acid	Acetazolamide
Isoniazid	Pyridoxine
Antineoplastic agents	Ergotamine tartrate
Vincristine	Sulindac
Procarbazine	
Cisplatin	
Cytosine arabinoside	

abuse. Abdominal or pelvic masses may produce pain that is referred to the back or the legs.

Neurologic examination:

Focus on the motor and sensory examinations in the location of the pain. A straight leg raise test should be done when there is low back or leg pain (Fig. 18–2). A straight leg raise test is positive when raising the leg reproduces the pain (by stretching the nerve root), particularly if the pain occurs with straight leg raise of the contralateral leg. Look for muscular atrophy in the distribution of the pain to suggest chronic sensorimotor neuropathy or local nerve entrapment or compression. Sensory loss will often map to the same territory as the pain. Hyporeflexia usually accompanies peripheral neuropathy.

■ MANAGEMENT

Management of individual pain syndromes is discussed later. There are, however, some general principles of pain management that apply in any symptomatic treatment of pain.

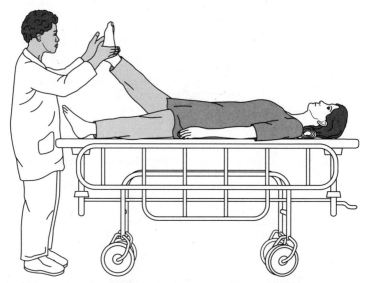

Figure 18–2 □ Straight leg raise. The physician raises each of the patient's legs, in turn, while the patient is supine. A positive test occurs when the pain is reproduced as a result of stretch on a nerve root. Pain of muscle stretch in the posterior thigh does not constitute a positive test.

1. **Treat acute pain aggressively and early.**

   A common error in managing pain is to wait to see whether the pain will go away or become less intense on its own. The problem with this approach is that peripherally induced central mechanisms may intensify and prolong the pain. Partial treatment of acute pain may also be counterproductive. **For severe, acute pain, opioids are the drug of first choice.** They are quick acting, and their actions may be reversed pharmacologically if necessary. Doses should be increased for maximal pain control and should be limited only by undesirable side effects. **Nonsteroidal anti-inflammatory drugs (NSAIDs), tricyclic antidepressants (TCAs), amphetamine, or hydroxyzine** may be useful adjuncts to opioids if only partial pain control is achieved.

2. **Avoid "as-needed" dosing for chronic or frequently recurring pain.**

   Regular dosing schedules achieve better pain control in chronic pain and minimize the anxiety from uncertainty about the next attack.

3. **Tailor the therapy to the type, location, and duration of pain.**

   Specific pharmacologic therapy remains the cornerstone of treatment, but nonpharmacologic treatment such as transcutaneous electric nerve stimulation (TENS), local or regional anesthetic blocks, or physical therapy may be useful in specific instances. Psychologic support is especially important in management of chronic pain.

■ SELECTED PAIN SYNDROMES

Sympathetically Maintained Pain (Reflex Sympathetic Dystrophy, Causalgia)

Clinical Presentation

This relatively rare entity usually occurs after trauma to a limb. The injury does not have to include neural injury. The natural history may be one of persistent pain, with the development of signs of sympathetic involvement occurring days to weeks later. Sympathetic signs may include vasoconstriction and sweating, with red, glossy skin and abnormalities of the hair and nails. Hyperpathia or allodynia to light touch or cold may be present on examination. Long-term consequences may be fixed joints and osteoporosis.

Diagnosis

The symptoms and signs resolve following sympathetic blockade. Blockade may be achieved by sympathetic ganglion blocks with local anesthetic, regional alpha-adrenergic blockade with guanethidine, or systemic alpha-adrenergic blockade with IV phentolamine.

Treatment

1. Pharmacologic: begin with **phenoxybenzamine** (systemic alpha-adrenergic blocker) **10 mg two times a day, tapering up to 120 mg per day** maximum or until unacceptable side effects (impotence, postural hypotension) occur. Alternatives are **clonidine 0.1 mg up to three times a day** or **prazosin 2 mg two times a day.**
2. Repeated regional sympathetic blockade with guanethidine.
3. Surgical sympathectomy.
4. Adjunctive therapy with phenytoin or carbamazepine may be helpful in any of the first three treatments.

Trigeminal Neuralgia (Tic Douloureux)

This disorder of the sensory division of the trigeminal nerve usually occurs in the middle and late stages of life. The cause is unknown. Degenerative or fibrotic changes in the gasserian ganglion have been reported. In some cases, the trigeminal nerve has been found to be compressed by a tumor or a blood vessel.

Clinical Presentation

Paroxysmal unilateral lightning-like jabs of pain occur in one or more divisions of the trigeminal nerve, most commonly in the second or third division. Paroxysms usually last 1 to 2 minutes but may last up to 15 minutes. The frequency of pain ranges from several times daily to once or twice a month. Typically, patients describe a trigger that induces the paroxysm, for example, chewing, facial movements, or light touch. Patients may avoid nourishment or conversation in a desperate attempt to avoid triggering an attack. There is generally no objective sensory loss or weakness in the distribution of the pain, although patients may refuse to be examined for fear of inducing a paroxysm.

Diagnosis

Because of an absence of signs, the diagnosis of trigeminal neuralgia is made on the basis of history and observation. The differential diagnosis includes dental and sinus pain, as well as herpes zoster. Herpes (and postherpetic neuralgia) most commonly involves the first division, however. The appearance of vesicles verifies the diagnosis of herpes infection.

Treatment

Carbamazepine 200 mg 2 to 5 times a day is the first-line treatment, and it induces remissions in a high percentage of patients. Phenytoin may be administered for additional benefit, if needed.

Herpetic Neuralgia (Shingles), Postherpetic Neuralgia

Clinical Presentation

Herpes zoster infection causes a painful neuropathy in a dermatomal distribution, thought to result from the reactivation of a latent infection of the virus in sensory ganglion cells (i.e., from childhood chickenpox). It occurs during the lifetime of 10 to 20% of the general population, but this incidence is mostly in the elderly and in those who are immunocompromised. A thoracic dermatome is the most common site of occurrence, followed by the cervical and then the lumbosacral dermatome. Herpes zoster ophthalmicus results from infection in the first division of the trigeminal ganglion, producing a painful vesicular eruption over the upper face and the eyes. The rash of herpes zoster appears 1 to 4 days after a prodrome of fever, malaise, and dysesthesias. The vesicular eruption becomes pustular in 3 to 4 days and then crusts over by 7 to 10 days. In the normal host, the lesions resolve without sequelae in 2 to 3 weeks. In immunocompromised hosts, however, the infection may linger.

Postherpetic neuralgia is the persistence of pain after the resolution of the rash. This occurs in 10 to 20% of patients with herpes zoster, with the bulk of occurrences in the elderly and the immunocompromised. Fifty percent of patients with postherpetic neuralgia will have a resolution of the pain in 2 months, and 70% of patients are better in 1 year. In some patients, however, the neuralgia may persist for many years.

Diagnosis

You can make the clinical diagnosis on the basis of the typical dermatomal rash. Pain and mild sensory loss should follow the same dermatomal distribution. For confirmatory diagnosis, consultation from the infectious disease or dermatology service may be helpful. Vesicles may contain polymorphonuclear leukocytes. A scrape biopsy may show giant cells and intranuclear inclusions. Varicella-zoster virus antibody titers may increase fourfold.

Treatment

1. **Acute herpes zoster infection**

   Acyclovir 5 mg/kg IV (infuse over 1 hour) three times a day for 7 days. This treatment will shorten the period of acute dermatomal pain and accelerate healing of the rash but will not reduce the incidence or severity of postherpetic neuralgia. A newer antiviral agent, **famciclovir, given orally for 7 days** may reduce the duration and severity of the neuralgia. **Prednisone 60 mg PO per day for 7 days** may reduce acute pain and potentially reduce the incidence of postherpetic neuralgia. Beware of using prednisone in immunocompromised hosts.

2. **Postherpetic neuralgia**

This condition is notoriously difficult to treat, and a variety of anticonvulsants and antidepressants have been tried. **Amitriptyline 50 to 150 mg PO per day in divided doses** may reduce the burning pain. **Carbamazepine 100 mg two times a day up to 600 or 800 mg per day** may be used as an alternative medication. Other anticonvulsants, such as phenytoin and gabapentin, may also be used.

Painful Peripheral Neuropathy

Clinical Presentation

Systemic disease affecting the peripheral nervous system produces symptoms in the longest nerves first. Dysesthesias and sensory loss in a symmetric, stocking-glove distribution are typical for early peripheral neuropathy. The patient may describe "burning" on the soles of the feet or hypersensitivity to touch in the feet more than in the hands. There may be gait disturbance from the pain of walking or from early sensory loss.

During the examination, look for wasting of the muscles, sensory loss (vibratory sense may be the first to be lost), and hyporeflexia in the distal extremities.

Diagnosis

The clinical diagnosis may often be made from the history and physical examination. Be sure to ask about diabetes mellitus, ethanol use, renal disease, and HIV risks. Occupational history may reveal exposure to toxins.

If the patient has an obvious cause (e.g., post–vincristine chemotherapy), no further workup may be needed. *Electromyography (EMG) and nerve conduction studies* can confirm a diagnosis of peripheral neuropathy and distinguish between demyelinating and axonal pathology (most painful neuropathies are axonal). Initial laboratory tests to order should include fasting glucose level with full chemistry panel including liver and thyroid function tests, rheumatologic screen (erythrocyte sedimentation rate [ESR], antinuclear antibodies [ANA], and rheumatoid factor [RF]) serum protein electrophoresis (SPEP [screen for multiple myeloma]), complete blood count (CBC), and serum vitamin B_{12} level.

Treatment

1. Treat any underlying metabolic disorder or malignancy or remove any offending neurotoxins.
2. Symptomatic treatment of painful peripheral neuropathy is with tricyclic antidepressants, which most likely act by potentiating central inhibitory signals mediated by norepineph-

rine and serotonin. Begin with **amitriptyline 10 to 25 mg daily** (lower dosage for elderly patients) and taper slowly up to 75 to 100 mg daily. Other tricyclic antidepressants may have less sedating effect and cardiac toxicity but may be less effective.

3. For topical treatment, use **capsaicin (0.075%) three to four times per day.**

4. Anti-inflammatory agents such as **ibuprofen 400 to 800 mg PO every 6 hours** may be a useful adjunct to more specific therapies, particularly when the cause of the neuropathy may be inflammatory. A 10- to 14-day tapering course of oral steroids such as **dexamethasone 6 mg PO four times a day** can be a useful analgesic while chemotherapy is being initiated.

5. Nonpharmacologic therapies such as TENS can supplement the treatment regimen.

Cervical or Lumbosacral Root Compression

Clinical Presentation

Acute low back or neck pain from root compression is often precipitated by a specific physical event such as lifting a heavy weight or twisting in an unusual way during housework or gardening. The differential diagnosis includes neck or back strain without neural injury. Radicular pain usually presents as shooting pain into an arm or leg. There is almost always perispinal pain because of reactive muscle spasm. With lumbosacral disk herniation, the pain is often increased by coughing or sneezing. Lumbar disks tend to herniate posterolaterally and cervical disks tend to herniate centrally. Disk herniation is therefore more likely to produce radicular syndromes in the low back as opposed to signs of myelopathy in the neck. Root compression in the neck, therefore, is more often seen with cervical degenerative disease. Osteoarthritis can produce cervical spondylitic ridges and osteophytes, facet joint arthritis, and neural foraminal narrowing.

Diagnosis

The typical symptom for lumbar radiculopathy is **sciatica**, or radiation of pain into the back and side of the leg. The most commonly affected roots are L5 (produced by herniation of the L4–L5 disk) and S1 (produced by herniation of the L5–S1 disk). Upper lumbar root compressions are less common. In the cervical region, C5 and C6 are the roots most affected by cervical spondylosis; C7 is the root most affected by disk lesions. Higher cervical involvement or thoracic radiculopathies warrant further investigation for neoplastic disease or neurofibromatosis. Table 18–2 lists the pain, sensory, and reflex changes for common cervical and lumbosacral radicular syndromes. Also see the **dermatome and myotome charts** in the Appendices A–1, A–2, and A–5.

Table 18–2 □ CLINICAL FEATURES OF CERVICAL AND LUMBOSACRAL ROOT COMPRESSION SYNDROMES

Root	Area of Pain	Sensory Loss	Motor Loss	Reflex
C5	Lateral upper arm and medial scapula	Lateral upper arm	Shoulder abduction, internal and external rotation, and elbow flexion	Biceps jerk
C6	Lateral forearm, thumb, and index finger	Lateral forearm and thumb	Elbow supination	Supinator jerk
C7	Over the triceps, mid-forearm, and middle finger	Middle fingers	Elbow extension and wrist extension	Triceps jerk
C8	Medial forearm and little finger	Medial forearm and little finger	Finger flexion and finger extension	Finger jerk
L4	Knee to medial malleolus	Medial knee and leg	Foot inversion and knee extension	Knee jerk
L5	Back of thigh, lateral calf, and dorsum of foot	Dorsum of foot	Foot and toe dorsiflexion	None
S1	Back of thigh, back of calf, and lateral foot	Behind lateral malleolus, sole of foot	Foot plantar flexion and foot eversion	Ankle jerk

Clinical diagnosis can usually be made from the history and examination. Be sure to check motor, sensory, and reflex function in the distribution of the pain. For lumbosacral pain, putting stretch on the root with a straight leg raise test (the exact pain syndrome should be reproduced by ipsilateral or contralateral straight leg raise) supports the diagnosis of radiculopathy (see Fig. 18–2). *Cervical or lumbosacral spinal magnetic resonance imaging (MRI)* is the diagnostic test of choice to visualize the spinal cord, the vertebrae, the disks, and the nerve roots. If there is any suspicion of a neoplastic or infectious lesion, a gadolinium MRI should be obtained.

Treatment

1. **Conservative management** with rest and analgesia usually suffices to achieve good recovery. Even if there is evidence for disk herniation, long-term recovery will be better if the condition resolves without operation. For cervical radiculopathy, a soft collar in combination with **ibuprofen 600 mg PO every 4 to 6 hours** may be enough to promote recovery. For cervical or lumbosacral root disease, the addition of narcotics such as **acetominophen with codeine 1 to 2 tabs PO every 4 to 6 hours** may be necessary, particularly in the first few days. The addition of **diazepam 2 to 5 mg every 6 hours** may also be helpful in the short term to relieve reactive muscle spasm.

2. **Surgical intervention** should be reserved for three indications: (1) bowel or bladder involvement with lumbosacral radiculopathy, (2) severe neurologic deficit, such as a complete footdrop or more than mild weakness in the upper extremity, and (3) failure to control pain or reverse a neurologic deficit with medical management for at least 3 weeks. Referral should be made to a neurosurgeon experienced with spine disease.

Brachial Neuritis (Neuralgic Amyotrophy, Brachial Neuralgia, Parsonage-Turner Syndrome)

Clinical Presentation

This rare syndrome typically begins with pain localized to the C5 and C6 dermatomes. Pain in the shoulder may have an aching quality that radiates into the arm. Some patients have mild sensory loss in the distribution of the axillary nerve. Within a few days, the shoulder girdle musculature becomes weak and atrophic, affecting the C5 and C6 myotomes. The disease is idiopathic and sporadic, affecting men more than twice as frequently as women. Most cases occur after the third decade. The syndrome may be associated with trauma, infection, or vaccination and is usually unilateral, rarely bilateral. Guarding of the shoulder may lead to a frozen shoulder.

Diagnosis

The clinical pattern of relatively rapid onset of pain followed by weakness is typical for brachial neuritis. The differential diagnosis at the early stage in which pain is the only complaint includes inflammatory and orthopedic involvement, as well as cervical radiculopathy and root compression from a rudimentary cervical rib. **EMG/nerve conduction studies usually show evidence of denervation in the affected myotomes and decreased amplitude of sensory nerve action potentials.** Subtle signs may also be present on the "unaffected" side in up to 25% of patients.

Treatment

Because the cause of brachial neuritis is unknown, there is no specific therapy. **Immobilization of the shoulder girdle** can help minimize the pain caused by movement, but gentle physical therapy with **passive range-of-motion exercises** should be used to avoid a frozen shoulder. **Ibuprofen 600 mg every 4 to 6 hours** may be used as the first therapy for analgesia. If there is no relief in 24 hours, **acetaminophen with codeine 1 to 2 tabs PO every 4 to 6 hours,** or a 2-week, tapering course of steroids, beginning with **prednisone 60 mg PO per day**, may be used. The prognosis is good, with 90% of patients making a good recovery. The prognosis is poor if the EMG shows no voluntary motor units.

19

AMNESIA AND DEMENTIA

Memory dysfunction may be variable in its presentation and ranges from the highly functioning senior citizen complaining of forgetfulness to the patient brought in by a relative for bizarre behavior and "confusion." **Amnesia** is defined as a pure loss of memory without other cognitive dysfunction. **Dementia** implies chronic, progressive cognitive loss including chronic loss of memory to a degree sufficient to interfere with occupational or social performance. Dementia should not be confused with delirium, which is an acute, global disorder of thinking and perception, characterized by impaired consciousness and inattention. **Retrograde amnesia** refers to loss of memory for events before a specific point in time. **Anterograde amnesia** is the inability to lay down new memory. Memory is often categorized into **immediate recall** (seconds), **short-term memory** (minutes to hours), and **long-term memory** (days to years), with short-term memory being the most vulnerable to pathologic processes, both in acute amnestic states and in dementia syndromes.

■ PHONE CALL

Questions

1. **What is the patient's predominant neurologic condition? In addition to memory loss, is there confusion, agitation, delirium, or stupor?**
   Although dementia or amnesia may be one element of a patient's presentation, memory loss may be part of an acute confusional state, decreased level of consciousness, or stroke.
2. **Is this new memory dysfunction, or does the patient have known dementia?**
   Much of your differential diagnosis will depend on the acuteness of onset. Acute-onset memory dysfunction suggests a vascular, epileptic, infectious, or toxic/metabolic etiology, whereas gradual onset suggests degenerative disease.
3. **How old is the patient?**
   The most common causes of dementia—Alzheimer's disease, vascular dementia, and Parkinson's disease with dementia—are diseases of the elderly. In patients younger than 60 years of age, Huntington's disease, acquired immu-

nodeficiency syndrome (AIDS), and a variety of metabolic disorders must be considered.

4. Does the patient have acute medical problems?

Although the evaluation of the dementia or amnesia may be your primary role in the patient's care and does not preclude your making an initial assessment, chronic dementia, in particular, is not a medical emergency. The acute medical illness may be a more pressing issue. Furthermore, treatment of an intervening illness may reverse a worsening of dementia.

Orders

1. Check the vital signs.
2. Obtain a finger stick glucose level.
3. If the patient is agitated, keep him or her under close observation. Avoid the use of sedative medications until an initial neurologic assessment can be made.
4. Make sure a family member or a health-care person is available to provide a history.

Inform RN

"Will arrive at the bedside in . . . minutes."

■ ELEVATOR THOUGHTS (DIFFERENTIAL DIAGNOSIS OF AMNESIA AND DEMENTIA)

V (vascular): cerebral infarction, multiple strokes, diffuse white-matter ischemia, bilateral thalamic infarctions, amyloid angiopathy

I (infectious): syphilis, chronic meningitis (tubercular or fungal), AIDS, progressive multifocal leukoencephalopathy, herpes simplex encephalitis, subacute sclerosing panencephalitis, Whipple's disease

T (traumatic): subdural hematoma, dementia pugilistica, head injury

A (autoimmune): central nervous system (CNS) vasculitis, multiple sclerosis

M (metabolic/toxic): renal failure, hepatic failure, hypothyroidism, hypercalcemia, benzodiazepine and other tranquilizer intoxication, chronic alcohol use (Wernicke-Korsakoff syndrome), vitamin B_{12} deficiency, nicotinic acid deficiency (pellagra), lead exposure, carbon monoxide exposure

I **(idiopathic/inherited):** transient global amnesia (TGA), Alzheimer's disease, Huntington's disease, Parkinson's disease, Lewy body disease, Pick's disease, progressive supranuclear palsy, amyotrophic lateral sclerosis-parkinsonism dementia complex of Guam, Wilson's disease

N **(neoplastic):** brain tumor, paraneoplastic limbic encephalitis, meningeal carcinomatosis, postradiation effects

S **(seizure, pSychiatric, structural):** complex partial seizure, postictal state, depression ("pseudodementia"), normal-pressure hydrocephalus

■ MAJOR THREAT TO LIFE

If the patient is awake, alert, and attentive, memory loss or other cognitive dysfunction is unlikely to indicate a life-threatening condition. For alterations in level of consciousness or delirium, see Chapter 6 or 9.

■ BEDSIDE

Quick Look Test

Is the patient agitated?

Patients with primary dementia can be agitated, particularly in the evening (evening disorientation and agitation is often referred to as "sundowning"), but you should be sure you are not dealing with delirium.

Does the patient look medically ill?

As mentioned earlier, medical illness can produce or exacerbate dementia. Attention may first need to be directed toward treating an acute medical condition such as hypoxia, hyperglycemia, or an infection.

Selective Physical Examination

HEENT:	Look for external signs of head trauma.
Cardiopulmonary:	Listen for rales to suggest congestive heart failure. Atrial fibrillation predisposes to cardioembolic stroke.
Abdomen:	Hepatomegaly and ascites may be signs of liver failure or chronic alcohol abuse.
Extremities:	Clubbing may indicate chronic disease. Asterixis is a nonspecific sign of metabolic disarray.

Neurologic examination:

1. **Mental status**

    Is the patient lethargic, inattentive, or aphasic? If there is a decreased level of consciousness, inattention, or aphasia, then memory deficits and other cognitive function cannot be accurately assessed. Dementia can be screened for with the standardized "Mini Mental State Examination" (MMSE) (Appendix A–6). A score less than 28 out of 30 in a younger person or less than 24 out of 30 in an older person is abnormal. The MMSE yields a quantitative score, which can be used to monitor the patient over time.

    a. **Alertness and attentiveness**

        Have the patient count backward from 20 to 1 or recite the months of the year backward. Serial sevens (serially subtracting 7 from 100) can be used also, but the test may be limited by education level.

    b. **Aphasia**

        Check for the following:

        (1) **Fluency**

            Listen for effortful, nonfluent speech with loss of grammar and syntax, not just word-finding difficulties.

        (2) **Naming**

            Anomia is a nonspecific finding common to all types of aphasia.

        (3) **Auditory comprehension of single and multistep commands**

            For example, commands such as "Show two fingers" or "With your eyes closed, tap your right knee with two fingers of your left hand."

        (4) **Repetition of unfamiliar phrases**

            When testing repetition, avoid stock phrases such as "no ifs, ands, or buts," which may be overlearned, practiced utterances.

        (5) **Reading aloud**

        (6) **Writing**

            Have the patient write his or her name, a dictated sentence, and a spontaneous sentence.

        (7) **Listen for phonemic paraphasias** (substitution of one phoneme for another within a word: e.g., "tadle" for "table") **or semantic paraphasias** (substitution of one semantically related word for another: e.g., "door" for "window").

    c. **Memory**

        Check for **immediate recall** by asking the patient to repeat number strings ("digit span"). Reciting less than six numbers forward or four numbers backward is abnormal for younger patients; reciting less than six numbers forward or three numbers backward is abnormal for patients over 65 years of age. Check **short-term memory** by asking the patient to repeat three words and then to recall them after 5 minutes. **Long-term memory** can be tested by asking the current month and year or the patient's address and phone number and by asking the patient to name present and past presidents, mayors, or sports players. Be sure to take into account education level and interests (the patient may follow sports but not politics, or vice versa).

d. **Calculations**

Ask the patient to do two-digit addition or multiplication, based on his or her education level, or to tell you how many quarters are in $1.75.

e. **Hemineglect**

Have the patient bisect a horizontal line. Average deviation from the true midline greater than 10% on six lines is abnormal. Ask the patient to perform a target cancellation task (e.g., to circle all letter As in an array of letters); look for left-right asymmetry in targets missed.

f. **Apraxia**

Apraxia is impairment of the execution of a learned or imitated movement in the absence of weakness, sensory loss, or incoordination. Ask the patient to pantomime striking a match or opening a lock with a key. Abnormal performance on this task (ideomotor apraxia) may be seen in Alzheimer's disease and other dementias. In more severe dementia, inability to use real objects in a motor sequence may be seen (ideational apraxia), for example, inability to open a milk carton or button a shirt.

g. **Drawing**

Have the patient copy a complex figure, for example, the Rey Complex Figure shown in Figure 19–1. Dyspraxia for drawing may be found in dementia. Evidence of hemineglect may also be picked up by this test.

2. **Motor**

Look for signs of hemiparesis that may suggest a focal lesion such as subdural hematoma, stroke, or tumor. **Adventitial movements** such as myoclonus, chorea, and tremor often accompany degenerative dementias, particularly in the later stages. Signs of parkinsonism may accompany Alzheimer's disease or be a part of the dementia of Lewy body disease, progressive supranuclear palsy, amyotrophic lateral sclerosis–parkinsonism–dementia complex of Guam, or idiopathic Parkinson's disease.

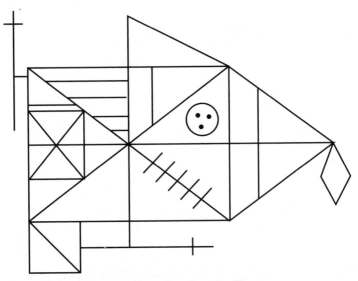

Figure 19–1 □ Rey Complex Figure.

3. **Coordination and gait**

 Ataxia may be present with **Wernicke-Korsakoff syndrome.** A **"magnetic gait,"** characterized by hesitancy and shuffling in initiation of gait and difficulty in turning 180 degrees, is seen in **normal-pressure hydrocephalus** (triad of urinary incontinence, gait dysfunction, and dementia).

4. **Frontal "release" signs**

 Frontal lobe dysfunction may produce a disinhibition of motor and behavioral functions, signaled by the appearance of the so-called frontal release signs. These include Myerson's or globellar sign and the snouting, rooting, and palmomental reflexes (Fig. 19–2).

■ **MANAGEMENT I**

1. **Check the vital signs.**

 If the patient is in respiratory distress, check an arterial blood gas measurement.

2. **Check the finger stick glucose level.**

3. **Order the following laboratory tests stat:**

 ▪ Complete blood count (CBC)
 ▪ Chemistry panel
 ▪ Erythrocyte sedimentation rate (ESR)

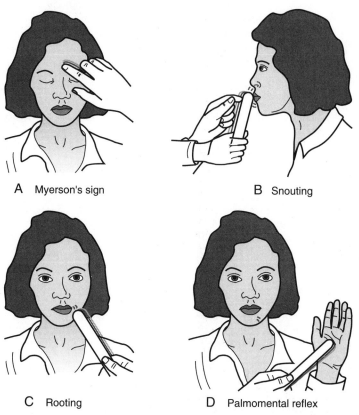

A Myerson's sign   B Snouting

C Rooting   D Palmomental reflex

Figure 19–2 □ Frontal release signs. *A*, Myerson's sign. Patient displays persistent blinking (does not habituate) to repeated taps to the brow above the bridge of the nose. *B*, Snouting. Patient purses lips reflexively in response to tapping with a pen or tongue blade. *C*, Rooting. Patient's lips and mouth deviate toward a light scratch to the side of the mouth. *D*, Palmomental reflex. Patient's chin twiches when the palm is scratched.

- Electrocardiogram (ECG)
- Chest x-ray
- Urinalysis
- Toxicology screen and ethanol level (if indicated)
4. **If the patient is too agitated to examine, follow the algorithm for delirium in Chapter 9.**

   Haloperidol (Haldol) 2 to 10 mg IM may be used unless there is alcohol use, benzodiazepine withdrawal, or hepatic encephalopathy, in which case, **lorazepam 1 to 2 mg IM or IV** may be used initially.

Selective History and Chart Review

Because of the nature of the disease, a detailed and reliable history is unlikely to come from the patient. A relative of the patient or a home health aide who knows the patient well is invaluable in helping to determine the diagnosis. Make the effort to locate such a person. If this individual is not available at the time of initial contact, try to reach that person at a later time.

1. **What was the time course of onset of the patient's memory dysfunction?**

   Has there been a gradual progression, for example, from minor forgetfulness to getting lost around town to being unable to fulfill basic needs? Or was the change relatively sudden, occurring over minutes, hours, or days? As discussed earlier, an insidious course suggests a chronic, degenerative process such as Alzheimer's disease. Be warned, however, that a patient may compensate in daily activities for some time before problems become manifest, particularly in the eyes of a loved one. If the onset was truly acute, consider a vascular, epileptic, infectious, or metabolic/toxic etiology.

2. **Has the patient started any new medications within the time frame of the memory loss?**

   Review the chart for any recent change in medications. Table 19–1 shows medications that may be associated with memory impairment.

3. **Is there any underlying medical illness?**

   Review the patient's medical history for underlying medical illness such as renal failure, hepatic failure, hypothyroidism, or other metabolic disorders.

4. **Have there been other cognitive or behavioral changes besides memory loss, such as difficulty making change in the grocery store, change in reading habits, or disorientation, particularly in the evening?**

   The differential diagnosis for an acute pure amnestic syndrome is limited. If the patient is awake, alert, and attentive and has no focal neurologic deficits, consider the diagnosis of TGA, particularly if there is no acute medical illness and no suspected drug toxicity.

Table 19–1 □ MEDICATIONS THAT MAY BE ASSOCIATED WITH MEMORY IMPAIRMENT

Corticosteroids	Chlorpromazine
Isoniazid	Anticonvulsants (overdose)
Benzodiazepines	Interleukins
Barbiturates	Methotrexate
Bromides	Clioquinol (antifungal)

5. **Is there any history of head trauma?**
   Boxers may develop chronic traumatic encephalopathy (dementia pugilistica). For the general population, head trauma may produce acute or chronic subdural hematoma, may predispose to the development of hydrocephalus, and may have an association with idiopathic Alzheimer's disease.

■ **MANAGEMENT II**

Diagnostic Testing

After acute medical illness has been eliminated as a cause of memory dysfunction, the evaluation of dementia should proceed with the following laboratory tests:
1. **Blood tests**
   - Thyroid function tests
   - Venereal Disease Research Laboratory (VDRL) test
   - Vitamin B_{12} level
   - HIV testing (if indicated)
2. **Imaging**
   - Computed tomography (CT) or magnetic resonance imaging (MRI) scan to identify structural and potentially treatable causes such as subdural hematoma, tumor, or hydrocephalus
   - Single photon emission computed tomography (SPECT) or positron emission tomography (PET) scan: Alzheimer's disease produces posterior parietotemporal hypometabolism; Pick's disease may show frontal hypometabolism; and TGA may show transient unilateral or bilateral hypoperfusion in the parieto-occipital region.
3. **Electroencephalogram (EEG)**
   EEG may help identify seizure or metabolic encephalopathy.
4. **Lumbar puncture**
   Lumbar puncture may be useful for diagnosing infection (e.g., syphilis, chronic meningitis, or herpes simplex encephalitis), carcinomatous meningitis, or hydrocephalus.

Treatment

Treatment of dementia may be possible by treating the underlying disease (infection, stroke, head trauma, intoxication, metabolic disarray, tumor, or seizure). For treating primary dementias, the management is two-pronged:

Treatment of Behavioral Dysfunction

1. **Agitation, delusions, or hallucinations/illusions**
   Treat initially with **haloperidol 0.5 to 2.0 mg PO every night or two times a day up to 10 mg per day** or **thioridazine 50 to 100 mg PO three times a day up to 800 mg per day.**
2. **Insomnia**
   Diphenhydramine 25 to 50 mg PO at night or **temazepam 7.5 to 15 mg at night** can be used.
3. **Anxiety**
   Treat with **lorazepam 0.5 to 1.0 mg PO up to three times a day** or **alprazolam 0.025 to 0.5 mg PO one or two times a day.**
4. **Depression**
   Nortriptyline 10 to 25 mg PO up to 75 mg every day, fluoxetine 20 mg per day, or **sertraline 50 to 100 mg per day** can be used.

Disease-Specific Treatment of the Pathophysiologic Process

1. **Alzheimer's disease**
   No agent has been proven effective in reversing the dementia of Alzheimer's disease. **Ergoloid mesylates (Hydergine) 3 to 6 mg daily** may produce subjective and minor objective improvement in memory, mood, and overall cognition in a small percentage of patients. **Tacrine 10 mg four times a day, tapering up to 30 mg four times a day** over several weeks, may produce some improvement in cognitive scores in some patients. **Donepezil hydrochloride 5 to 10 mg PO per day,** a newer acetylcholinesterase inhibitor, appears to slow the progression of mild to moderate Alzheimer's disease with minimal side effects.
2. **Parkinson's disease, Lewy body disease, and progressive supranuclear palsy**
   A common feature of these diseases is extrapyramidal signs from dopamine depletion. Motor dysfunction responds better than cognitive deficits to dopamine agonists. **Bromocriptine 1.25 mg PO every day** tapering slowly up to a maximum of 10 to 25 mg and **pergolide 0.05 mg every day** tapering up to 2 to 3 mg daily can be used. **Selegiline 5 to 10 mg daily** may be effective in idiopathic Parkinson's disease. Anticholinergics should be avoided in all patients with dementia in this category. Administration of dopamine agonists may be limited by the development of psychosis.
3. **Normal-pressure hydrocephalus**
   A ventriculoperitoneal shunt may produce a reversal of the urinary incontinence and gait disturbance. Reversal of the dementia is less common. Improvement of symptoms, particularly the gait, may be seen minutes to hours after a

large-volume tap—removal of 25 to 40 ml of CSF. A positive response to the lumbar puncture may indicate a better response to ventriculoperitoneal shunting.

4. **Huntington's disease**

No specific treatment is available for this disease. Antidepressants can be helpful. Propranolol may be helpful in reducing impulsive behavior.

5. **AIDS dementia complex**

Zidovudine (AZT) 200 mg every 4 hours has been shown to improve cognitive function better than placebo can. Treatment with tricyclic antidepressants and psychostimulants such as **methylphenidate 10 to 30 mg daily** in divided doses and **dextroamphetamine tapering up from a dose of 5 mg daily** in divided doses may help with the symptoms of withdrawal and abulia.

6. **Transient global amnesia**

Patients with TGA are middle-aged or older, often with hypertension, prior ischemic episodes, or atherosclerotic heart disease, but otherwise healthy. Typically, they are brought in by a relative or friend because they are "confused." On examination, there are no focal neurologic deficits. Cognitive function and language are intact, except for a profound anterograde amnesia and a retrograde amnesia for the preceding several hours or days. Patients typically appear agitated and will repeat the same question over and over, such as "What am I doing here?" The anterograde amnesia clears gradually after minutes to hours and usually resolves completely within 24 to 48 hours. A residual retrograde amnesia for the hours immediately surrounding the event is often permanent. TGA often appears in the setting of an emotional or physical stress. The pathophysiology is unknown; both epileptic mechanisms and vascular mechanisms have been proposed but have not been proved. The differential diagnosis includes unwitnessed head trauma or seizure, drug intoxication, stroke, dissociative states, and Wernicke-Korsakoff syndrome. The EEG is usually negative. The condition is self-limiting and there is no specific treatment, although some physicians have advocated using **aspirin 325 mg per day** for secondary prophylaxis. Recurrence occurs in less than one fourth of the patients.

7. **Wernicke-Korsakoff syndrome**

Wernicke-Korsakoff syndrome is a nutritional thiamine deficiency occurring in chronic alcoholics. The acute component (Wernicke's encephalopathy) is characterized by inattentiveness, lethargy, truncal ataxia, and ocular dysmotility (nystagmus—horizontal with or without a vertical or rotary component; and gaze palsy—horizontal or lateral rectus palsy, progressing to complete external ophthalmoplegia).

Other signs of nutritional deficiency may be present, such as skin changes or redness of the tongue. If left untreated, the condition is fatal in 10% of patients. Treatment is **thiamine 100 mg IV, IM, or PO daily for 3 days**, along with magnesium and multivitamins. Although the ataxia, inattentiveness, and ocular dysmotility may resolve, the more purely amnestic Korsakoff's syndrome persists in greater than 80% of patients. Korsakoff's syndrome is characterized by moderate to severe anterograde amnesia and patchy long-term memory loss. Unlike patients with TGA, patients with Korsakoff's syndrome are not distressed by their amnesia. Confabulation is often present. Even with good nutrition, the amnesia of Korsakoff's syndrome rarely resolves. Histopathology shows cell loss and degenerative changes in the dorsomedial thalami, the mamillary bodies, the periaqueductal midbrain, and the Purkinje cell layer of the cerebellar vermis.

20

BRAIN DEATH

Brain death describes a condition of complete and irreversible cessation of all cortical and brain stem activity. Although death has traditionally been defined by the irreversible cessation of cardiorespiratory function, technologic advances have led to formal recognition of death on the basis of complete and permanent brain destruction in individuals on life support. In turn, legislative and hospital policies recognizing cerebral death as the equivalent of cardiac death have enabled physicians to save thousands of lives through organ transplantation.

The most common causes of brain death are trauma, intracranial hemorrhage, and hypoxic-ischemic injury from cardiac arrest. Whatever the inciting cause, in the end, brain death ultimately results from widespread cerebral necrosis and edema, herniation, increased intracranial pressure (ICP), and the complete absence of cerebral blood flow.

■ CLINICAL SIGNIFICANCE OF BRAIN DEATH

It is important to identify and diagnose brain death **quickly** for the following reasons:
1. To prevent prolonged anguish and suffering on the part of the patient's loved ones.
2. To avoid the needless waste of valuable medical resources in an unequivocal no-win situation.
3. To create an opportunity for organ donation. Because circulatory collapse and homeostatic disarray begin as soon as brain death occurs, delays in declaration of brain death can lead to the loss of organ viability.

Although the clinical criteria for brain death outlined below are widely agreed upon, policies vary by state and institution regarding (1) the need for examination by a concurring physician, (2) the timing of examinations or a required observation period, and (3) the requirements for confirmatory testing. If you are unsure of the policy at your institution, find out. The declaration of death is a serious issue and must be made with care and precision.

■ CRITERIA FOR THE CLINICAL DIAGNOSIS OF BRAIN DEATH

To make the clinical diagnosis of brain death, the following conditions must be met:

1. **Cerebral function must be absent.**

    This means that the patient must be in deep coma, with no behavioral or reflex responses to painful stimuli mediated above the level of the foramen magnum. Triple flexion responses, deep tendon reflexes, or other primitive movements (back arching, extensor plantar responses) may be seen because of spinal reflex activity and are compatible with brain death. In most cases, the patient with brain death is in a state of flaccid and areflexic paralysis, with minimal lower-extremity triple flexion responses to deep pain. Decerebrate or decorticate posturing is incompatible with brain death, because these reflexes are mediated at the brain stem level. Seizures are incompatible with brain death as well.

2. **Brain stem functions must be absent.**

    a. **Pupils**

      The pupils must be unreactive to bright light. Size is not critical, as pupils may be small, midposition, or large. Exposure to mydriatic agents must be excluded.

    b. **Ocular movements**

      Ocular responses must be absent to passive head turning (the oculocephalic or "doll's eye" reflex) and caloric irrigation of the ear canals with 50 ml of ice water (the oculovestibular reflex). Care must be taken that the stimulus reaches the tympanic membrane. Testing using passive head turning alone is not adequate.

    c. **Facial sensation and motor response**

      Corneal reflexes should be tested with a cotton swab. Reflex or spontaneous facial or eyelid movements must be completely absent.

    d. **Pharyngeal and tracheal reflexes**

      Cough and gag responses must be absent in response to manipulation of the endotracheal tube or bronchial suctioning.

3. **The patient must be apneic.**

    Spontaneous respirations must be absent in response to a hypercarbic stimulus, as documented by formal apnea testing (Box 20–1).

4. **A proximate and untreatable cause of brain death must be established.**

    a. **The cause of coma should be clearly evident and sufficient to account for the loss of brain function.**

      Examples include documented structural disease (e.g., massive intracranial hemorrhage) or severe brain anoxia resulting from cardiopulmonary arrest.

    b. **Potentially reversible conditions must be excluded.**

      These conditions may include hypothermia (core temperature less than 32°C), drug intoxication or poisoning, hypo-

Box 20–1. PROTOCOL FOR APNEA TESTING

1. Adjust minute ventilation to attain partial pressure of carbon dioxide (P_{CO_2}) levels of 35 to 45 mm Hg and document with a **baseline arterial blood gas measurement.**
2. **Preoxygenate** with 100% oxygen for 5 minutes.
3. Place the patient on a **T-piece with 100% oxygen flow-by** at 6 to 10 L/min for 6 to 10 minutes. Because P_{CO_2} increases 3 to 4 mm Hg per minute of apnea, a *6- to 10-minute period of observation* should allow the P_{CO_2} to rise to levels of hypercarbia (greater than 55 mm Hg) sufficient to provide an adequate respiratory stimulus.
4. **Observe for respiratory movements.** Abort the test and place the patient back on mechanical ventilation if cardiac arrhythmia, hypotension, or significant oxygen desaturation occurs.
5. At the end of the observation period, **perform a second ABG measurement** to document the level of hypercarbia attained and place the patient back on **mechanical ventilation.**
6. **Write a note** in the chart documenting that no respiratory movements were observed. Record the duration of the observation period and the postobservation arterial blood gas level.

tension (systolic blood pressure [BP] less than 90 mm Hg), and severe acid-base or electrolyte abnormalities. If these conditions are present, the patient may require rewarming, treatment with IV pressors, or correction of acid-base and electrolyte disorders in order to proceed with the declaration of brain death. A toxicology screen should be performed in all patients.

c. **Loss of all brain function should persist for an appropriate period of observation.**

If the cause of coma is established and is adequate to account for brain death, an extended period of observation is not required. A period of observation of 6 to 24 hours may be appropriate if the cause of brain death is not absolutely clear (for example, suspected but unwitnessed cardiac arrest). Some institutions require a period of observation of 6 to 24 hours in all patients.

■ CONFIRMATORY TESTING

Brain death is a clinical diagnosis. *Confirmatory tests such as EEG are not essential to the declaration of brain death but may be required according to state laws or institutional policy.* In circumstances in which the clinical diagnosis of brain death cannot be made with certainty, a confirmatory test may be needed. Examples may include severe facial or limb trauma, pre-existing pupillary abnormalities, or severe pulmonary disease resulting in chronic retention of carbon dioxide.

Tests Commonly Used for the Confirmation of Brain Death

1. **Electroencephalography (EEG)**

   Confirmation of neocortical death should be documented by at least 30 minutes of electrocerebral silence, using a 16-channel instrument with increased gain settings, according to guidelines developed by the American Electroencephalographic Society. If any brain wave is present, the diagnosis of brain death cannot be made.

2. **Angiography**

   Complete absence of intracranial blood flow in a four-vessel angiogram confirms the diagnosis of brain death.

3. **Radioisotope cerebral imaging**

   The complete absence of cerebral perfusion can also be established using radionuclide angiography or single photon emission computed tomography (SPECT).

4. **Transcranial Doppler ultrasonography**

   A velocity profile showing systolic spikes with absent or reversed diastolic flow is consistent with the cessation of cerebral blood flow and brain death.

■ PSYCHOSOCIAL ISSUES

The emotional and psychosocial impact of death is always stressful for those who survive the patient; this can be even more difficult in the setting of brain death. Communication of the concept and meaning of brain death to the patient's family is paramount. This communication, however painful, should be initiated as early as possible in order to give those involved time to adjust to the situation. Although family permission is generally *not* required to discontinue life support once a patient is declared legally brain dead, their consent and understanding is extremely important. Misunderstanding, bereavement, emotional upset, and religious or moral beliefs may lead family members to object to "pulling the plug" in some cases. In these instances, third-party mediation by a medical ethics consultant or member of the clergy may be desirable.

■ MANAGEMENT OF THE POTENTIAL ORGAN DONOR

Brain death eventually leads to severe homeostatic derangements and cardiac arrest, despite mechanical ventilation and aggressive life-support measures. This inexorable progression toward multisystem organ failure creates a challenge in managing the potential organ donor, in whom the goal is to maintain and optimize organ viability for transplantation.

Most patients become hypotensive and require IV pressors at the time brain death occurs, and soon thereafter they develop diabetes insipidus (because antidiuretic hormone secretion ceases). As the situation deteriorates, hypothermia, refractory hypoxia, disseminated intravascular coagulation, and metabolic acidosis can occur. The key to management is to be ready for these complications. Even with meticulous attention to cardiovascular, acid-base, and electrolyte homeostasis, organ viability in most patients with brain death can be maintained for only 72 to 96 hours.

Protocol for Management of the Potential Organ Donor in the Intensive Care Unit

1. Insert a central venous catheter or two large-bore peripheral IV lines.
2. Insert an arterial line for continuous BP monitoring.
   a. Maintain systolic BP at or higher than 100 mm Hg with stepwise intervention:
      (1) **500 ml 0.9% saline fluid bolus (two times at 10-minute intervals)**
      (2) **Dopamine 800 mg/500 ml NS (start at 13 ml/hour, 5 μg/kg/min), titrated to maintain systolic BP at or higher than 100 mm Hg**
      (3) If refractory hypotension (systolic BP less than 90 mm Hg) or tachyarrhythmia occurs with dopamine treatment, start Pitressin drip (see below)
3. Start baseline IV flow: **0.9% saline at 150 to 200 ml/hour.**
   a. Check serum sodium levels every 6 hours:
      (1) If sodium level is 150 to 159 mmol/L, change baseline IV to 0.45% saline
      (2) If sodium level is at or higher than 160 mmol/L, change baseline IV to 0.25% saline
4. Transfuse if hematocrit is lower than 25%.

5. Adjust fraction of inspired oxygen and positive end expiratory pressure to maintain oxygen saturation at or higher than 90%.
6. Insert a Foley catheter. Measure fluid input and urine output and monitor urine specific gravity every 2 hours.
   a. If the urine output over 2 hours is greater than 500 ml with specific gravity of 1.005 or lower:
      (1) Administer **aqueous Pitressin 10 U IVP every 6 hours.**
      (2) Replace hourly urine output milliliter for milliliter with D5W
   b. If the urine output persistently remains higher than 200 ml/hour:
      (1) Stop the aqueous Pitressin IVP
      (2) Start **Pitressin 200 U/500 ml D5W; begin at 10 ml/hour (4 U/hour) and titrate to maintain urine output to less than 200 ml/hour**
7. Check the finger stick glucose level every 4 hours.
   If finger stick glucose level is higher than 350 mg/dl ×2 (over 8 hours), begin **insulin drip (100 U regular insulin in 1000 ml 0.9% saline), starting at 20 ml/hour (2 U/hour).**

SELECTED NEUROLOGIC DISORDERS

21

NERVE AND MUSCLE DISEASES

Louis H. Weimer

Patients with neuromuscular disease generally present with weakness, sensory loss, or both of these conditions. Your approach should initially focus on localizing the problem to a specific component of the peripheral nervous system that is involved (e.g., neuropathy or myopathy) and then be directed toward identifying a specific disease process. The major anatomic components of the peripheral nervous system are listed in Table 21–1.

■ APPROACH TO THE PATIENT WITH SUSPECTED NEUROMUSCULAR DISEASE

History

1. **Clarify the pattern of weakness.** Proximal weakness suggests myopathy; distal weakness suggests neuropathy.
2. **Characterize any sensory symptoms.** Have the patient identify the exact region involved.
3. **Ask about cramps and muscle twitches (fasciculations).** These symptoms point to disease of the motor neuron (amyotrophic lateral sclerosis [ALS]) or muscle (myopathy).
4. **Ask about pain.** Pain may be related to a musculoskeletal structure (e.g., herniated disk), or it may be neuropathic or muscular.
5. **Is there any autonomic involvement?** Ask about orthostatic dizziness, anhidrosis, visual blurring, urinary hesitancy or incontinence, constipation, and impotence.

Examination

1. **Determine whether the patient has true weakness.** Decreased strength needs to be differentiated from limitation arising from pain, and from submaximal effort. Effort-limited weakness is inconsistent and tends to "give way" suddenly.
2. **Map out any sensory deficits.** Think in terms of identifying *diffuse, distal sensory loss* (stocking-glove pattern), as seen in polyneuropathy; *focal sensory loss* restricted to a single root dermatome or peripheral nerve; or *multifocal sensory loss,* which suggests mononeuropathy multiplex or a plexus lesion (Fig. 21–1).

249

Table 21–1 □ BASIC ANATOMIC SUBTYPES OF NEUROMUSCULAR DISEASE

Anatomic Site	Typical Pattern of Motor and Sensory Deficit	Examples
Motor neuron disease	Weakness, wasting, fasciculations; no sensory deficits; hyperreflexia with ALS	Amyotrophic lateral sclerosis, spinal muscular atrophy, polio
Monoradiculopathy	Distribution of a single nerve root (dermatomal pattern)	L5 or S1 root compression from herniated disk
Polyradiculopathy	Distribution of multiple nerve roots	Cauda equina syndrome; carcinomatous meningitis
Plexopathy	Distribution of a nerve plexus	Acute brachial neuritis
Mononeuropathy	Distribution of a single peripheral nerve	Carpal tunnel syndrome
Mononeuropathy multiplex	Multifocal process affecting several discrete peripheral nerves	Vasculitis, leprosy
Polyneuropathy	Diffuse, symmetric, distal stocking-glove pattern; distal hyporeflexia	Diabetic polyneuropathy
Neuromuscular junction disease	Fluctuating weakness with fatigability; no sensory deficits; reflexes preserved	Myasthenia gravis
Myopathy	Diffuse proximal muscle weakness; no sensory deficits; preserved reflexes until late	Polymyositis; muscular dystrophy

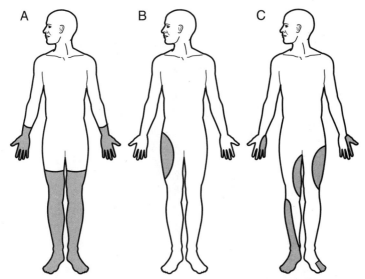

Figure 21–1 □ Patterns of sensory loss in patients with neuropathy. *A,* Polyneuropathy: diffuse stocking-glove pattern. *B,* Mononeuropathy: focal involvement corresponding to a single peripheral nerve. *C,* Mononeuritis multiplex: pattern of multiple, asymmetric regions of sensory loss, corresponding to multiple peripheral nerves.

3. **Test the reflexes.** Loss of deep tendon reflexes suggests peripheral nerve involvement.
4. **Undress the patient to check for wasting and fasciculations** (irregular individual muscle twitches). These indicate lower motor neuron disease.

■ MOTOR NEURON DISEASE

The clinical hallmarks of anterior horn cell disease are the lower motor neuron signs of **weakness, wasting (atrophy), and fasciculations.** These signs may be seen alone or in combination with upper motor neuron signs (hyperreflexia, upgoing toes) in the case of ALS. Sensory disturbances are absent. There are several distinct forms of motor neuron disease:

1. **Amyotrophic lateral sclerosis**

   Also known as Lou Gehrig's disease, ALS is the most common form of motor neuron disease. It is easily recognized on the basis of progressive weakness, wasting, fasciculations, and upper motor neuron signs. It is familial in 5 to 10% of cases. The presence of bulbar involvement (dysarthria, dysphagia) carries a worse prognosis. Median survival after diagnosis is 3 years. Approximately 5% of patients have a circulating paraprotein, and in these cases an underlying lymphoma or plasma cell dyscrasia may be detected. ALS is a clinical diagnosis, which is supported by the finding of diffuse, chronic denervation in at least three limbs on electromyography (EMG).

2. **Spinal muscular atrophy**

    This condition resembles ALS but is limited to pure lower motor neuron degeneration (e.g., no upper motor neuron signs are seen). Spinal muscular atrophy may have an earlier onset and slower progression than ALS and is more often hereditary.

3. **Multifocal motor neuropathy**

    This is an immune-mediated motor neuropathy, differentiated by the presence of **conduction block** on nerve conduction studies. The course is slowly progressive, and the weakness is often asymmetric. Some patients have anti-GM1 antibodies. The disorder is important to recognize because it is treatable with intravenous immune globulin (IVIG).

4. **Other motor neuron diseases**

    These include poliomyelitis, hereditary neurodegenerative diseases, and metabolic systemic storage disorders.

Diagnosis

Diagnostic testing for suspected motor neuron disease should include the following: EMG/nerve conduction studies (NCS), thyroid function tests, serum and urine electrophoresis, serum immunoelectrophoresis, quantitative immunoglobulins, anti-GM1 antibody levels, and cervical spine magnetic resonance imaging (MRI). In patients with a paraprotein, bone marrow biopsy should be performed.

Treatment

ALS is incurable, but two new treatments may slow the progression of the disease: **riluzole 50 mg PO twice per day**, a glutamate antagonist; and **myotrophin** (not yet approved), an insulin-like growth factor. Patients with multifocal motor neuropathy may improve with treatment with **IVIG 0.4 g/kg given every 6 to 12 weeks.**

■ MONORADICULOPATHY AND POLYRADICULOPATHY

Monoradiculopathies typically result from disk herniation and nerve root compression. They present with a radicular distribution of pain and are discussed in Chapter 18. *Polyradiculopathy* involving multiple lumbosacral nerve roots (cauda equina syndrome) presents with low back pain, urinary disturbances, and gait failure.

■ PLEXOPATHY

Diseases that cause diffuse injury to either the brachial or the lumbosacral plexus lead to **regional motor, sensory, and reflex disturbances in one limb.** The key to identifying the syndrome is to find a pattern of deficits that cannot be explained by involvement of one nerve root or a single peripheral nerve. EMG and NCS are helpful in confirming and defining the syndrome. See Appendices A–3 and A–4 for the anatomy of the brachial and lumbosacral plexus.

Brachial Plexopathy

Upper brachial plexus injury (arising from C5 to C7) results in weakness and atrophy of the shoulder and upper arm muscles (Erb's palsy). Lower brachial plexus injury (arising from C8 and T1) leads to weakness, atrophy, and sensory deficits in the forearm and hand (Klumpke's palsy). The main causes of brachial plexopathy include the following:

- **Trauma**
- **Idiopathic brachial neuritis (Parsonage-Turner syndrome)**

    This underrecognized syndrome presents with the sudden onset of pain in the shoulder and arm; as the pain resolves over 2 to 4 weeks, weakness and muscle wasting become evident.
- **Tumor infiltration**

    Metastatic disease and neurofibroma are most common.
- **Radiation plexopathy**

    High-dose irradiation for lymphoma or breast cancer can lead to painless progressive brachial plexopathy 1 to 5 years later. *Myokymia* is often a feature.
- **Cervical rib or bands (thoracic outlet syndrome)**

    This rare condition is caused by compression of the lower trunk of the brachial plexus as it passes over an abnormal first cervical rib or fibrous band. Patients complain of pain and paresthesias in the C8/T1 distribution of the hand and medial forearm when carrying heavy objects or when raising the arm above shoulder level. Surgical decompression may be helpful in rare cases.

Diagnosis

In many cases, the cause of brachial plexopathy is readily apparent (e.g., trauma or radiation). If not, chest and cervical spine x-rays, lumbar puncture (LP), and MRI of the plexus should be considered.

Treatment

Physical therapy can help speed recovery, minimize muscle wasting, and prevent contractures.

Lumbosacral Plexopathy

Unilateral lumbosacral plexopathy is rare. The main diagnostic considerations include idiopathic neuritis, diabetic infarction, and compression from a retroperitoneal abscess, hemorrhage, or neoplasm. MRI or CT of the pelvis should be performed to exclude a compressive mass lesion.

■ MONONEUROPATHIES

Mononeuropathies result from injury, compression, or entrapment of a single nerve, usually at a specific site. There are several different syndromes.

Carpal Tunnel Syndrome

Carpal tunnel syndrome is by far the most common cause of mononeuropathy; it results from compression of the median nerve at the wrist and usually presents with wrist pain and tingling of the first three digits. The pain may radiate proximally to the elbow and is almost always worse at night. Examination may reveal Tinel's sign (radiation of pain into the first three digits when the wrist is tapped with a hammer), thenar muscle wasting, and sensory deficits in the distribution of the median nerve (Fig. 21–2). Risk factors include repetitive "overuse" injury, thyroid disease, pregnancy, acromegaly, diabetes, and amyloidosis.

Diagnosis

EMG and NCS show focal sensory and/or motor slowing across the wrist in the median nerve. Check thyroid function tests and fasting glucose level to screen for hypothyroidism and diabetes.

Treatment

Mild disease can be treated with a neutral position wrist splint; more severe disease may require surgical decompression. Repetitive stress to the wrist can be minimized with special occupational devices.

Facial Palsy (Bell's Palsy)

Facial palsy (Bell's palsy) is the most common cranial mononeuropathy. Patients present with acute unilateral facial paralysis, with equal involvement of the forehead and lower half of the face. The disorder is thought to result from compression of CN 7 within the facial canal. In some patients, an antecedent viral infection is identified, and approximately 25% of cases are associated with pain in the ipsilateral ear. If the injury to the facial

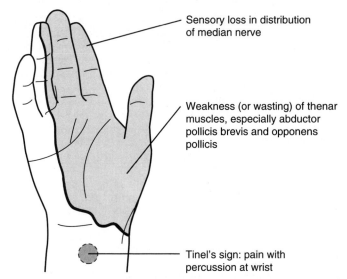

Sensory loss in distribution of median nerve

Weakness (or wasting) of thenar muscles, especially abductor pollicis brevis and opponens pollicis

Tinel's sign: pain with percussion at wrist

Figure 21–2 □ Sensory and motor involvement in carpal tunnel syndrome.

nerve is proximal to the chorda tympani in the facial canal, loss of taste occurs on the anterior two thirds of the tongue ipsilaterally. Complete or near-complete recovery occurs in 85% of cases.

Diagnosis

The majority of cases are idiopathic (Bell's palsy). Examination should focus on searching for signs of other treatable diseases that can present with facial paralysis:

- Decreased hearing or a decreased afferent corneal reflex is suggestive of a cerebellopontine angle tumor (e.g., acoustic neuroma), which should be excluded by MRI with gadolinium.
- Vesicles in the external auditory canal are indicative of the Ramsay Hunt syndrome, which results from herpes zoster infection of the ipsilateral geniculate ganglion.
- An antecedent annular rash or tick bite is suggestive of Lyme disease. Serum Lyme antibody titers and LP with testing for cerebrospinal fluid (CSF) Lyme antibodies are required to establish the diagnosis.
- Interstitial lung disease with hilar adenopathy, uveitis, or parotitis may be clues to neurosarcoidosis. CSF examination may reveal a lymphocytic pleocytosis; biopsy of involved tissue is required to establish the diagnosis.

Treatment

Recovery from idiopathic Bell's palsy can be accelerated by treatment with **prednisone 80 mg PO daily for 5 days,** followed by a 7-day taper. Ramsay Hunt syndrome is treated with **acyclovir 800 mg PO five times daily for 7 days** in addition to prednisone. The likelihood of complete recovery is increased when treatment is started within 7 days of onset. Treatment for Lyme disease (see Chapter 23) and neurosarcoidosis (see Chapter 22) is discussed elsewhere. Patients with incomplete eye closure should use an ophthalmic ointment (e.g., Lacri-Lube) and a protective eye shield at night to prevent corneal abrasions.

Other Common Nerve Entrapment Syndromes

The nerves implicated in selected other entrapment syndromes are the following:
- Ulnar nerve at the medial epicondyle of the humerus
- Median nerve at the pronator teres (pronator syndrome)
- Radial nerve at the spiral groove of the humerus (Saturday night palsy)
- Obturator nerve at the obturator foramen (childbirth)
- Peroneal nerve at the fibular head (leg crossers and surgical malpositioning)
- Lateral femoral cutaneous nerve (meralgia paresthetica)
- Posterior tibial nerve at the tarsal tunnel

■ MONONEUROPATHY MULTIPLEX

Diseases that affect multiple peripheral nerves at different sites result in the syndrome of *mononeuropathy multiplex.* The presence of **asymmetric and multifocal motor, sensory, and reflex deficits** is the key to identifying the syndrome. The patient's history may reveal a stepwise progression of deficits. The differential diagnosis of mononeuropathy multiplex includes the following:
- Vasculitis
    Polyarteritis nodosa is the most common vasculitis associated with this condition. Systemic lupus erythematosus, rheumatoid arthritis, and cryoglobulinemia may, on rare occasions, produce the condition.
- Diabetes mellitus
- Leprosy
- Sarcoidosis
- Human immunodeficiency virus (HIV) infection
- Lymphoma
- Hereditary liability to pressure palsies
- Multifocal motor neuropathy (pure motor)
- Chronic inflammatory demyelinating polyneuropathy (CIDP)

Diagnosis

Initial blood tests should include fasting glucose level with chem-20 screen, complete blood count (CBC), erythrocyte sedimentation rate (ESR), antinuclear antibody (ANA), rheumatoid factor (RF), antineurotrophil cytoplasmic antibody (ANCA), HIV testing, hepatitis serologies, cryoglobulins, and serum angiotensin converting enzyme (ACE) activity. LP should be considered to rule out inflammatory conditions (e.g., chronic inflammatory demyelinating polyneuropathy, neurosarcoidosis) and carcinomatous meningitis. A comprehensive EMG and NCS examination is often needed to prove multifocal involvement. Muscle or nerve biopsy is usually necessary to rule out vasculitis, sarcoidosis, leprosy, and lymphoma.

Treatment

Therapy is directed toward treating the underlying disease.

■ POLYNEUROPATHY

The prototypical polyneuropathy patient presents with gradual **distal, symmetric sensorimotor deficits and hyporeflexia.** Typically, the longest nerves in the body are affected first, resulting in a stocking-glove distribution of symptoms and signs (see Fig. 21–1). Dysesthetic sensory changes are often the first symptom, with weakness developing later.

The number of entities that can cause peripheral neuropathy is vast (Table 21–2), and pinpointing a precise cause can be difficult. An organized and stepwise approach is essential. **Consideration of the following points can help narrow the possibilities and allow you to screen for the most common and important (i.e., treatable) causes.**

Clinical Approach to the Patient with Polyneuropathy

1. **History**
   - **Is the neuropathy acute or chronic?** Acute polyneuropathy (Guillain-Barré syndrome) is discussed in Chapter 16.
   - **Ask a carefully directed set of questions to identify an obvious cause.** Ask about diabetes, renal disease, HIV infection, current medications, alcohol use, potential exposure to toxins, and family history. *The majority of polyneuropathies are complications of previously evident medical disorders, medications, or alcohol.*
   - **Do the symptoms fluctuate?** Fluctuations suggest a relapsing demyelinating neuropathy (CIDP) or repeated exposures to toxins.
2. **Examination**
   - **Determine the predominant systems involved.** Most neuropathies are sensorimotor, with the sensory component predominant. Identifying a predominantly motor, pure sensory, or particularly painful neuropathy helps to limit the differential diagnosis considerably (Table 21–3).

Table 21–2 □ CAUSES OF PERIPHERAL POLYNEUROPATHY

Metabolic and endocrine diseases
Diabetes mellitus*
Renal failure*
Hepatic failure
Porphyria
Hypothyroidism
Critical illness polyneuropathy*
Vitamin deficiency states
Beriberi (thiamine deficiency)
Vitamin B_6 (pyridoxine) deficiency
Vitamin B_{12} deficiency .
Vitamin B complex deficiency
Pellagra (niacin deficiency)
Vitamin E deficiency
Toxins and poisons
Alcohol
Heavy metals: arsenic, lead, mercury, thallium
Organic and industrial solvents: carbon disulfide, hexane, acrylamide, methyl-N-butyl ketone
Pyridoxine (vitamin B_6) overdose
Nitrous oxide (also causes myopathy)
Medications
Antibiotics: dapsone, nitrofurantoin, isoniazid, ethambutol, metronidazole, stavudine (d4T), 3TC, didanosine (ddI), dideoxyctidine (ddC), zidovudine
Antiarrhythmics: amiodarone, procainamide
Chemotherapeutic agents*: vincristine, vinblastine, cisplatin, paclitaxel (Taxol), adriamycin
Cimetidine
Chloroquine (also causes myopathy)
Colchicine (also causes myopathy)
D-Penicillamine
Disulfiram

Table continued on opposite page

- **Determine whether the findings are asymmetric.** Patchy and asymmetric motor, sensory, and reflex deficits suggest *mononeuropathy multiplex* or *polyradiculopathy* (see above).
- **Check for palpably enlarged nerves.** Although unusual, this finding can help pinpoint the diagnosis (see Table 21–3).

3. **EMG and NCS**
   - **Determine whether the neuropathy is axonal or demyelinating.** Electrodiagnosis is critical for making this distinction, which can help to narrow your differential diagnosis. *Distal axonal sensorimotor neuropathies* are the most common. *Demyelinating neuropathies* have a much smaller differential diagnosis (see Table 21–3).

Table 21–2 □ **CAUSES OF PERIPHERAL POLYNEUROPATHY** *Continued*

Medications *Continued*
Gold salts
Hydralazine
Ipecac
Phenytoin
Thalidomide

Immunologic or paraprotein-mediated diseases
Acute inflammatory polyneuropathy (Guillain-Barré syndrome)*
Chronic inflammatory polyneuropathy (chronic inflammatory demyelinating polyneuropathy)*
Paraneoplastic disease (sensorimotor or pure sensory)*
Multiple myeloma
Anti–myelin-associated glycoprotein antibody-mediated disease
Amyloidosis
Lymphoma with paraprotein
Monoclonal gammopathy
Cryoglobulinemia
Collagen vascular disease (systemic lupus erythematosus, rheumatoid arthritis, etc.)
Sarcoidosis

Genetic/hereditary diseases
Charcot-Marie-Tooth disease*
Refsum's disease
Storage diseases (metachromatic leukodystrophy, adrenomyeloneuropathy, etc.)
Inherited metabolic enzyme defects

Infectious diseases
Human immunodeficiency virus infection*
Cytomegalovirus infection*
Leprosy
Lyme disease
Human T-cell leukemia virus type I (HTLV-1) infection (also causes myelopathy)

* Common

Management

Laboratory Testing for Evaluation of Polyneuropathy

1. If an obvious cause for the neuropathy exists (e.g., post–vincristine chemotherapy), no further workup may be needed. Otherwise proceed with the next steps.
2. The following initial laboratory tests should be performed: fasting glucose with full chemistry panel including liver function tests (LFTs), CBC, TFTs, initial rheumatologic screen (ESR, ANA, RF), serum protein electrophoresis, vitamin B_{12} level.
3. Other tests to consider include LP, testing of urine for paraproteins, serum immunofixation electrophoresis, quantitative

Table 21–3 □ **FEATURES HELPFUL IN NARROWING THE CAUSE OF PERIPHERAL NEUROPATHY: SYNDROMES OTHER THAN DISTAL AXONAL NEUROPATHIES**

Pure (or predominantly) motor neuropathy	Lymphoma, multifocal motor neuropathy (with or without anti-GM1 antibodies) *Toxic:* dapsone, lead, organophosphates Porphyria Guillain-Barré syndrome Tick paralysis Diphtheria
Pure (or predominantly) sensory neuropathy*	Acute idiopathic sensory neuropathy Primary biliary cirrhosis Sjögren's syndrome Diabetes mellitus Human immunodeficiency virus infection Hereditary sensory and autonomic neuropathies Uremia Paraneoplastic sensory ganglioneuritis (anti-Hu antibodies) *Toxic:* thallium, pyridoxine (vitamin B_6) intoxication
Palpably enlarged nerves	*Genetic:* Charcot-Marie-Tooth disease, Dejerine-Sottas disease, Refsum's disease, neurofibromatosis, hereditary liability to pressure palsies Leprosy Chronic inflammatory demyelinating polyneuropathy
Demyelinating neuropathies	*Immunologic:* Guillain-Barré syndrome, chronic inflammatory demyelinating polyneuropathy, paraproteinemia, anti-MAG (myelin-associated glycoprotein) antibodies *Toxic:* diphtheria, buckthorn toxin, amiodarone, perhexiline *Genetic:* Charcot-Marie-Tooth type I disease, storage diseases, hereditary liability to pressure palsies

*Usually small-fiber sensory loss (pain, temperature) with prominent autonomic dysfunction.

immunoglobulins, testing urine for heavy metals, tests for HIV, CMV, human T-cell leukemia virus type I (HTLV-1), Lyme antibody, other vitamin levels (vitamins B and E), ANCA, ACE level, homocysteine/methionine levels (vitamin B_{12} deficiency), genetic testing (Charcot-Marie-Tooth disease), special antibody assays (anti-Hu, anti-GM1, anti-MAG, anti-sulfatide), and bone marrow biopsy.

4. Nerve and muscle biopsy is helpful for confirming several diagnoses (Table 21–4), but it is most useful in evaluating *mononeuropathy multiplex.*

Selected Causes of Neuropathy

- **Diabetes mellitus**

  Diabetes is the most common cause of neuropathy in the

Table 21–4 □ CAUSES OF PERIPHERAL NEUROPATHY THAT CAN BE DIAGNOSED BY NERVE BIOPSY

Vasculitis
Leprosy
Lymphoma
Cytomegalovirus (causes polyradiculopathy or mononeuropathy multiplex)
Storage diseases (metachromatic leukodystrophy [MLD],
    adrenomyeloneuropathy [AMN], Krabbe's disease)
Sarcoidosis
Amyloidosis
Immune-mediated diseases (IgM and complement deposition)

United States. Several different forms of neuropathy may occur, and an individual may have more than one type:

1. **Distal axonal sensorimotor neuropathy** is most common. Sensory symptoms (small fiber) usually predominate, including painful dysesthesias.
2. **Autonomic neuropathy** is commonly seen in combination with axonal small-fiber sensory neuropathy. Symptoms may include anhidrosis, orthostatic hypotension, impotence, gastroparesis, and bowel and bladder disturbances.
3. **Mononeuropathy** may occur from either nerve infarction or entrapment (e.g., carpal tunnel syndrome).
4. **Mononeuropathy multiplex**
5. **Diabetic amyotrophy (asymmetric proximal motor neuropathy)** presents with dull, aching proximal pain, followed by asymmetric proximal leg weakness and wasting not limited to a root, plexus, or nerve territory.

- **Ethanol**
  Ethanol is a very common cause of axonal sensorimotor neuropathy with prominent distal paresthesias and numbness. Vitamin B complex supplements and alcohol cessation can lead to improvement.
- **Uremia**
  Renal failure often leads to a distal, axonal, sensorimotor neuropathy with prominent cramps and unpleasant dysesthesias. Improvement may occur with dialysis or kidney transplantation.
- **Chronic inflammatory demyelinating polyneuropathy**
  CIDP presents as a chronic relapsing sensorimotor polyneuropathy or, rarely, as mononeuropathy multiplex. The diagnosis is confirmed by *elevated CSF protein* and *a demyelinating pattern on EMG/NCS*. In some cases, a plasma cell dyscrasia or paraprotein may be identified. **Prednisone, starting at 60 mg/day,** is the treatment of first choice. Long-term daily maintenance doses of 5 to 20 mg may be required in

responders. **Plasmapheresis, IVIG (0.4 g/kg per treatment),** and **azathioprine 150 mg per day** are other treatment options.

- **Paraprotein-associated neuropathy**
    These neuropathies can result in a demyelinating or axonal sensorimotor neuropathy. CSF protein is elevated in 80% of demyelinating cases. The protein can be identified by either serum or urine protein electrophoresis or immunofixation electrophoresis. Bone marrow biopsy may be helpful in the two thirds of cases with plasma cell dyscrasia; in the remaining patients, multiple myeloma (in 12%), amyloidosis (in 9%), lymphoma (in 5%), leukemia (in 3%), or Waldenstrom's macroglobulinemia (in 2%) may be identified. **Prednisone 40 to 100 mg per day** or **azathioprine 150 mg per day** may benefit some patients; **plasmapheresis** and **IVIG** are other treatment options.
- **Critical illness polyneuropathy**
    This polyneuropathy is associated with sepsis and multisystem organ failure. It usually presents as failure to wean from mechanical ventilation. EMG/NCS is consistent with severe sensorimotor axonal neuropathy. There is no specific treatment, but if the patient survives, recovery is the rule.
- **Paraneoplastic neuropathy**
    Paraplastic neuropathy most often manifests as an *axonal sensorimotor neuropathy,* but it can also take the form of a *large-fiber pure sensory neuropathy,* a *demyelinating sensorimotor neuropathy,* or a *pure motor neuronopathy* (usually seen with lymphoma). These and other paraneoplastic syndromes (see Chapter 24) are mediated by autoimmune responses against peripheral nerve.
- **Genetic (hereditary) neuropathies**
    These neuropathies are unusual except for **Charcot-Marie-Tooth disease,** which comes in two forms: type I (demyelinating) and the less common type II (axonal). The disease is autosomal dominant, with variable expression from one generation to the next. Patients present with insidious distal lower extremity weakness and wasting ("stork leg deformity"), high arches, pes cavus, and minimal sensory symptoms.

General Care of the Patient with Neuropathy

1. **Remove any potential neurotoxic medications,** even if these are not the primary cause (see Table 21–2 for a list).
2. **Treat neuropathic pain** with tricyclic antidepressants **(amitriptyline 25 to 100 mg daily** or **nortriptyline 10 to 25 mg daily), carbamazepine 200 mg three to four times a day,** or **capsaicin cream 0.075% three to four times a day.**
3. **Initiate occupational and physical therapy** in patients with

moderate to severe disability for gait training, prevention of contractures, orthoses, and assistive devices.

4. **Skin care** is important in patients with severe sensory neuropathy to prevent trophic ulcers, infections, and neuropathic (Charcot) joints.

5. **Autonomic neuropathy** may require treatment for orthostatic hypotension **(fludrocortisone 0.1 mg one to three times a day)** and gastroparesis **(metoclopramide 5 to 10 mg three times a day).**

■ NEUROMUSCULAR JUNCTION DISEASE

Myasthenia gravis and **botulism,** both of which can lead to respiratory failure, are discussed in Chapter 16.

■ MYOPATHY

Diseases of muscle typically lead to **proximal, symmetric weakness** without sensory deficits or bowel or bladder symptoms. The patient may complain of difficulty reaching above the head, getting out of a chair, or climbing stairs.

Questions to Ask the Patient with Suspected Myopathic Disease

1. Does the patient have muscle aches or tenderness, suggestive of muscle inflammation or necrosis?
2. Has the patient noticed darkened, cola-colored urine *(myoglobinuria)*?
3. Does the weakness fluctuate or worsen with exercise, suggestive of myasthenia gravis or periodic paralysis?
4. Are there any sensory or bowel or bladder symptoms? (Such symptoms would make a myopathic disease unlikely.)
5. Have there been any new cardiac symptoms? (Many entities affect both skeletal and cardiac muscle.)

Examination

1. Map out the pattern of weakness (proximal versus distal). Most myopathies cause proximal weakness; exceptions include myotonic dystrophy, inclusion body myositis, and rare genetic causes.
2. Check for *myotonia* (prolonged muscle contraction after voluntary contraction or percussion), which can be tested by handgrip, forced eye closure, or muscle percussion.
3. Palpate for muscle tenderness.
4. Undress the patient to evaluate for a pattern of muscle wasting.

Management

Diagnostic Testing

1. **Initial laboratory tests.** Creatine phosphokinase (CPK) level, chem-20 screen, TFTs, sedimentation rate, ECG
2. **EMG/NCS.** Needle electromyography in patients with myopathy shows abnormal, short-duration, low-amplitude, polyphasic motor unit potentials and overly rapid recruitment of motor units with an excessively low amplitude interference pattern (see Chapter 4).
3. **Muscle biopsy** is often needed to establish a diagnosis.
4. **Other tests to consider** include ACE level, serum cortisol level, serum and CSF lactate (mitochondrial myopathy), forearm ischemic exercise test (for McArdle's disease), genetic testing (for muscular and myotonic dystrophy), and toxicology screen.

Causes of Myopathy

Causes of myopathy can be categorized into five main groups: **inflammatory, endocrine, toxic, hereditary, and infectious.**

1. **Inflammatory myopathies**
   a. **Polymyositis**
      This is an inflammatory autoimmune muscle disease characterized by chronic and relapsing proximal limb weakness. Although the eyes and face are almost never affected, pharyngeal and neck weakness is common (in approximately 50% of patients). Cardiomyopathy, interstitial lung disease, and other systemic autoimmune diseases (e.g., systemic lupus erythematosus, Crohn's disease) are also found in a significant proportion of patients.
      (1) Diagnosis: CPK levels are elevated in almost all cases, and EMG shows myopathic findings with denervation secondary to segmental muscle necrosis. Muscle biopsy reveals endomesial lymphocytic infiltrates, necrotic and atrophic muscle fibers, and connective tissue deposition.
      (2) Treatment: **Prednisone 60 to 100 mg daily** leads to improvement in most patients within 2 to 3 months and is most effective early in the disease course. **Azathioprine 1 to 3 mg/kg per day** or **methotrexate 25 to 50 mg per week** can be used for disease suppression in steroid nonresponders.
   b. **Dermatomyositis**
      Dermatomyositis is similar to polymyositis but is accompanied by a characteristic rash that precedes or accompanies muscle weakness. Skin manifestations include a heliotrope (bluish) rash on the upper eyelids, erythematous rash on the face and trunk, violaceous scaly eruptions on the knuckles (Gottron's papules), and subcutaneous calcifications.
      (1) Diagnosis: Muscle biopsy findings differ from polymyo-

sitis in showing perivascular inflammation and *perifascicular atrophy*. A malignancy screen is prudent with a later age of onset.

(2) Treatment: Treatment is the same as for polymyositis.

c. **Inclusion body myositis**

This entity differs from polymyositis in that it tends to produce distal and asymmetric weakness, it occurs primarily at an older age, and it responds poorly to steroids. Muscle biopsy reveals rimmed vacuoles and eosinophilic cytoplasmic inclusions with amyloid. **IVIG (0.4 mg/kg per treatment)** may improve strength. Finger flexor and quadriceps weakness is a hallmark.

d. **Sarcoidosis**

Patients with sarcoidosis can develop focal or generalized myopathy. Biopsy shows noncaseating granulomas. Steroids usually produce clinical improvement.

2. **Endocrine myopathies**

Patients with endocrine myopathy usually show systemic signs of endocrine disease before the onset of weakness, but in some instances, myopathy is the presenting feature. CPK levels are usually normal or only mildly elevated. In all cases, weakness is reversed by treating the underlying endocrinopathy, which includes **thyroid disease, Cushing's disease (hyperadrenalism),** or **parathyroid disease.**

3. **Toxic myopathies**

a. Medications

Drugs and medications produce subacute, generalized proximal muscle weakness through a variety of mechanisms. Table 21–5 lists some medications and toxins commonly associated with myopathy.

b. **Critical illness myopathy**

This myopathy presents as a failure to wean from mechan-

Table 21–5 □ DRUGS THAT CAN CAUSE MYOPATHY

Rhabdomyolysis	Procainamide
Amphotericin B	Cimetidine
ε-aminocaproic acid	**Myopathy (weakness and myalgia)**
Fenfluramine	Colchicine
Heroin	Zidovudine
Phencyclidine	Steroids
Alcohol	Clofibrate
Barbiturates	Chloroquine
Cocaine	Emetine
Hypokalemic myopathy	Labetalol
Diuretics	Perhexiline
Azathioprine	Propranolol
Myositis (inflammatory)	Vincristine
Penicillamine	

ical ventilation in ICU patients treated with steroids and nondepolarizing paralyzing agents (e.g., vecuronium). Muscle biopsy shows selective loss of thick myosin filaments.

c. **Neuroleptic malignant syndrome**

Dopamine blockers (e.g., haloperidol, chlorpromazine [Thorazine]) can produce this rare, idiosyncratic response characterized by generalized muscle rigidity with rhabdomyolysis, fever, altered mental status, tremor, and autonomic instability (especially hypertension). CPK levels are always elevated; white blood cell counts are usually increased. Treatment includes discontinuation of the offending agent, surface cooling, **dantrolene 1 to 10 mg/kg per day IV every 4 to 6 hours** as needed to attain muscle relaxation, and **bromocriptine 2.5 to 5 mg three times a day.**

d. **Malignant hyperthermia**

This is an autosomal dominant condition that predisposes to severe muscle rigidity, rhabdomyolysis, fever, and metabolic acidosis following exposure to inhalation anesthetics or succinylcholine. Treatment is with **dantrolene 1 to 2 mg/ kg IV in repeated doses.**

4. **Hereditary myopathies**

a. **Muscular dystrophy**

This is a progressively degenerative genetic myopathy. Weakness is usually present in early life, gets worse over time, and often leads to early death.

(1) **Duchenne muscular dystrophy** (X-linked). The onset is by age 5 with inability to walk occurring by age 10 and with eventual respiratory failure. Features include calf pseudohypertrophy, cardiomyopathy, and occasional mental impairment. *Becker muscular dystrophy* is a later-onset form of the disease with less severe manifestations. **Prednisone 20 to 40 mg per day** can increase strength and function, but it does not alter the overall course. Diagnosis is confirmed by abnormal dystrophin staining on biopsy.

(2) **Myotonic dystrophy** (autosomal dominant). This is the most common form of muscular dystrophy. It leads to progressive *distal* myopathy. The disease occurs earlier and is more severe with successive generations (genetic anticipation). Besides myotonia, features include a distinctive facies with ptosis and frontal balding, cataracts, cardiac conduction defects, gonadal atrophy, and mental impairment. **Phenytoin 300 mg per day PO** and **procainamide 20 to 50 mg/kg per day three times a day** occasionally are used to treat the myotonia, if clinically necessary. ECGs performed at least yearly are prudent to assess for evolving heart block.

(3) **Other myopathies.** These include facioscapulohumeral

(autosomal dominant), limb girdle (autosomal recessive), oculopharyngeal (autosomal recessive), and Emery-Dreifuss (X-linked) myopathies.

b. **Metabolic myopathies**

Seen mostly in the pediatric population, these diseases result from deficiencies of specific enzymes involved in utilization of glucose or lipid (the two main sources of skeletal muscle energy). Besides muscle weakness, patients with metabolic myopathies often experience *rhabdomyolysis* and *myoglobinuria*. Muscle biopsy is necessary to establish the diagnosis. The most common metabolic myopathy is **McArdle's disease,** an autosomal recessive disorder resulting from myophosphorylase deficiency. It presents in childhood with painful muscle cramps and myoglobinuria after intense exercise. A lack of increase in lactate levels with ischemic forearm testing is characteristic.

c. **Periodic paralysis**

These rare disorders are caused by genetic abnormalities of membrane ion channels. The majority are inherited in autosomal dominant fashion. Patients are usually normal between attacks of severe weakness. **Hypokalemic** and **hyperkalemic** forms have been described.

d. **Congenital myopathies**

This group of rare disorders presents mostly at birth with floppy infant syndrome, and the disorders are usually nonprogressive. Examples include nemaline (rod) body myopathy, myotubular (centronuclear) myopathy, and central core disease.

e. **Mitochondrial myopathy**

These diseases result from defects in the mitochondrial genome and hence are maternally inherited. Muscle biopsy shows "ragged red fibers." Suspicious signs for mitochondrial diseases include ptosis, ophthalmoparesis, and high serum lactate levels. Variants include myoclonic epilepsy with ragged red fibers, MELAS (mitochondrial encephalomyopathy, encephalopathy, lactic acidosis, and stroke-like episodes), and Kearns-Sayre syndrome (pigmentary retinopathy, cardiac conduction defects, high CSF protein). Genetic analysis is available for many types of mitochondrial myopathies.

5. **Infectious myopathies**

Muscle infiltration with the organisms that cause *trichinosis, toxoplasmosis,* and *cysticercosis* can lead to a widespread or a localized inflammatory myopathy. Acute rhabdomyolsis and myoglobinuria can occur as a result of infection with influenza virus, rubella virus, coxsackievirus, echoviruses, and mycoplasma. HIV myopathy is not uncommon and must be distinguished from zidovudine toxicity.

DEMYELINATING AND INFLAMMATORY DISORDERS OF THE CENTRAL NERVOUS SYSTEM

Timothy Lynch

Several diseases affecting the central nervous system (CNS) involve destruction of myelin. Diseases in which normal myelin is disrupted are considered demyelinating, whereas diseases in which an intrinsic abnormality of myelin exists are considered dysmyelinating. The best example of demyelinating disease (loss of myelin with relative preservation of the axons) is multiple sclerosis (MS). Dysmyelinating disorders almost always present in childhood and will not be discussed in this chapter.

Diseases affecting myelin can be classified as follows:

1. **Acquired inflammatory or infectious demyelination** (e.g., MS, acute disseminated encephalomyelitis, acute necrotizing hemorrhagic encephalomyelitis, progressive multifocal leucoencephalopathy)
2. **Hereditary metabolic disorders of myelin** (e.g., metachromatic leukodystrophy, adrenoleukodystrophy, Canavan's disease, Alexander's disease)
3. **Acquired toxic/metabolic disorders of myelin** (e.g., central pontine myelinolysis, hexachlorophene exposure, Marchiafava-Bignami disease)
4. **Nutritional disorders of myelin** (e.g., vitamin B_{12} deficiency)
5. **Traumatic disorders of myelin** (e.g., traumatic compression)

Table 22–1 lists the pathologic features of myelin disorders.

■ MULTIPLE SCLEROSIS

MS commonly occurs in young adulthood and is characterized by acute focal neurologic deficits appearing irregularly throughout the CNS both in place and in time, with spontaneous or partial remission. The disease may present acutely, subacutely, intermittently, or insidiously. Although relapses and remissions occur in two thirds of patients, it often adopts a slower progressive form in the older patient. The 25-year mortality in older patients is about 26%, compared to 14% in the general population. The likelihood of a more benign prognosis is greater if (1) there is an early age of onset, (2) there is a relapsing and remitting

Table 22–1 □ PATHOLOGIC CHARACTERISTICS OF MYELIN DISORDERS

	Demyelinating	Dysmyelinating	Myelinolytic
Disease	Multiple sclerosis	Leukodystrophy	Aminoaciduria
Etiology	Acquired	Hereditary	Acquired or hereditary
Symmetry	Rare	Usual	Usual
Plaque edge	Sharp	Blunt	Blunt
U fiber involvement	Involved	Spared	Spared or selective
Axonal involvement	Spared	Involved	Involved
Myelin degeneration	Sudinophilic	Variable	Sudinophilic or spongy

course, or (3) the onset is with optic neuritis or with sensory or motor symptoms rather than with brain stem or cerebellar signs. When retrobulbar neuritis is the initial lesion there may a long latent period (15 to 20 years) before further neurologic symptoms occur.

Clinical Features

When the symptoms appear, they often develop steadily over a period of days. The most common complaints are blurring of vision with impaired visual acuity or color desaturation; diplopia; dizziness and imbalance; band-like paresthesias; sphincter disturbance (urinary retention or urgency, fecal incontinence); and impotence. At no stage does any single symptom or sign establish the diagnosis. In chronic disease, the diagnosis becomes obvious, with evidence of disturbances in the spinal cord and brain stem (diplopia, facial myokymia, tic douloureux) and occurrence of hemispheric disease (behavioral change, depression).

Pathologically, the disease affects the following sites (in order of decreasing frequency):

1. **CNS motor tracts (upper motor neuron),** producing weakness (paraparesis, hemiparesis, monoparesis), spasticity, and sensory changes.
2. **Optic nerve,** causing retrobulbar neuritis or papillitis. Ocular pain and dimming of vision are the complaints. Optic disk pallor or atrophy can be seen on fundoscopy. MS develops in approximately 34% of men and 74% of women presenting

with retrobulbar neuritis. Forty percent of MS patients have had at least one attack of optic neuritis.

3. **CNS sensory tracts.** Symptomatically, there may be paresthesias or proprioceptive loss in a limb or in half of the body. Lhermitte's sign (development of electric-like shocks down the body when the patient flexes the head) may be an indication of spinal cord involvement.

4. **Spinal cord urinary autonomic tracts.** Disturbed micturition may occur in 50% of patients; frequency and urgency are common.

5. **Cerebellar white matter.** Signs of cerebellar involvement include nystagmus, intention tremor and dysmetria on the finger-nose-finger test, dysdiadochokinesis, rebound, ataxia, and dysarthria (slow, slurred, jerky, explosive, staccato, or scanning speech). There may be inspiratory whoops, indicating the lack of coordination between respiration and phonation. Hypotonia and pendular reflexes are rarely found. The rare combination of nystagmus, scanning speech, and intention tremor is called Charcot's triad.

6. **Upper brain stem tracts.** Internuclear ophthalmoplegia from involvement of the medial longitudinal fasciculus is a common presenting sign. Diplopia is the symptom.

7. **Lower brain stem white matter.** Acute vertigo and vomiting may be seen from demyelination in the medulla, pontocerebellar tracts, or cerebellar white matter.

8. **Subcortical white matter.** Cognitive change is common, particularly in the latter stages of the disease, with personality change, depression, or euphoria. Seizures may occur in 2 to 3% of patients.

Pathogenesis

The name "multiple sclerosis" is derived from the multiplicity of lesions with sclerotic appearance on cut sections. The patches of demyelination occur solely in white matter of the brain and spinal cord. The lesions occur only in the CNS. Clinical manifestations result from disruption of central nerve transmission. Remyelination is incomplete, and thus, a steady accumulation of neurologic deficits may occur over the course of the disease.

There is considerable evidence to suggest that MS is a complex genetic condition, probably autoimmune in nature, and that both genetic susceptibility and environmental factors contribute to its clinical expression. The disease is rare in tropical climates and more common in temperate zones. Symptoms are commonly exacerbated by fatigue, infection, exertion, and heat—for example, the patient may be able to get into, but not out of, a hot bath. The female/male ratio is 2:1. Relatives of patients are at greater risk than is the general population, the risk being highest (40%)

in monozygotic twins, although the absolute risk is considerably less than the 100% risk expected in a purely genetic condition. Many other autoimmune disorders (e.g., juvenile diabetes) show similar twin concordance rates and relative risk ratios. The prevalence varies from 5 per 100,000 in Africa and Asia to 80 per 100,000 in northern Europe and 1 per 200 on the Shetland Islands. It is likely that at least two genes will be found to influence susceptibility to this disease. There is a genetic association with certain human leukocyte antigen (HLA) class II molecules on chromosome 6. The at-risk alleles vary between populations and include the Dw2, DR15, and DQw6 alleles.

Although the cause of MS is unknown, the possibility that infection interacts with or stimulates an altered immunologic mechanism is suggested by the unusual epidemiology, genetic susceptibility, alterations in immune cell reactivity, and presence of increased immunoglobulin G (IgG) and oligoclonal IgG in spinal fluid and within the plaques themselves. There is evidence for a T cell immunopathology, with activated T cells in plaques, supporting the concept of T cell–mediated autoimmune response directed at myelin antigens.

Diagnosis

MS is a **clinical diagnosis.** For a diagnosis of clinically definite MS, there must be a minimum of two clinical episodes separated in time characteristic of an MS attack. The term "multiple sclerosis" should not be used until the diagnosis is certain. Table 22–2 outlines the criteria for clinically definite, probable, or possible MS. In addition to the clinical picture, laboratory data can support the diagnosis. Characteristic white matter lesions on magnetic resonance imaging (MRI), prolonged P100 on visual evoked potentials, and positive oligoclonal bands (OCBs) from the cerebrospinal fluid (CSF) should be sought. A diagnosis of "laboratory-supported definite" MS may be made if there was only one characteristic MS attack but the laboratory data, including OCBs, are positive.

Laboratory Investigations
Lumbar Puncture

The spinal fluid is abnormal in 90% of patients and the white blood cell count is increased up to $50/mm^3$ in 50% of patients. The pleocytosis is a measure of disease activity and tends to be more marked during acute exacerbations. CSF may show an increase in total protein, usually less than 100 mg/dl (in 40% of patients). An elevated (greater than 12% of total protein) gamma-globulin subfraction is found in 60 to 75% of patients with clinically obvious MS. The OCB pattern is more sensitive and occurs in 90% of established cases but is not specific to MS. OCBs

Table 22–2 □ **CRITERIA FOR CLINICAL DIAGNOSIS OF MULTIPLE SCLEROSIS**

Clinically definite MS	Consistent course
	Relapsing, remitting course; at least two bouts separated by at least 1 month
	Slow or stepwise progressive course for at least 6 months
	Documented neurologic signs of lesions in more than one site, either in brain or spinal cord white matter
	Onset of symptoms between ages of 10 and 50 years
	No better neurologic explanation
Probable MS	History of relapsing, remitting symptoms, but signs are not previously documented and there is only one current sign commonly associated with MS
	Documented single bout of symptoms with signs of more than one white matter lesion; good recovery, then variable symptoms and signs
	No better neurologic explanation
Possible MS	History of relapsing, remitting symptoms without documentation of signs
	Objective signs insufficient to establish more than one lesion of central white matter
	No better neurologic explanation

From Rose AS, Ellison GW, Meyers LW, Tourtellotte WW. Criteria for the clinical diagnosis of multiple sclerosis. Neurology 1976;26:20. © Amer. Academy of Neurology.

may be seen in other neurologic conditions including syphilis, subacute sclerosing panencephalitis, fungal meningitis, and rubella panencephalitis. Elevated CSF myelin basic protein has been demonstrated in 70% of cases of acute MS; however, this finding is nonspecific.

Evoked Potentials

The visual evoked potentials are useful in those patients with an isolated lesion caused by MS, for example, spastic paraparesis, CN6 palsy, trigeminal neuralgia, facial palsy, and postural vertigo. Visual evoked potentials can demonstrate a delay and abnormality in central conduction of the chessboard pattern presented to the eyes and are positive in 90% of patients with clinically obvious MS, in 50% of those with probable MS, and in 25% of those with possible MS. Brain stem auditory evoked potentials are abnormal in 50% of patients with definite MS and in 20% of patients with probable MS. Somatosensory evoked potentials are abnormal in 70% of patients with probable or definite MS.

Neuroimaging

Computed tomography (CT) can detect abnormalities in one third of MS patients, but it has been superseded by MRI, which can be used to predict whether a patient with a single episode of demyelination is likely to progress to clinically definite MS. Those patients with greater than 1.23 cm^3 of plaque at initial presentation have a 90% chance of progressing to MS within 5 years. Those patients whose MRI was normal at presentation have only a 6% chance of progressing to MS at 5 years. T2–weighted images demonstrate demyelination and edema, and gadolinium-enhancing T1 lesions indicate the presence of inflammation in all new MS lesions. The enhancement disappears in two thirds of the lesions by 4 to 6 weeks. Most gadolinium-enhancing lesions are clinically silent, but clinical changes tend to be associated with bursts of gadolinium enhancement. MRI has demonstrated that MS is much more dramatic and dynamic than previously thought (subclinical burden), with the disease process being a continuous one and active in most patients long before diagnosis. However, the greater the number of lesions, the more likely significant disability. Table 22–3 outlines the guidelines for MRI diagnosis of MS.

Differential Diagnosis

The **VITAMINS** mnemonic may be helpful in remembering a differential diagnosis for multiple sclerosis.

V (vascular): lacunar disease with multiple infarcts

I (infectious): human immunodeficiency virus (HIV) infection/acquired immunodeficiency syndrome (AIDS), progressive multifocal leukoencephalopathy, Lyme disease, syphilis, parainfectious meningoencephalomyelitis, human T cell lymphotropic virus type I (HTLV-1) infection

---

Table 22–3 □ MAGNETIC RESONANCE IMAGING CRITERIA FOR DIAGNOSIS OF MULTIPLE SCLEROSIS

MRI strongly suggestive of MS
    Four lesions present (each lesion must be at least 3 mm in size)
    Three lesions present (one must be periventricular)
MRI suggestive of MS
    Three lesions present
    Two lesions present (one must be periventricular)
MRI possibly suggestive of MS
    Two lesions present
    One periventricular lesion

Adapted from Paty DW, Oger JJF, Kastrukoff LF, et al. MRI in the diagnosis of MS: A prospective study with comparison of clinical evaluation, evoked potentials, oligoclonal bonding, and CT. Neurology 1988;38:180. © Amer. Academy of Neurology.

T **(traumatic):** trauma can be associated with a relapse

A **(autoimmune):** vasculitis including systemic lupus erythematosus (SLE), polyarteritis nodosa (PAN), and Behçet's disease; sarcoidosis

M **(metabolic/toxic):** Canavan's disease, adrenoleukodystrophy, metachromatic leukodystrophy, vitamin B_{12} deficiency resulting in subacute combined degeneration, vitamin B_6 deficiency resulting in optic neuritis, radiation

I **(idiopathic/iatrogenic):** Friedreich's ataxia, spinocerebellar degeneration, motor neuron disease, Arnold-Chiari malformation

N **(neoplastic):** multiple metastases, CNS lymphoma, paraneoplastic syndrome, cord compression resulting in spastic paraparesis, pituitary tumor resulting in visual loss

S **(pSychiatric):** conversion disorder, malingering

Management

The relapsing and remitting quality of the disease and individual variation in therapeutic response make it difficult to assess effectiveness of therapy. Some pharmacologic treatments have been shown to be effective for certain aspects of the disease.

Treatment of Disease Progression

Subcutaneous interferon beta-1b 0.25 mg (8 million IU) every other day is the first therapeutic intervention that has been shown to be effective in altering the natural history of *relapsing-remitting MS.* Two double-blind multicenter studies demonstrated that interferon beta decreases the number and severity of exacerbations in relapsing-remitting MS. One study demonstrated slowing of the disease progression. In addition, the number of gadolinium-enhancing MRI lesions is decreased. Interferon is proposed to work by modifying the effects of endogenous interferon beta on the immune system. Some patients (approximately 56%) develop a transient influenza-like illness associated with interferon beta use. Treatment for *chronic progressive MS* is limited, and supportive therapy and treatment of complications are the main therapeutic options. **Oral methotrexate 7.5 mg weekly** slows progression. Psychologic support, physical therapy, and occupational therapy are essential throughout the illness.

Treatment of Acute Exacerbations

The most commonly used agents are corticosteroids, the aim being to reduce the edema and inflammatory aspects of the acute lesion. A short course of high-dose **methylprednisolone**

(1 g IV per day for 7 to 10 days) can help to reverse acute symptoms, and it is usually followed by a tapering course of oral steroids **(prednisone 100 mg per day tapered over 6 to 8 weeks)**. Adrenocorticotropic hormone (ACTH) does not alter the course of MS but helps shorten acute symptoms. The side effects of ACTH treatment can be significant, however. Other immunosuppressive agents include azathioprine, cyclophosphamide, cyclosporine, levamisole, methotrexate, cladribine, mitoxantrone, and total lymphoid irradiation. These agents have been used with some success but have limited duration of efficacy and significant side effects. A meta-analysis of azathioprine trials suggested a possible minor benefit if the drug was started early in the disease course. Tolerance therapy, for example, subcutaneous copolymer-1, may be of benefit if used early in the disease course. It results in a statistically significant reduction in the MS relapse rate and acts by inducing antigen-specific suppressor cells and interfering with the activation of T cells. Oral myelin is currently undergoing trials.

Treatment of Spasticity and Pain

Exercise, physical therapy, and occupational therapy with pharmacologic support are the main approaches. Medications used for spasticity, pain, and spasms include **baclofen 10 to 40 mg PO three times a day, cyclobenzaprine 10 mg one to three times a day, diazepam 5 to 10 mg PO two times a day,** and **dantrolene 25 to 50 mg two to four times a day.** When rehabilitation and medication fail, spinal cord stimulation, intrathecal baclofen, anterior rhizotomy, and peripheral nerve block may be considered.

Treatment of Bladder Dysfunction

Urodynamic (cystometric) studies are important for clarifying the cause of incontinence. For the 30% of patients with incontinence because of involuntary bladder contractions (spastic bladder), parasympatholytic agents **(propantheline 15 mg PO three times a day** or **oxybutynin 5 mg PO two to three times a day)** can aid in the retention of urine. For the 20% who have difficulty emptying their bladder, **bethanecol chloride** (a cholinergic agonist) **10 to 50 mg PO two to four times a day** or **phenoxybenzamine** (an alpha blocker that relaxes the urethral sphincter) **20 to 40 mg three times a day** may be of benefit, in addition to Credé's or Valsalva's maneuvers. The remaining 50% of patients have a combination of the two problems (detrussor dysynergia), and in these cases, regular intermittent self-catheterization or permanent catheterization may be required. Since asymptomatic bacterial colonization of the bladder is common, antibiotics should be reserved for active infection to prevent the selection of highly resistant organisms.

Treatment of Tremor

Coarse cerebellar and rubral tremor are common in patients with MS. Medical therapy including weighting the limb, **clonazepam 0.5 to 2 mg three times a day, propranolol 10 to 40 mg four times a day, glutethimide 250 mg two to three times a day** and **isoniazid 100 to 300 mg one to three times a day** rarely provides complete relief, and ventrolateral thalamic ablation may have to be considered in severe cases. Subthalamic electrical stimulation is a novel promising therapy.

Psychiatric Complications

Depression, euphoria, emotional lability, and psychosis may require psychiatric management.

Treatment of Pain and Fatigue

Paroxysmal pain of MS can respond to **carbamazepine 200 mg two to three times a day, phenytoin 100 to 300 mg per day, amitriptyline 25 to 150 mg per day,** and **baclofen 10 mg three times per day.** The fatigue associated with MS may respond to **amantadine 100 mg two times a day, pemoline 37.5 mg every morning,** and the potassium channel blockers **4-aminopyridine 0.5 mg/kg daily in three divided doses** and **3,4-diaminopyridine 1.0 mg/kg daily in three divided doses.**

■ OPTIC NEURITIS

Optic neuritis produces unilateral impairment of vision in young and middle-aged adults. Although this condition may appear as part of MS (see above) or other generalized demyelinating diseases, it may also occur in isolation. The onset is rapid with blindness, blurred vision, or achromatopia in the affected eye. Retrobulbar neuritis occurs in 50% of the patients, and the other 50% have papillitis on fundoscopy. There is an edematous disk, but venous engorgement is less than that in papilledema. Moreover, in papilledema, visual acuity is good, and pupillary responses to light and consensual reflex are normal. In optic neuritis, visual acuity is diminished (40% have visual acuity less than 20/200), and there may be no direct light reflex with sparing of the consensual reflex. Alternatively, there may be a relative afferent pupillary defect (Marcus Gunn pupil) on the affected side. Half of the patients suffer only unilateral optic neuritis. Functional vision is restored within 2 weeks in 25% of the patients and within 2 months in another 50% of patients but requires 1 year for the remaining patients. Recurrence occurs in approximately 10 to 15% of patients within the first year.

Differential Diagnosis

V **(vascular):** ischemia (e.g., retinal ischemia), central retinal artery occlusion, ischemic optic neuropathy

I **(infectious):** infections affecting vision can be local (retinitis, periostitis, meningitis) or systemic (syphilis, toxoplasmosis, typhoid fever, leptospirosis). These rarely cause such rapid visual loss without other symptoms.

T **(traumatic):** rare

A **(autoimmune):** giant cell arteritis or temporal arteritis causes sudden visual loss in the elderly and often affects the second eye within days (therefore, if there is a suspicion of this diagnosis, start high-dose steroids and arrange for temporal artery biopsy); multiple sclerosis

M **(metabolic/toxic):** diabetes mellitus; severe anemia especially after hemorrhage; vitamin B_{12} and vitamin B_1 deficiency, tropical ataxic neuropathy (cassava diet); methyl alcohol, lead, benzene, tobacco use associated with a defect in cyanide detoxification

I **(idiopathic/hereditary):** Friedreich's ataxia, Leber's optic atrophy (suspicion is raised when new vessel formation is noted on fundoscopy or when the visual acuity fails to improve after 3 months; the condition progresses to affect the second eye after an interval of weeks to months)

N **(neoplastic):** orbital tumor (usually slower progression to visual loss)

Diagnosis and Management

The CSF in optic neuritis, as in MS, may show pleocytosis and increased IgG levels. **Intravenous methylprednisolone 250 mg every 6 hours for 3 days** followed by **prednisone PO 1 mg/kg per day for 11 days** speeds the recovery of visual loss in severe optic neuritis but, after 1 year, results in similar vision compared to treatment with placebo or oral steroids alone. In addition, the combination reduces the rate of development of MS over a 2-year period, especially in those patients with an abnormal MRI scan.

■ OTHER DEMYELINATING DISORDERS

Devic's Disease (Neuromyelitis Optica)

Considered by some physicians to be another MS variant, this condition is characterized by acute bilateral optic neuritis and transverse myelitis. Eye and spinal involvement may occur together or may be separated by days or weeks. Devic's disease may occur as a phase in a typical MS case, or it may be a manifestation of postinfectious encephalomyelitis. The pathology parallels the severe clinical outcome, demonstrating necrosis of axons as well as of myelin. The prognosis is poor. It is most common in Asia.

Acute Disseminated Encephalomyelitis (ADEM, Postvaccinal Encephalomyelitis, Postinfectious Encephalomyelitis)

This disease is an acute demyelinating disorder with diffuse involvement of the brain, spinal cord, and meninges. The onset is acute with confusion, somnolence, seizures, headache, fever, meningismus, and complete or partial paraplegia or quadriplegia with bladder and bowel involvement. Ataxia, myoclonus, chorea, and decerebrate posturing can occur. It can occur following measles, rubella, chickenpox, mumps, influenza, or *Mycoplasma pneumoniae* infection or after vaccination or inoculation. Foci of demyelination surrounding small and medium-sized vessels are scattered throughout the brain and spinal cord. It is thought that an immune-mediated complication of infection is responsible, possibly via a delayed hypersensitivity mechanism. The laboratory model of demyelinating disease (experimental allergic encephalomyelitis) supports this concept. The mortality is high, and significant neurologic deficits commonly persist in survivors. **Methylprednisolone IV 1 g per day** or plasmapheresis can be used to modify the severity of ADEM, but experience is limited.

Acute Necrotizing Hemorrhagic Encephalomyelitis

This fulminant demyelinating disease affects children and young adults and is probably a variant of acute disseminated encephalomyelitis. The onset is abrupt following a respiratory illness. The presentation is similar to that of acute disseminated encephalomyelitis, but the CSF, under increased pressure, shows marked pleocytosis (approximately 3000 to 30,000 cells/mm^3), red blood cells, normal glucose levels, and high protein levels. The erythrocyte sedimentation rate (ESR) is high, and neuroimaging demonstrates extensive white matter destruction with secondary hemorrhages. It is important to consider herpes simplex virus infection, brain abscess, and subdural empyema in the differential diagnosis. The prognosis is poor.

Marchiafava-Bignami Disease

This disorder is a primary degeneration of the corpus callosum characterized by necrosis of the medial zone. It occurs in elderly, alcoholic Italian men. The mechanism behind this degeneration is unknown, but it appears to be associated with intake of crude

Italian wine, although there have been reports of its occurrence in teetotalers. The insidious onset of a nonspecific dementia is the initial sign of the disease, and this is followed by mania, paranoia, depression, and extreme apathy. Seizures, tremors, aphasia, apraxia, and transient hemiparesis may occur. It is slowly progressive and results in death within 3 to 6 years. Neuroimaging can demonstrate callosal atrophy and symmetric frontal demyelinating lesions.

Central Pontine Myelinolysis

This condition is characterized by symmetric destruction of the myelin sheaths in the basis pontis. It occurs in patients with a history of alcoholism, malnutrition, multiorgan (liver, kidney, brain) disease, and electrolyte imbalance (hyponatremia, hypokalemia, hypochloremia, low serum osmolality). Rapid correction of hyponatremia is associated with the onset in many cases. The lesion destroys the myelin sheath, sparing neurons and axons. Destruction begins in the median raphe. It presents as a rapid flaccid tetraplegia with facial, glottal, and pharyngeal paralysis in a debilitated patient suffering from an acute illness. The patient may become locked-in, not comatose but mute and paralyzed. Neuroimaging may demonstrate characteristic changes in the pons. Death generally ensues within days or weeks of the onset. A variant with involvement of white matter in the basal ganglia (extra-pontine myelinolysis) has been described.

■ INFLAMMATORY DISORDERS OF THE CENTRAL NERVOUS SYSTEM

Sarcoidosis (Besnier-Boeck Disease)

Sarcoidosis is a systemic disease characterized by a granulomatous reaction to an unknown stimulus involving any organ. The cause remains unknown but may be an infectious one. It most commonly affects the lungs, mediastinal lymph nodes, and skin. Systemic features include fever, malaise, lassitude, erythema nodosa, polyarthralgia, mediastinal hilar lymphadenopathy, uveoparotid fever (Heerfordt's syndrome: parotitis, uveitis, and facial palsy), keratoconjunctivitis sicca, hepatosplenomegaly, anemia, cardiac conduction defects, phalangeal bone cysts, and hypercalcemia. It affects the nervous system in 5% of patients, primarily the leptomeninges, especially at the base of the brain. The clinical presentation, related to the site of involvement, may include headache, vertigo, impaired vision, isolated cranial nerve lesions (e.g., bilateral facial palsy), intracranial mass lesions, hemiparesis, ataxia, paresthesias, diabetes insipidus from pituitary and hypothalamic dysfunction, seizures, encephalopathy, psychosis, dementia, hydrocephalus, peripheral neuropathy, or myopathy. Rarely is the spinal cord involved. Sarcoidosis is five times more common in women and is found worldwide, with a prevalence of 3 to 50 per 100,000. The median age of onset of sarcoidosis is 27 to 30 years; however, the range is broad.

Laboratory investigations in sarcoidosis may reveal hypercalcemia, hyperuricemia, an elevated serum globulin level, and increased serum angiotensin converting enzyme (ACE) activity. The CSF ACE is positive in 55% of patients with neurosarcoidosis but is negative in those without CNS involvement. The CSF may be abnormal, with raised pressure, a slight pleocytosis, an absence of organisms, markedly increased protein levels, and hypoglycorrhachia in 20 to 30% of patients. An elevated IgG index is found in one third of patients. Cutaneous anergy is common and a Kveim test, if available, can be of diagnostic help. An association with HLA-B8 has been reported. Brain imaging may show leptomeningeal enhancement and parenchymal lesions. The diagnosis is made clinically and is confirmed by a biopsy of a suitable granuloma, the examination revealing a focal collection of epithelioid histiocytes surrounded by a rim of lymphocytes, endothelial cells, and giant cells (Langhans' giant cells) without organisms or caseation. Isolated neurosarcoidosis, seen in only 2 to 3% of patients with CNS involvement, is difficult to diagnose. Its differential diagnosis includes leprosy, cryptococcosis, syphilis, and tuberculosis. ACTH and high-dose steroids are the only known treatments of benefit.

Behçet's Disease (Adamantiades-Behçet Syndrome)

This is an inflammatory disorder of unknown etiology characterized by a relapsing iritis and uveitis associated with oral (in 100% of cases) and genital (in 75% of cases) aphthous ulceration. Systemic features include recurrent fevers, keratoconjunctivitis, hypopyon, migrating superficial thrombophlebitis (in 25% of cases) that may present as deep venous thrombosis, erythema nodosum (in 65% of cases), furunculosis, intestinal ulceration, epididymitis, systemic and pulmonary arterial aneurysms, and arthralgia of large joints (in 60% of cases). Neurologic manifestations, including abrupt onset of recurrent meningoencephalitis and cranial nerve palsies, occur in 5 to 30% of patients. Papilledema (intracranial hypertension due to venous sinus occlusion), hemiparesis, quadriparesis, pseudobulbar palsy, basal ganglia, or cerebellum or spinal cord involvement can occur. Its cause is presumed to be viral or immunologic. It is more common and more severe in men, and the peak age of onset is in the 20s. The diagnosis is chiefly clinical and is based on the occurrence of meningoencephalitis in combination with the characteristic cutaneous and ocular lesions. It may mimic MS or stroke, with transient or persistent multifocal involvement of the nervous system. There is no single confirmatory test, but an ESR over 50 mm/hour is common. CSF studies show a mild pleocytosis with a moderate increase in protein. Brain imaging may show infarction (in 25% of cases), hypodense or hypointense enhancing lesions, and leptomeningeal enhancement. Pathologically, inflammatory changes are found in the iris, choroid, retina, optic nerve, meninges, perivascular spaces of the cortex (vasculitis), basal ganglia, brain stem, and cerebellum. Focal areas of necrosis may also be seen. Treatment may include use of analgesics, anticoagulants, colchicine, dapsone, levamisole, thalidomide, steroids, and immunosuppressives (azathioprine, chlorambucil, or cyclophosphamide). Posterior uveal tract and neurologic lesions, if untreated, may lead to blindness or death.

23

INFECTIONS OF THE CENTRAL NERVOUS SYSTEM

Most infections of the central nervous system (CNS) are life-threatening. For this reason, prompt diagnosis and treatment are essential to prevent death or permanent neurologic disability. **The possibility of CNS infection is usually raised by the combination of fever, headache, and neurologic signs or symptoms.** After your initial history and examination, the goal is to identify the possible causative organisms and treat them empirically. Definitive treatment will later be based on the results of cultures or other diagnostic tests.

■ APPROACH TO THE PATIENT WITH SUSPECTED CNS INFECTION

History and Examination

1. **Check for the following symptoms:** fever, headache, change in mental status, focal weakness, or back pain.
2. **Identify any predisposing causes of immunosuppression:** diabetes, alcoholism, malignancy, steroids, chemotherapy, human immunodeficiency virus (HIV) infection, or acquired immunodeficiency syndrome (AIDS).
3. **Check for evidence of infection elsewhere in the body:** endocarditis, pneumonia, osteomyelitis, or tick bite.
4. **Always be sure to check for the following:** papilledema, meningismus, skin rash, sinus tenderness, otitis media, or spine tenderness.

Lumbar Puncture

Lumbar puncture (LP) is the single most important test for establishing the presence of a CNS infection and for identifying the causative organism. The technique for performing LP is covered in Chapter 4. Herniation is a serious but rare complication of LP. **If CNS infection is suspected, when deciding whether to perform an LP, the following clinical rule may be helpful:**

1. Fever
2. Headache
3. Change in mental status

Any 2 of these 3 require LP

Computed tomography (CT) scan is required prior to LP if ANY of the following are present:
1. Papilledema
2. Depressed level of consciousness (lethargy, stupor, or coma)
3. Focal neurologic deficit
4. Known intracranial mass lesion
5. AIDS

■ ACUTE MENINGITIS

Bacterial Meningitis

Bacterial meningitis typically presents as the classic triad of *fever, headache, and stiff neck.* The presentation is usually dramatic but may be less obvious at the extremes of age (in infants and in the elderly), in whom change in mental status is often the only symptom. Seeding of the leptomeninges usually results from hematogenous spread of the infecting organism (e.g., pneumococcal pneumonia complicated by meningitis), but it can also result from a parameningeal infection (e.g., otitis media) or following trauma or neurosurgery (e.g., cerebrospinal fluid [CSF] leak).

Diagnosis

The diagnosis is established by LP, which demonstrates polymorphonuclear pleocytosis, elevated protein level, and reduced glucose level (Table 23–1). The organism is identified on the basis of CSF cultures.

Treatment

The prognosis in bacterial meningitis depends on the interval between onset of disease and initiation of therapy. Selection of antibiotics for empirical coverage depends on age and risk factors, as shown in Table 23–2. Most adults should be treated with **ampicillin and ceftriaxone** pending the results of CSF cultures (see Table 23–2). **Dexamethasone 10 mg IV every 6 hours for 4 days** may also be given in severe cases to reduce the severity of residual neurologic and cranial nerve damage.

Viral (Aseptic) Meningitis

Viral meningitis is a self-limited illness seen most frequently in children and young adults. The presentation is similar to bacterial meningitis, except that neurologic dysfunction (e.g., change in mental status, neurologic focality) does not occur, and the overall prognosis is excellent. The diagnosis is suggested by lymphocytic pleocytosis with a normal glucose level in the CSF (see Table 23–1) and is confirmed by negative bacterial cultures. In some

Table 23-1 □ CEREBROSPINAL FLUID FINDINGS IN SELECTED INFECTIONS OF THE CENTRAL NERVOUS SYSTEM

	No. of White Blood Cells (per mm^3)	Cell Type	Concentration of Protein (mg/dl)	Concentration of Glucose (mg/dl)	Pressure (cm H$_2$O)
Normal	≤5	Lymphocytes and monocytes only	15 to 45	45 to 80	80 to 180
Bacterial meningitis	5 to 10,000	Polymorphonuclear leukocytes	Increased	Decreased	Increased
Viral meningitis	5 to 1000	Lymphocytes	Increased	Normal	Normal, occasionally increased
Tubercular meningitis	5 to 500	Lymphocytes	Increased	Decreased	Increased
Cryptococcal meningitis	5 to 100	Lymphocytes	Increased	Normal, occasionally decreased	Increased
Active neurosyphilis	5 to 500	Lymphocytes	Increased	Normal, occasionally decreased	Normal

Table 23–2 □ EMPIRICAL ANTIBIOTIC THERAPY FOR BACTERIAL MENINGITIS

Risk Group	Etiologies	Antibiotic Coverage
Neonates (less than 1 month)	Group B or group D streptococci Gram-negative rods (e.g., *Escherichia coli*) *Listeria monocytogenes*	Ampicillin 50 to 100 mg/kg per day every 12 hours Ceftriaxone 100 mg/kg per day every 12 hours
Children (3 months to 7 years)	*Haemophilus influenzae* *Streptococcus pneumoniae* *Neisseria meningitides*	Ceftriaxone 100 mg/kg per day every 12 hours
Adults (7 to 50 years)	*S. pneumoniae* *N. meningitides* *L. monocytogenes*	Ampicillin 2 g IV every 4 hours Ceftriaxone 2 g IV every 12 hours
Adults older than 50 yrs; alcoholics; patients with a debilitating medical condition	*S. pneumoniae* Gram-negative rods *H. influenzae*	Ampicillin 2 g IV every 4 hours Ceftriaxone 2 g IV every 12 hours
Patients with postneurosurgical procedure or head trauma	*Staphylococcus aureus* Gram-negative rods *S. pneumoniae*	Vancomycin 1 g IV every 12 hours Ceftazidime 1 to 2 g every 8 hours

instances, the virus can be cultured from CSF, from blood, or from nasal, pharyngeal, or rectal swabs. Treatment is supportive.

■ CHRONIC MENINGITIS

Tuberculosis

Meningitis caused by *Mycobacterium tuberculosis* is a severe infection that carries a high morbidity and mortality. *Cranial nerve palsies* and *vasculitic small-vessel infarctions* occur frequently and result from severe granulomatous inflammation of the basal meninges. Tuberculosis can also produce a *miliary encephalitis* or *focal tuberculoma*, with or without meningitis. Although immunosuppressed patients (patients with AIDS or alcoholic patients) are particularly at risk, the disease can strike anyone. Evidence of active pulmonary disease is found in only 30% of the cases, and only 50% of the cases are purified protein derivative (PPD)–positive. *Hydrocephalus* is a frequent late complication.

Diagnosis

The CSF shows lymphocytic pleocytosis, elevated protein level, and reduced glucose level (see Table 23–1). The diagnosis is established by observing *acid-fast* mycobacteria in the CSF; the yield exceeds 50% when multiple large-volume taps (10 to 25 ml) are examined. *M. tuberculosis* can also be *cultured* from the CSF, but the yield is low, and 4 to 6 weeks are needed for the organism to grow. *Polymerase chain reaction (PCR)* testing can establish the diagnosis by amplifying small amounts of tubercle bacillus DNA.

Treatment

Until antibiotic sensitivity is known, treatment with four drugs is recommended for the first 2 months. A full course of treatment requires 9 to 12 months. Options include **isoniazid 300 mg per day** (also give **pyridoxine 50 mg per day**), **rifampin 600 mg per day, pyrazinamide 15 to 30 mg/kg per day, ethambutol 15 to 20 mg/kg per day, streptomycin 15 mg/kg per day IM,** and **ciprofloxacin 750 mg two times a day.**

Cotreatment with **dexamethasone 10 mg IV every 6 hours** may also be used in severe cases (with depressed level of consciousness, focal deficits, or multiple cranial nerve palsies) to inhibit the inflammatory response and limit damage.

Neurosyphilis

Syphilis is a chronic systemic infection caused by the spirochete *Treponema pallidum*. **Primary infection** is characterized by a chancre (firm, painless genital ulcer). A **secondary bacteremic stage** may occur 2 to 12 weeks later, and this results in generalized mucocutaneous lesions (palmar and plantar rash) and lymphadenopathy. In 40% of the cases, the CNS is asymptomatically seeded at this point, and mild CSF changes (elevation of cells and protein) can be detected. Two percent of patients with secondary infection experience acute *meningovascular syphilis.*

Following a latent period of 15 to 20 years, tertiary syphilis manifests as a slowly progressive systemic inflammatory disease of the skin (gummas), heart (aortitis), eyes (chorioretinitis), or CNS. *Tertiary neurosyphilis* develops in 7% of patients with untreated primary syphilis and results from chronic meningeal and parenchymal inflammation. The classic manifestations include the following:

1. General paresis
    This condition results from diffuse infection of brain parenchyma and manifests as dementia with prominent psychiatric features and bilateral upper motor neuron signs.
2. Tabes dorsalis
    Tabes dorsalis results from chronic spinal polyradiculitis with secondary dorsal root and column degeneration. Symptoms may include neuropathic shooting pains in the lower extremities, loss of posterior column sensation, and areflexia.
3. Argyll Robertson pupils
    These are small irregular pupils that react to accommodation but not to light and reflect chronic optic neuritis. Optic atrophy and blindness may also occur.

Diagnosis

Neurosyphilis is defined by a positive serologic test (Venereal Disease Research Laboratory [VDRL] test) in the CSF and may be latent (normal CSF) or active (elevation of white blood cell count and protein level). Patients with active neurosyphilis are often asymptomatic. **LP is required to rule out neurosyphilis in all patients with positive serologies (RPR, VDRL) and inadequately treated syphilis of greater than 1 year's duration.** Also, note that in late syphilis, serum VDRL and rapid plasmin reagin (RPR) reactivity (nontreponemal tests) often falls to 70%, whereas fluorescent treponemal antibody absorption (FTA-ABS) reactivity remains positive in 90 to 95% of patients.

Treatment

Primary and secondary syphilis can be treated with **benzathine penicillin, 2.4 million units IM weekly for 3 weeks.** Neurosyphilis, whether latent or active, is treated with **penicillin G 2 to 4 million units IV every 4 hours for 10 days.**

Lyme Disease

Lyme disease is caused by the spirochete *Borrelia burgdorferi,* which is inoculated into humans by the bite of an infected deer tick *(Ixodes dammini)*. A characteristic expanding erythematous "target" lesion, erythema chronicum migrans, develops at the site of the tick bite, and this is often accompanied by fever, fatigue, arthralgias, and headache. Chronic infection can lead to arthritis, carditis, and CNS involvement (Table 23–3).

Diagnosis

The CSF shows a mononuclear pleocytosis with elevated protein levels, and the diagnosis is confirmed by detecting intrathecal production of IgG antibodies to *Borrelia* (CSF titer is higher than the serum titer). A PCR test for *Borrelia* DNA in CSF is also available. *Positive serologic blood testing alone is not enough to confirm the diagnosis in patients with suspected neurologic Lyme disease.*

Treatment

For patients with Lyme meningoradiculitis, treat with **ceftriaxone 2 g IV per day** or **penicillin G 4 million units IV every 4 hours for 2 to 4 weeks.** Early Lyme disease (less than 30 days) without neurologic manifestations or isolated facial palsy can be treated with **doxycycline 100 mg PO two times a day** or **tetracycline 250 mg PO four times a day for 10 to 30 days.**

Fungal Meningitis

Fungal infection of the CNS typically occurs in immunocompromised hosts (patients with AIDS, malignancy, diabetes, or alcoholism), but exceptions may occur. The vast majority of cases in the United States result from *Cryptococcus neoformans;* other causes include *Coccidioides immitis* (southwestern United States), *Candida albicans, Histoplasma capsulatum,* and *Blastomyces* species. *Aspergillus* and *Mucor* species are unique in their tendency to invade local tissues and cause vasculitic infarction.

Table 23–3 □ **NEUROLOGIC MANIFESTATIONS OF LYME DISEASE**

Stage 1 (less than 1 month after infection)
    Headache, neck stiffness (CSF normal)
Stage 2 (occurs in 15% of patients 1 to 6 months after infection)
    Meningitis
    Cranial neuritis, single (e.g., facial) or multiple nerves
    Polyradiculopathy
    Plexopathy
    Mononeuritis multiplex
    Acute polyneuropathy (resembles Guillain-Barré syndrome)
Stage 3 (months to years after infection)
    Chronic encephalopathy
    Demyelinating syndrome (multiple sclerosis–like)
    Chronic myelitis

Diagnosis

The CSF shows mononuclear pleocytosis, elevated protein level, and normal or reduced glucose level. Diagnosis is based on demonstrating the organism by wet smear or culture. *Cryptococcus* infection can also be diagnosed using the India ink stain or by detecting capsular antigen in the CSF with latex agglutination.

Treatment

All forms of fungal meningitis are treated with **amphotericin B 0.5 to 1.5 mg/kg per day IV for 4 to 6 weeks.** *Cryptococcus* is also treated with **flucytosine (5-FC) 150 mg/kg PO per day,** which allows a lower dose of amphotericin B (0.5 mg/kg per day) to be used. **Dexamethasone 10 mg IV every 6 hours** can be used to limit cranial nerve damage or reduce intracranial pressure (ICP) in severe infections.

■ BRAIN ABSCESS AND PARAMENINGEAL INFECTIONS

Bacterial Abscess

Brain abscess most commonly presents with subacute progression of headache (in 75% of patients), altered mental status (in 50% of patients), focal neurologic signs (in 50% of patients), and fever (in 50% of patients). The infection usually begins as a focus of cerebritis, which develops into a localized collection of pus with a surrounding fibrovascular capsule. Most abscesses are formed by contiguous spread from a parameningeal infection (otitis media, osteomyelitis, sinusitis) or by hematogenous spread in patients with endocarditis, bronchiectasis, or congenital cyanotic heart disease. The most common organisms encountered are streptococci, *Staphylococcus aureus*, gram-negative bacilli, and anaerobes such as *Bacteroides fragilis*. Polymicrobial infections are common.

Diagnosis

The diagnosis is suggested by a ring-enhancing lesion (Fig. 23–1) in the brain on CT or MRI. The CSF may be normal or may show a mild pleocytosis; a pathogen can be isolated from CSF cultures in less than 10% of cases. Blood cultures, echocardiography, chest x-ray, HIV testing, and a skull CT scan (to rule out sinusitis, otitis, or tooth abscess) should be performed in addition to LP in all patients with brain abscess of unknown etiology. Culture of pus obtained from a surgical drainage procedure is often the only way to establish the diagnosis, but even these cultures are negative in 20% of cases.

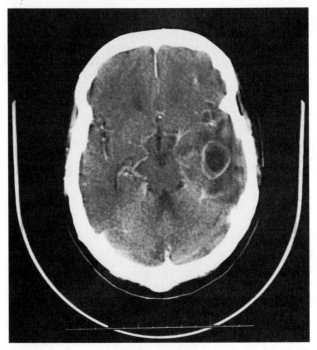

Figure 23–1 □ Ring-enhancing lesion on CT scan, characteristic of bacterial abscess.

Treatment

For broad-spectrum empirical coverage of suspected bacterial abscess, treat with (1) **oxacillin 2 g IV every 4 hours or penicillin G 4 million units IV every 4 hours;** (2) **metronidazole 500 mg IV every 6 hours,** and (3) **ceftriaxone 2 to 4 g IV every 12 hours.** If the patient fails to respond, consideration should be given to administering **amphotericin B** to treat a possible fungal infection. Complete treatment takes 4 to 8 weeks. **Surgical options** include stereotactic needle aspiration, abscess drainage, and abscess excision (e.g., removal of capsule). Patients with depressed level of consciousness should also be treated with **dexamethasone 4 to 10 mg IV every 6 hours for 4 to 6 days** to reduce edema.

Subdural Empyema

Subdural empyema is a closed-space infection between the dura and arachnoid, usually over the hemispheric convexity. In adults, spread of infection from a contiguous source (e.g., sinusitis or otitis) is the cause in most cases, whereas in children, subdural empyema often occurs as a complication of meningitis. The organisms most often cultured are similar to those for brain abscess, and empirical antibiotic coverage is the same. Surgical drainage at the earliest opportunity is essential for successful treatment.

Cranial and Spinal Epidural Abscess

Epidural CNS infection almost always results from infection from a contiguous source and is often seen in combination with osteomyelitis. The CSF often shows mild signs of inflammation (elevated WBC and protein levels) but is sterile.

Cranial epidural abscess usually presents with localized pain and tenderness and can lead to cranial nerve deficits. For example, infection of the petrous temporal bone (Gradenigo's syndrome) often results in CN 5 and CN 6 deficits. Common infecting organisms are the same as for brain abscess, and empirical antibiotic treatment is the same.

Spinal epidural abscess is most common in the thoracic region and often occurs in diabetics and intravenous drug users. Symptoms may include intense local pain and tenderness, local root irritation with referred pain, and cord compression, which is a neurologic emergency. *S. aureus* and streptococci account for 75% of the infections, and gram-negative organisms account for 20%; unusual causes include *M. tuberculosis* (Pott's disease) and fungi. MRI of the spine is the diagnostic technique of choice. Treatment with high-dose steroids **(dexamethasone 60 to 100 mg IVP, followed by 10 to 20 mg IV every 6 hours)** and **surgical drainage** should be performed immediately to prevent cord compression. **Oxacillin** and **ceftriaxone** usually provide adequate empirical antibiotic coverage for bacterial infection.

Toxoplasmosis

Toxoplasmosis is the most common opportunistic infection affecting the CNS in patients with AIDS. *Toxoplasma gondii* is an intracellular protozoan; infection usually results in necrotic abscess formation, but disseminated meningoencephalitis can develop in some cases.

Diagnosis

The diagnosis is suggested by one or more ring-enhancing lesions in the brain on CT or MRI. The CSF may show mild elevation of the WBC count or protein level. The presence of serum antibodies to *Toxoplasma* is evidence of prior exposure to the organism, but it does not prove active infection. Demonstration of the organism by biopsy is required for definitive diagnosis and differentiation from CNS lymphoma but is generally required only in patients who fail a 7- to 10-day trial of empirical treatment.

Treatment

Patients with suspected toxoplasmosis should be treated empirically with **sulfadiazine 25 mg/kg PO every 6 hours** and **pyrimethamine 100 to 150 mg PO on day 1, followed by 50 to 75 mg per day for 6 to 8 weeks. Folinic acid 5 to 10 mg PO every day** should also be given to minimize hematologic toxicity. **Clindamycin 600 mg PO four times a day** can be used instead of sulfadiazine in patients who are allergic to sulfa drugs. **Dexamethasone 6 to 10 mg IV every 6 hours** should be restricted to patients with large mass lesions and reduced level of consciousness, because it increases the rate of false-negative results for lymphoma, should biopsy be performed at a later date.

Cysticercosis

Cysticercosis is the most common parasitic CNS disease. Ova shed by the intestinal tapeworm *Taenia solium* in human feces can contaminate food ingested by the host or others, which leads to hematogenous dissemination of encysted larvae throughout the body, including the CNS. Most cases occur in Latin America (e.g., Mexico) and Southeast Asia.

Diagnosis

CT and MRI scans are usually highly characteristic: *uninflamed cysts* appear as small (less than 1 cm), fluid-filled cysts; *active inflamed cysts* are identified by the presence of contrast enhancement; *inactive cysts* appear as small, punctate calcified lesions. Detection of *serum antibody titers* to *Cysticercus* can confirm the diagnosis, but sensitivity is less than 100% in patients with inactive disease or with a single enhancing lesion. Patients and family members should undergo stool examinations for ova and parasites, because treatment can prevent reinfection.

Treatment

Patients with inactive (calcified) neurocysticercosis or with a single enhancing lesion and minimal symptoms (e.g., seizures controlled with anticonvulsants and a nonfocal examination) do not require treatment. In the latter case, follow-up neuroimaging 6 to 10 weeks later usually shows progression of the enhancing lesion to a small, calcified nodule. **Praziquantel 50 mg/kg per day** or **albendazole 15 mg/kg per day, split into three divided doses for 14 days,** will kill surviving larvae in patients with active infestation. Treatment results in active inflammation from dying organisms, which can be limited by a brief course of **dexamethasone (4 to 6 mg every 6 hours for 5 days)** in patients with severe disease.

■ VIRAL ENCEPHALITIS

Herpes Simplex Encephalitis

Herpes simplex virus type 1 (HSV-1) encephalitis is the most common cause of viral encephalitis (approximately 15% of all cases) and is fatal in up to 40% of untreated patients. Patients present with fever, altered mental status, headache, and seizures. The disease results from reactivation of dormant HSV-1 within the trigeminal ganglion, with viral spread via sensory pathways into the brain, rather than the more common picture of retrograde viral expression leading to perioral herpetic lesions.

Diagnosis

The CSF may show mild lymphocytic pleocytosis, increased red blood cells, and increased protein, but it may be normal, particularly early in the disease. CSF cultures usually do not yield the virus. Focal necrotizing lesions of the inferior frontal and temporal lobes are highly characteristic and are best seen with contrast MRI. An electroencephalogram (EEG) often shows periodic lateralized epileptiform discharges, consistent with structural temporal lobe lesions. Definitive diagnosis is made by brain biopsy, which demonstrates eosinophilic intracellular (Cowdry type I) inclusions. Biopsy may not be necessary if the clinical, radiologic, and EEG findings are highly characteristic.

Treatment

All patients with suspected viral encephalitis should be treated empirically with **acyclovir 10 to 12.5 mg/kg IV every 8 hours for 14 days.** *Because efficacy depends on early treatment, acyclovir should be started as soon as possible and should never be withheld pending the results of diagnostic studies.* Steroids should not be used unless signs of herniation are present. Anticonvulsants (e.g., **phenytoin**) should be given to all patients and discontinued after 2 weeks if no seizures occur. An ICP monitor is recommended in patients who are comatose (Glasgow Coma scale score less than 8).

Other Causes of Encephalitis

The infectious agent in patients with encephalitis is usually identified *after* the acute illness on the basis of rising acute to convalescent antibody titers. With the exception of HSV and cytomegalovirus (CMV), no specific treatment is available. Causes of viral encephalitis other than HSV-1 are listed below. Serologic testing for these agents, as well as viral cultures of the CSF, pharynx, urine, and stool, may be helpful in establishing the diagnosis.

1. **Mumps virus**

   Infection with mumps virus is unusual now since most children are vaccinated.

2. **Enteroviruses**

   This group includes coxsackievirus, echovirus, and poliovirus. Encephalitis occurs during summertime epidemics of gastroenteritis.

3. **Arboviruses (arthropod-borne viruses)**

   These viruses are spread by mosquitoes. They can also infect horses and birds, and they are most prevalent in the late summer and early fall.

   - **Equine encephalomyelitis viruses.** Eastern equine encephalomyelitis virus (Atlantic and Gulf coasts) is the most severe form and infection carries a mortality of 50%. Others include western equine encephalomyelitis virus (in the Western United States and the Midwest) and Venezuelan equine encephalomyelitis virus.
   - **St. Louis encephalitis virus.** This disease occurs in epidemics in the rural Midwest.
   - **California encephalitis virus**
   - **Colorado tick fever virus**
   - **Japanese encephalitis virus**

4. **Measles virus**

   Besides causing acute encephalitis 1 to 14 days after a viral exanthem (rubeola), measles virus can cause (1) a relentlessly progressive subacute encephalitis in immunosuppressed patients, (2) postinfectious immune-mediated demyelinating encephalomyelitis, and (3) **subacute sclerosing panencephalitis (SSPE)**, a "slow" viral infection characterized by progressive dementia, ataxia, myoclonus, periodic sharp waves on EEG, elevated titers of anti–measles virus antibodies in the CSF, and pathologic intracellular viral inclusion bodies.

5. **Rabies virus**

   Rabies is spread by the bite of an infected (rabid) animal. After a variable incubation period (1 to 3 months), rabies encephalomyelitis invariably leads to delirium, seizures, paralysis, and death. After inoculation, the virus travels to the CNS via retrograde axonal transport. Negri bodies, dark intracellular viral inclusions, are the characteristic pathologic lesion.

6. **Lymphocytic choriomeningitis (LCM) virus**

   This usually causes viral (aseptic) meningitis. Infection comes from exposure to mice and hamster feces.

7. **Epstein-Barr virus (EBV)**

   EBV produces a systemic viral infection known as *mononucleosis* (pharyngitis, malaise, fever, adenopathy, liver function test abnormalities, splenomegaly, and atypical lymphocytes on blood smear), which may be complicated by encephalitis.

8. **Cytomegalovirus**

CMV causes a systemic infection similar to EBV that can be complicated by encephalitis but that more often manifests as ventriculitis or encephalitis in immunosuppressed patients (see below).

■ NEUROLOGIC COMPLICATIONS OF AIDS

Opportunistic Infections

Patients with AIDS are at risk for the following opportunistic infections of the CNS, particularly when CD4+ T helper lymphocyte counts are less than 200. The approximate percentage of AIDS patients affected is shown in parentheses. *Patients with AIDS are at risk for multiple, simultaneous opportunistic infections.*

1. **Toxoplasmosis (10%)**

Toxoplasmosis usually presents as single or multiple brain abscesses or as meningoencephalitis.

2. **Cryptococcus (10%)**

Cryptococcus presents as acute or chronic meningitis.

3. **Progressive multifocal leukoencephalopathy (PML) (5%)**

PML presents with multiple, relentlessly progressive demyelinating lesions within the CNS. It is caused by papovaviruses (JC and SV-40 viruses), which can be demonstrated by biopsy. Progressive neurologic deficits are the rule, and death usually ensues within a few months. There is no treatment.

4. **CMV infection (5% excluding retinitis)**

CMV infection most often presents as *ventriculitis* but can also manifest as *encephalitis, myelitis,* and *lumbosacral polyradiculopathy.* CMV retinitis is extremely common (it occurs in 20% of all AIDS patients). The diagnosis of ventriculitis is suggested by ependymal enhancement on MRI. All forms of infection may be treated with **gancyclovir 5 mg/kg IV every 12 hours for 14 to 28 days,** but efficacy has been shown only with retinitis and polyradiculopathy. **Foscarnet 60 mg/kg IV every 8 hours for 14 days** can be used as a second-line agent. Because CMV infection is difficult to diagnose in the setting of an acute illness, therapy should be started empirically prior to culture results.

5. **Herpes zoster (5%)**

Herpes zoster radiculitis can be treated topically with acyclovir cream. **IV treatment (acyclovir 10 to 12.5 mg/kg every 8 hours)** is necessary only if multiple dermatomal levels are involved.

6. **Syphilis (less than 5%)**
   The course of syphilis is often accelerated in HIV-infected patients, the CSF VDRL test may be negative, and treatment may require a prolonged course of antibiotics.

Nonopportunistic Nervous System Complications of AIDS

Besides opportunistic infections, patients with AIDS are subject to peripheral neuropathy, dementia or myelopathy from the direct effects of HIV infection, and CNS lymphoma. The frequency among AIDS patients is shown in parentheses.

1. **HIV sensory neuropathy (30%)**
   A small-fiber sensory neuropathy is seen frequently in advanced AIDS. Common findings include painful dysesthesia and hyperesthesia of the feet and loss of ankle reflexes. Treatment of the neuropathic pain is symptomatic (see Chapter 18).

2. **AIDS dementia complex (15 to 20%)**
   Progressive dementia occurs frequently in HIV-infected patients, and it is an AIDS-defining illness. In addition to cognitive deficits, pyramidal and extrapyramidal signs (rigidity, tremor, cogwheeling) may be seen. MRI shows diffuse atrophy, and the CSF is usually normal. Some patients may respond to antiretrovirus therapy early in the course of the illness **(zidovudine 200 mg every 8 hours or didanosine [Videx] 125 to 250 mg two times a day).**

3. **HIV myelopathy (15 to 20%)**
   A progressive vacuolar myelopathy resulting in spastic paraparesis, sensory ataxia, and bowel or bladder incontinence is seen frequently in combination with AIDS dementia complex. A spinal cord compressive lesion, vitamin B_{12} deficiency, human T cell lymphotropic virus type I (HTLV-1) infection (tropical spastic paraparesis), and CMV or HSV myeloradiculitis should be excluded. There is no treatment.

4. **Primary CNS lymphoma (5%)**
   CNS lymphoma presents as one or more enhancing mass lesions in the CNS and can be impossible to differentiate from toxoplasmosis with radiographic findings. In most patients, the diagnosis is established by biopsy after failure to respond to empirical treatment for toxoplasmosis. Steroids cause tumor necrosis and reduce the diagnostic yield of biopsy tissue; hence, if biopsy is being considered, **dexamethasone should be withheld** unless absolutely necessary. Most lymphomas respond radiographically and clinically to whole-brain radiation; however, the effects are palliative, and survival rarely exceeds 3 to 6 months.

5. **HIV (aseptic) meningitis (1 to 2%)**

   Acutely infected patients occasionally develop a self-limited aseptic meningitis, in combination with constitutional symptoms of viral infection (fever, malaise, adenopathy).

6. **Acute demyelinating polyneuropathy (less than 1%)**

   This complication is clinically indistinguishable from Guillain-Barré syndrome (see Chapter 16).

24

NEOPLASMS OF THE CENTRAL NERVOUS SYSTEM

Casilda Balmaceda and J. Torres Gluck

Most brain tumors are diagnosed when computed tomography (CT) or magnetic resonance imaging (MRI) shows an enhancing intracranial mass lesion in a patient with new progressive neurologic symptoms that have developed over weeks to months. Figure 24–1 lists the most common primary central nervous system neoplasms in adults by location. Except in patients with known systemic cancer and presumed metastases, tissue biopsy is mandatory for establishing the diagnosis.

Dexamethasone, 4 to 10 mg IV or PO every 6 hours, is a potent glucocorticoid that can dramatically reduce vasogenic peritumoral edema associated with CNS neoplasms. It is indicated in all patients who are symptomatic from a mass effect related to a brain tumor, but, if possible, it should be withheld prior to biopsy if primary CNS lymphoma is a consideration, because its use tends to produce nondiagnostic results. Diagnostic and management considerations for specific tumors are provided below.

■ INTRACRANIAL METASTATIC DISEASE

Brain metastases occur in 15 to 20% of patients with cancer and represent the most common form of intracranial neoplasm. Brain metastases usually occur in patients with widely disseminated disease and can take one of three forms: *parenchymal metastases, leptomeningeal metastases* (i.e., meningeal carcinomatosis or carcinomatous meningitis), and *skull base metastases*. Systemic cancer can also affect the nervous system through the remote effects of cancer, which are also known as paraneoplastic syndromes (Table 24–1).

Parenchymal Metastases

Epidemiology. Approximately 40% of patients have a *solitary metastasis.* Gastrointestinal (e.g., colonic) and gynecologic (e.g., ovarian, endometrial, and cervical) malignancies are the most common source of a solitary metastasis. Tumors that are most prone to present with multiple metastases include lung tumors, breast tumors, and melanoma.

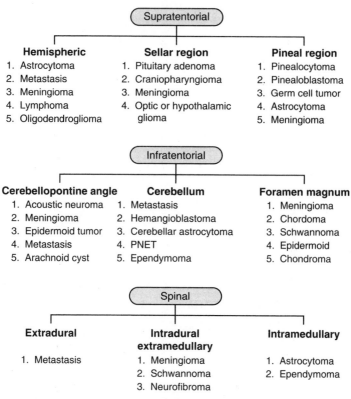

Figure 24–1 □ Radiographic differential diagnosis of solitary CNS neoplasms in the adult patient by location. PNET, Primitive neuroectodermal tumor.

Pathophysiology. Brain metastases are usually well-demarcated and amenable to surgical resection. Extensive surrounding edema is common. Metastases most often reach the brain hematogenously and tend to deposit at the *gray-white junction.*

Presentation. Symptoms usually develop over weeks to months. Headache (in 60%), motor weakness (in 60%), mental status changes (in 35%), and seizures (in 20%) are the most common presenting complaints. A *sudden focal deficit* resembling stroke can occur with intratumoral hemorrhage in highly vascular or necrotic tumors (melanoma, choriocarcinoma, and renal cell tumors).

Table 24–1 □ PARANEOPLASTIC SYNDROMES

Syndrome	Common Tumors	Comments
Sensorimotor neuropathy	Lung (small cell) tumors, lymphoma, many others	Most common syndrome; axonal or demyelinating
Pure motor neuronopathy	Myeloma, lymphoma	Paraprotein (IgG, IgM) often present
Pure sensory neuropathy (ganglioneuritis)	Lung (small cell) tumors	Primarily small fiber; anti-Hu antibodies may be present
Limbic encephalitis	Lung (small cell) tumors, lymphoma	Agitation, confusion, amnesia, dementia
Cerebellar degeneration	Ovarian, breast, or lung (small cell) tumors, lymphoma	Anti-Yo and anti–Purkinje cell antibodies may be present
Opsoclonus-myoclonus	Neuroblastoma, lung or breast tumors	Anti-Ri antibodies may be present; may improve with tumor resection or steroids
Necrotizing encephalomyelitis	Lung (small cell) or breast tumors, lymphoma	Anti-Hu antibodies may be present; poor prognosis
Dermatomyositis	Lung, breast, or ovarian tumors, lymphoma	Treat with steroids
Lambert-Eaton myasthenic syndrome	Lung (small cell), ovarian breast, prostate, stomach tumors	Autonomic dysfunction and limb weakness common
Carcinoma-associated retinopathy	Lung (small cell) or cervical tumors	Anti-retinal antibodies may be present

Diagnosis. *MRI with gadolinium* is more sensitive than CT for detecting multiple metastases and thus is the imaging test of choice. Contrast enhancement may be uniform or in a ring pattern when the metastasis has a necrotic center.

Treatment. *Surgery followed by radiation* is the treatment of choice for patients with a single, accessible metastasis. Surgery for multiple brain metastases is generally contraindicated, unless one of the metastases is imminently life-threatening because of its size or location. Surgical excision or biopsy is also indicated in patients with one or more brain lesions of unknown primary origin. *Whole-brain radiation therapy* is recommended in patients with multiple metastases. A total dose of approximately 3000 cGy is typically administered in 10 fractions over a 2-week period. Fractionation and concomitant administration of corticosteroids lowers the cerebral toxicity of the radiation. Radiation leads to neurologic improvement in approximately 60% of cases. *Chemotherapy* for brain metastases has yielded disappointing results.

Leptomeningeal Metastases

Epidemiology. Also known as carcinomatous meningitis, leptomeningeal metastasis results most often from carcinoma of the breast and lung, non-Hodgkin's lymphoma, and malignant melanoma.

Pathophysiology. Cancer cells reach the leptomeninges hematogenously and then travel via the CSF to distant areas of the neuraxis, causing widespread dissemination. Neoplastic infiltration frequently leads to multifocal cranial and spinal nerve deficits.

Presentation. A combination of *headache* and *somnolence* with *multifocal neuropathies* should alert the physician to the possibility of meningeal carcinomatosis. In advanced cases, meningeal carcinomatosis may present with hydrocephalus or seizures.

Diagnosis. *Lumbar puncture* (LP) for analysis of the CSF is the mainstay of diagnosis. In most cases, the CSF reveals lymphocytic pleocytosis, elevated protein levels, and low glucose levels. CSF cytology reveals neoplastic cells and confirms the diagnosis. The sensitivity of three LPs is 90%. *MRI* may reveal leptomeningeal enhancement or nodules.

Treatment. The prognosis of patients with leptomeningeal metastasis is dismal, with median survival ranging from 3 to 6 months. *Chemotherapy* is given intrathecally via LP or, preferably, via an Ommaya reservoir. The most commonly used agents are **methotrexate (12 mg biweekly)** and **ara-C (50 mg biweekly).** These are given two times a week at first, then less frequently as the CSF begins to clear. *Craniospinal radiation* (4000 cGy to the brain, 3000 cGy to the spine) may also be offered in an attempt to reduce the tumor burden.

Skull Base Metastases

Epidemiology.   The most common hematogenously spread primary tumors are breast, lung, and prostate cancers. At the time of presentation with skull base metastases, about 50% of patients have bony metastases elsewhere in the body.

Presentation.   Five typical clinical syndromes may occur. *Orbital syndrome* presents with dull supraorbital pain, blurred vision, and diplopia. Examination may reveal proptosis, ophthalmoplegia, and decreased sensation along V1. *Parasellar syndrome* presents with frontal headache and ophthalmoparesis but usually not with proptosis. *Middle cranial fossa syndrome* presents as numbness along the distribution of V2 and V3 (numb chin syndrome). *Jugular foramen syndrome* is caused by tumor compressing CN 9, CN 10, and CN 11 as they exit the skull through the jugular foramen. This entity presents with unilateral occipital or glossopharyngeal pain, followed by hoarseness and dysphagia. *Occipital condyle syndrome* presents with orbital pain that worsens with neck flexion. On examination, patients tend to hold the neck stiffly and have tenderness on palpation over the occiput.

Diagnosis.   *CT* is more useful than MRI in evaluating bone destruction of the skull base.

Treatment.   Surgical resection should be performed when feasible, followed by focal radiation. The syndromes that are most likely to respond to radiation are the orbital syndrome, parasellar syndrome, and middle cranial fossa syndrome.

■ GLIOMAS

Approximately 13,000 new cases of **glioma** are diagnosed each year in the United States, a statistic that is dwarfed by that for CNS metastases. Nevertheless, their relentless course, resistance to treatment, and capacity to cause significant morbidity make these neoplasms among the most feared by both patients and physicians. Gliomas are generally classified according to the cell of origin: *astrocytomas, oligodendrogliomas,* and *ependymomas.*

Astrocytomas

Astrocytomas, the most common form of primary brain tumor (approximately 80%), are characterized by their infiltrative nature and heterogeneity, with different regions of the same tumor frequently harboring low-grade, anaplastic, and highly malignant tumor cells. Astrocytomas tend to develop increasingly malignant features over time.

Glioblastoma Multiforme (GBM, Grade III Astrocytoma)

GBM is the most malignant and common form of astrocytoma.

Epidemiology.   GBM represents 60% of all gliomas. The peak incidence of GBM is between 50 and 60 years of age, and the incidence is slightly higher in men than in women.

Pathology.   The main histologic features of GBM are hypercellularity, nuclear atypia and multiple mitotic figures, neovascular endothelial proliferation, and necrosis. This leads to a pattern of necrotic tissue surrounded by ribbons of hypercellularity, a phenomenon termed "pseudopalisading."

Presentation.   Patients present most often with headache (80%), mental status changes (50%), focal motor deficits (40%), and seizures (30%).

Diagnosis.   The imaging test of choice is *MRI*, which shows heterogeneous enhancement with gadolinium, poorly demarcated borders, and hyperintensity on T2-weighted images. *Biopsy* is required to confirm the diagnosis.

Treatment.   *Surgical resection* is the fastest and most effective means to achieve substantial tumor load reduction (debulking). Biopsy is performed in patients with inaccessible tumors or in patients in whom the tumor is in close proximity to eloquent brain areas. *External beam radiation* directed with wide margins is effective in temporarily curbing tumor growth. A dose of up to 6000 cGy is administered. *Chemotherapy* may be used in conjunction with radiation; the most commonly used agents are the nitrosoureas (bischloroethylnitrosourea [BCNU], chloroethylcyclohexlnitrosourea [CCNU]), cisplatin, and procarbazine.

Prognosis.   The majority of patients survive less than 1 year, and 5-year survival is less than 10%. Favorable prognostic factors include age less than 40, good performance status, histologic features, and gross total surgical resection. With multimodality therapy, the median survival improves incrementally:

- Corticosteroids alone: less than 3 months
- Surgery: 4 to 5 months
- Surgery plus radiation: 10 to 12 months

Anaplastic Astrocytoma (Grade II Astrocytoma)

Anaplastic astrocytoma is a glioma of intermediate malignancy between GBM and low-grade astrocytoma.

Epidemiology. Anaplastic astrocytoma accounts for approximately 30% of gliomas. The peak incidence is between 40 and 50 years of age.

Pathology. These are hypercellular tumors, with variable amounts of nuclear pleomorphism and mitoses. As in GBM, there may be neovascular proliferation, but necrosis is distinctly absent.

Presentation. The average duration of symptoms at the time of diagnosis is 15 months, compared to 5 months for GBM. Seizures are the most common presentation, occurring in at least 50% of the cases.

Diagnosis. *MRI* is the imaging test of choice. The tumor may or may not enhance with contrast, and the borders of the tumor are generally poorly defined. *Biopsy* is required to make the diagnosis.

Treatment. *Surgery* is usually not helpful owing to the highly infiltrative nature of these tumors, unless decompression from mass effect is required. The mainstay of treatment is *focal radiation* (5000 to 6000 cGy), but the efficacy of this treatment has never been proven.

Prognosis. Median survival with treatment is approximately 2 years.

Low-Grade Astrocytoma (Grade I Astrocytoma)

Low-grade astrocytoma is a slow-growing, infiltrating tumor. Most tumors harbor functional brain tissue within the gross tumor margin.

Incidence. Low-grade astrocytoma constitutes 20% of all gliomas. It occurs primarily in children and young adults.

Pathology. The tumor cells resemble reactive astrocytes with abundant cytoplasm. They demonstrate a low degree of cellularity and no mitoses, nuclear atypia, or endothelial proliferation.

Presentation. The presentation is typically indolent and of long duration. The most common presentation is *seizures* (65%), which in many cases may be present for years prior to the diagnosis.

Diagnosis. *MRI* is the imaging test of choice. The tumor does not enhance with gadolinium and is poorly defined. Mass effect is a late finding. *Biopsy* is required to make the diagnosis.

Treatment. The highly infiltrative nature of low-grade glioma with functional brain elements within the tumor generally precludes gross total resection. The benefit of radiotherapy versus expectant follow-up has not been established. Radiation should be given, however, if there is clinical progression, or if there are uncontrollable seizures.

Prognosis. Median survival is 8 to 10 years. Older age, change in mental status, and focality on neurologic examination are poor prognostic factors.

Oligodendrogliomas

These uncommon tumors arise from oligodendrocytes, the cells that form axonal myelin sheaths within the CNS.

Epidemiology. Oligodendrogliomas represent approximately 5% of all gliomas, with a peak incidence between 40 to 50 years of age.

Pathology. The tumor cells have a characteristic "fried egg" appearance, with an area of clear cytoplasm surrounding the nucleus.

Presentation. *Seizures* are the most common presenting complaint (in approximately 60% of patients). Focal symptoms are uncommon.

Diagnosis. MRI reveals a tumor with indistinct margins and variable amounts of contrast enhancement. *Calcification* is present in nearly 75% of patients.

Treatment. *Surgery* for biopsy or resection is helpful in establishing a diagnosis and debulking the tumor. In contrast to other gliomas, oligodendrogliomas are exquisitely sensitive to chemotherapy. The most effective chemotherapeutic regimen (termed PCV) combines procarbazine, CCNU, and vincristine. The role of radiation in the treatment of oligodendroglioma is controversial; some experts advocate its use only after subtotal resection of the neoplasm, whereas others recommend it regardless of resection.

Prognosis. As with all gliomas, oligodendroglioma tends to become increasingly malignant over time. Median survival is approximately 3 years.

Ependymomas

These rare neoplasms arise from ependymal cells and can arise anywhere within the neuraxis.

Epidemiology. Ependymomas comprise less than 5% of all gliomas. They are most common in children and young adults, with two peak ages of incidence, at 5 years and at 25 years. They comprise only 3% of intracranial gliomas and approximately 60% of spinal cord gliomas.

Pathology. *Papillary ependymomas* are most common, with well-differentiated cuboidal cells that form "rosettes" (around a central blood vessel) or perivascular "pseudorosettes." *Myxopapillary ependymomas* are more benign and occur exclusively in the sacral filum terminale. *Ependymoblastomas* are more malignant and tend to occur in children. Drop metastases, which result from seeding via the CSF, occur in approximately 10% of patients.

Presentation. In children, the tumor most often arises from the floor of the fourth ventricle, where it can cause symptoms of brain stem dysfunction (ataxia, cranial nerve deficits) or hydrocephalus (headache, vomiting). In approximately one third of cases, ependymomas arise from the supratentorial ventricular system. These patients tend to be young adults who present with signs of increased intracranial pressure (ICP).

Diagnosis. *MRI* is the imaging test of choice. The tumor enhances irregularly with gadolinium, and some degree of calcification is present in more than 50% of the cases. In patients with supratentorial tumors, *spinal MRI* and *LP* are mandatory for the detection of drop metastases.

Treatment. *Surgical resection* is indicated to confirm the diagnosis and debulk the tumor. *Focal radiation* (approximately 4500 cGy) should be directed postoperatively to the tumor bed, and *craniospinal radiation* should be performed if CSF cytology is positive or if drop metastases are detected.

■ NONGLIAL BRAIN TUMORS
Primitive Neuroectodermal Tumors

Epidemiology. Primitive neuroectodermal tumors (PNETs) occur almost exclusively in children or adolescents.

Pathology. PNETs arise from primitive neuroectodermal cells and are malignant, aggressive tumors with rapid growth and a high recurrence rate. They also have the tendency to spread throughout the CSF (drop metastases). Histologically, they consist of small, darkly staining cells that show evidence of neuronal differentiation on immunocytochemistry.

Presentation. Common forms of PNET include the following:
- *Hemispheric PNET.* These are aggressive, highly infiltrative tumors.
- *Medulloblastoma.* This is the most common malignant brain tumor in children (20% of all pediatric brain tumors). Usually localized to the midline cerebellum, medulloblastoma typically presents with ataxia and symptoms of hydrocephalus (headache, vomiting). Nearly one third of the tumors have seeded the CSF at the time of diagnosis.

- *Pineoblastoma.* These tumors occur in the pineal region and are highly responsive to radiation and chemotherapy. They present with hydrocephalus and Parinaud's syndrome (impaired upgaze, loss of pupil reactivity, retraction nystagmus).
- *Neuroblastoma.* Neuroblastoma may arise in the cerebral hemispheres or be intrathoracic (sympathetic ganglia); it sometimes presents with paraneoplastic opsoclonus.
- *Retinoblastoma.* Retinoblastoma presents as an intraocular mass in infants. It is often bilateral and can be familial.
- *Esthesioneuroblastoma.* This tumor arises from the olfactory neuroepithelial tissue in the nasal passages and extends to the base of the brain.

Symptoms depend on tumor location. Extraneural metastases (to bones, lymph nodes, liver, and lungs) occur more often with PNETs than with any other CNS neoplasm.

Treatment. Complete *surgical resection* should be performed in all patients. Most PNETs are responsive to *radiation* (5000 cGy and higher), but recurrence is common. Even if seeding of the CSF is not documented, many practitioners advocate prophylactic craniospinal irradiation.

Prognosis. The overall prognosis is poor. Even with surgery, radiation, and chemotherapy, average survival is 2 years. Surgery combined with radiation is sometimes curative with highly localized tumors; patients surviving for a period of time equal to age at diagnosis plus 9 months can be considered cured.

Primary Central Nervous System Lymphoma

Epidemiology. Primary CNS lymphoma (PCNSL) accounts for 1 to 2% of all primary brain tumors, but the incidence is rising. Patients who are immunocompromised (e.g., patients with acquired immunodeficiency syndrome [AIDS] or organ transplant recipients) are at particularly high risk.

Pathology. PCNSLs are non-Hodgkin's lymphomas, usually of B cell origin, occurring in the absence of systemic lymphoma.

Presentation. There are four distinct clinical presentations of PCNSL:
- *Solitary or multiple discrete tumors.* This is the most common form of presentation; approximately 50% are multifocal.
- *Diffuse infiltrative PCNSL.* This tumor presents as a widespread infiltrative process throughout the brain or as carcinomatous meningitis.
- *Ocular PCNSL.* Retinal or vitreous infiltration antedates or follows the development of CNS lesions in 10% of patients.
- *Spinal PCNSL.* An isolated intramedullary spinal cord lesion is rare.

Diagnosis. *MRI* is the imaging test of choice, because PCNSL may appear isointense on CT. The tumor is often periventricular and usually enhances uniformly with gadolinium, although ring enhancement may occur with larger tumors. The diagnosis is established by *biopsy.* Because steroids have a strong tumoricidal effect and greatly increase the likelihood of a nondiagnostic biopsy, every attempt should be made to prevent treatment with dexamethasone prior to tissue diagnosis. *LP* should be performed unless mass effect is present to detect CSF dissemination, which occurs in up to 35% of patients. *Slit-lamp examination* is required in all patients to detect ocular involvement. In patients with ocular symptoms, a vitreous biopsy should be performed.

Treatment. The role of surgery is limited to tissue diagnosis. **Dexamethasone 10 mg four times a day** leads to temporary tumor regression in many patients, but *radiation* (up to 5000 cGy) is the mainstay of treatment. *Chemotherapy* with methotrexate or cytosine arabinoside (ara-C) may be given postirradiation, and intrathecal methotrexate via an Ommaya reservoir is sometimes used to treat patients with diffuse meningeal disease.

Prognosis. Mean survival with corticosteroids and irradiation is 1 to 2 years in immunocompetent patients and much shorter in immunosuppressed patients. Neuraxis dissemination ultimately occurs in 60% of patients, and systemic lymphoma is present in 10% of patients who survive 1 year, suggesting that systemic chemotherapy should be used as a primary treatment for this disease.

Meningioma

Epidemiology. Meningiomas account for 20% of all intracranial tumors and, after gliomas, are the second most common type of brain tumor in adults. They are twice as common in women as in men; the peak incidence is in the 40s and 50s.

Pathology. Meningiomas are usually histologically benign tumors that arise from arachnoidal cells. They do not invade cerebral tissue but cause symptoms by compressing surrounding structures. The more benign histologic subtypes (meningothelial, fibroblastic, transitional, and psammomatous) behave similarly. The more malignant subtypes (sarcomatous, angioblastic, and hemangiopericytomatous) are prone to recur.

Presentation. The most frequent sites of occurrence of meningioma, in order of decreasing frequency, are hemispheric sites (parasagittal or convexity), sphenoid wing, olfactory groove, suprasellar site, and posterior fossa.

Diagnosis. MRI and CT reveal a homogeneous, sharply demarcated tumor that is dural based and that uniformly enhances with contrast. CT or plain x-rays of the skull may often show overlying areas of calvarial thickening and sclerosis (hyperostosis).

Treatment. *Surgical resection* is the treatment of choice but may not be necessary for incidental, asymptomatic tumors that can be followed expectantly. The rate of recurrence after surgery varies between 10% and 30%, depending on the extent of resection. *Radiotherapy* may be given for tumors with multiple recurrences or for histologically malignant tumors.

Prognosis. Prolonged survival after surgical resection is the rule.

Acoustic Neuroma

Acoustic neuroma arises from the Schwann cells of the vestibular division of CN8; hence, a more appropriate name is vestibular schwannoma. This benign tumor arises within the internal acoustic canal and follows the path of least resistance, growing into the cerebellopontine angle.

Epidemiology. These tumors account for 8% of all brain tumors and occur mainly in middle-aged adults. About 5 to 10% of patients have neurofibromatosis type 2 and may harbor bilateral acoustic neuromas, cranial tumors, or spinal tumors.

Presentation. The most common presenting symptom is unilateral tinnitus or hearing loss. As the tumor grows, it compresses the adjacent cranial nerves, including the trigeminal nerve (leading to facial numbness, reduced corneal reflex), facial nerve, and vestibular nerve (leading to vertigo). Ataxia from compression of the pons and cerebellum is a late sign.

Diagnosis. *Gadolinium-enhanced MRI* can reveal even small intracanalicular tumors. Both *audiography* and *brain stem auditory evoked potentials* are important for quantifying the extent of damage to the cochlear nerve.

Treatment. *Surgical resection* is curative in most cases, particularly when the tumor is small (less than 2 cm in diameter). The main complication of surgery is damage to the cochlear or facial nerves. Radiation is not effective. Stereotactic radiosurgery (gamma knife) shows promise for treating patients with medical conditions that would increase the risk of surgery.

Pituitary Adenoma

Epidemiology. Pituitary adenomas comprise 10% of all brain tumors and occur most frequently in young adults (in their 20s and 30s).

Pathology. These histologically benign tumors tend to be slow growing, and they compress, rather than invade, surrounding neural tissue. Anatomically, pituitary adenomas can be categorized as *microadenomas* (less than 10 mm in diameter), *diffuse adenomas* (surrounded by dura but with some suprasellar extension), and *invasive adenomas* (infiltrating dura, bone, or brain). Histologically, cells may appear chromophobic (most common), acidophilic, or basophilic (least common). However, the light microscopic appearance correlates poorly with secretory activity. The majority of pituitary adenomas are nonsecretory or are prolactinomas.

Presentation. Pituitary adenomas may present via one of three mechanisms:
- *Excessive hormonal secretion*
    Functional or secretory pituitary adenomas may present as (1) Cushing's disease, from ACTH secretion, (2) amenorrhea-galactorrhea, from prolactin secretion, or (3) acromegaly-giantism, from growth hormone secretion. These tumors tend to be small (less than 1 cm) upon diagnosis.
- *Mass effect*
    Besides headache, common syndromes include (1) visual loss with bitemporal hemianopia, (2) panhypopituitarism (hypothyroidism, hypoadrenalism, hypogonadism, diabetes insipidus), and (3) cavernous sinus infiltration (ptosis, proptosis, diplopia).
- *Pituitary apoplexy*
    This syndrome results from acute infarction or hemorrhage into a large, highly vascular tumor and can be life-threatening. Patients present suddenly with headache, visual loss, ophthalmoparesis, and mental status changes. Emergency decompression may be required.

Diagnosis. *MRI* is more sensitive than CT for detecting microadenomas and is the imaging study of choice. Gadolinium normally causes enhancement of the pituitary gland, making adenomas hard to detect. *Visual field testing* is mandatory in all patients. *Endocrinologic investigation* should include the following: T_3, T_4, thyroid-stimulating hormone, growth hormone, prolactin, luteinizing hormone, follicle-stimulating hormone, fasting glucose, serum cortisol, and estradiol (in women) or testosterone (in men) levels.

Treatment.   With the exception of prolactinomas, *transsphenoidal surgery* is generally indicated if signs of mass effect on the optic chiasm or cranial nerves are present. It is often impossible to completely remove a tumor with suprasellar extension, and in these cases, the tumor usually recurs. Focused *radiation* (4000 to 6000 cGy over 4 to 6 weeks) reduces the postoperative recurrence rate and is indicated if the tumor cannot be completely resected. **Bromocriptine 2.5 to 5 mg three times a day,** a synthetic dopamine agonist that inhibits pituitary secretion of prolactin, is the first line of treatment for prolactinomas regardless of size. Large prolactinomas may shrink dramatically with bromocriptine therapy, making surgery unnecessary.

Prognosis.   The overall recurrence rate following surgical resection of pituitary adenoma is approximately 12%, with most recurrences occurring after 4 years.

Craniopharyngioma

Craniopharyngiomas arise from squamous cell nests in the region of the pituitary stalk (Rathke's pouch) and present as suprasellar lesions.

Epidemiology.   Craniopharyngiomas occur both in childhood and in adulthood; they represent 3% of all brain tumors. They are slightly more common in men.

Pathology.   The tumors are biologically and histologically benign but have the tendency to recur if incompletely resected.

Presentation.   As with other suprasellar tumors, craniopharyngiomas cause symptoms by compressing the optic tracts, by depressing hypothalamic or pituitary function, or by increasing ICP.

Diagnosis.   The tumor is often irregular and well demarcated from surrounding structures. Enhancement with contrast is irregular, and many tumors are cystic. Calcification is common (in approximately 50%).

Treatment.   *Surgery* and postoperative *radiation* are the treatments of choice.

25

CEREBROVASCULAR DISEASE

Cerebrovascular disease includes a wide spectrum of disorders, all sharing an acquired or inherited pathology of the cerebral vasculature. Stroke syndromes range in scope from a minor hemisensory loss in a single limb to hemiplegia, cognitive changes, and coma. The onset of deficits usually occurs in seconds to minutes. The **physical examination** can give an impression of the size and a fair estimate of the location of the infarct and can thus guide the urgency of subsequent management steps. **Brain imaging** will be necessary in almost all evaluations of stroke. Magnetic resonance imaging (MRI) should identify all but the smallest lesions and is superior to computed tomography (CT) for brain stem and small, deep, so-called lacunar infarcts. CT is the equal of MRI in detecting acute hemorrhage and is superior for assessing bony abnormalities. Either technology may miss an infarct within the first several hours of onset. Because the brain can tolerate only a few hours of ischemia before becoming irreversibly infarcted, the window of opportunity for acute intervention is narrow. This chapter will focus on the presentation of acute stroke, with attention to the pathophysiologic mechanisms that drive the management decisions discussed in Chapter 7.

■ CLASSIFICATION

Acute stroke comprises three broad categories: **subarachnoid hemorrhage (SAH), ischemic stroke, and intracerebral hemorrhage (ICH).** The clinical presentations may be similar, yet the pathophysiology and consequent management algorithms are distinct.

Subarachnoid Hemorrhage

Clinical Presentation

Sudden, severe ("thunderclap") headache is the classic presentation of SAH from a ruptured cerebral aneurysm. When asked, patients will usually classify the headache as the worst they have ever had or rate it a 10 on a scale of 1 to 10. Stiff neck and photophobia are often present, requiring a consideration of acute bacterial meningitis in the differential diagnosis. Preceding minor headache may occur from a "sentinel bleed" as a preamble to a major hemorrhage. Trauma is a more common cause of hemorrhage in the subarachnoid space, but the clinical presentation is then usually obvious. The most common neurologic finding in SAH is altered mental status. If local signs or symptoms appear, it is often because of the presence of a focal, intracerebral clot or because of direct compression of the aneurysm on a cranial nerve (causing, for example a CN 3 palsy). Missing the diagnosis of SAH can be disastrous. Untreated SAH may be fatal in up to 50% of patients. A large percentage of the deaths may be an immediate consequence of the hemorrhage, but secondary vasospasm, rerupture of the aneurysm, and obstructive hydrocephalus can add significantly to the morbidity and mortality. The rate of rerupture may be as high as 1 to 2% per day for the first 2 weeks. Early diagnosis and surgical clipping of the aneurysm are therefore essential.

Diagnosis

1. **An anatomic brain image should be obtained as soon as possible.**

   Both CT and MRI are good at detecting acute hemorrhage. CT hyperdensity in the sulci, major fissures, or around the brain stem is diagnostic. Particular attention should be paid to the basal cisterns. Subarachnoid blood pooling in the quadrigeminal plate cistern, for example, may appear only as a subtle hyperdensity in this space and may even appear isodense with brain if the blood is 5 to 7 days old. Figure 7–1 shows an example of SAH on CT. Other causes of SAH that may be detectable on CT or MRI include vascular malformation, venous thrombosis, and tumor.

2. **A negative CT or MRI scan does not rule out the diagnosis of SAH.**

   If there is clinical suspicion, and if CT or MRI is negative, a lumbar puncture should be performed. Cerebrospinal fluid will show greater than 1000 red blood cells (RBCs) per mm^3 that do not clear in later tubes. Pathognomonic for SAH is **xanthochromia,** a straw-colored appearance of the CSF supernatant after centrifugation. Lumbar puncture can also rule out a diagnosis of bacterial meningitis.

3. **Patients should be classified according to the SAH grading scale of Hunt and Hess (Table 25–1).**

   Grading SAH patients not only will help monitor the clinical course but will allow more accurate determination of prognosis and will guide management decisions. SAH of Hunt and Hess grades 1 and 2 has a relatively good prognosis and will be managed more aggressively. Patients with grades 3 and 4 have a worse prognosis, and grade 5 patients

Table 25–1 □ **CLINICAL GRADING OF SUBARACHNOID HEMORRHAGE ACCORDING TO THE CLASSIFICATION OF HUNT AND HESS**

Grade	Description
0	Unruptured aneurysm
1	Minor headache, mild nuchal rigidity
2	Severe headache, nuchal rigidity, no focal deficits other than cranial nerve palsy
3	Lethargy, confusion, or mild focal deficit
4	Stupor, moderate to severe hemiparesis
5	Deep coma, decerebrate rigidity, moribund

are moribund. Aggressive, early intervention will usually yield good results only if the initial presentation is at grades 1 to 3.

4. **Once a diagnosis of SAH is made, a four-vessel cerebral angiogram should be performed as soon as possible.**

MR angiography is not indicated because it has a lower sensitivity; whether or not it is positive, an angiogram will still be necessary. The most common sites for aneurysm formation are at vascular branching points around the circle of Willis (Fig. 25–1). Fifteen percent of patients have more than one aneurysm. Nonaneurysmal causes for SAH that may be detectable on angiogram include arteriovenous malformation (AVM), angiopathies such as vasculitis and fibromuscular dysplasia, and venous thrombosis.

5. **If both MRI and angiogram are negative, the SAH may have arisen from a venous bleed around the midbrain.**

A chemistry panel, coagulation profile, and toxicology screen for cocaine should also be obtained if the diagnosis is still unclear.

Management

For patients with aneurysm identified by angiography, management is two-pronged. First, early operative intervention to clip the aneurysm will improve short- and long-term morbidity and mortality. Because the rerupture rate is as high as 20% in the first 2 weeks, clipping the aneurysm will remove a substantial secondary risk. Second, fluid management is crucial both preoperatively and postoperatively to maintain adequate cerebral blood flow in the presence of cerebral ischemia from vasospasm.

1. **Surgery**

Surgical clipping of the aneurysm is generally done as early as possible after the hemorrhage, but it cannot be done

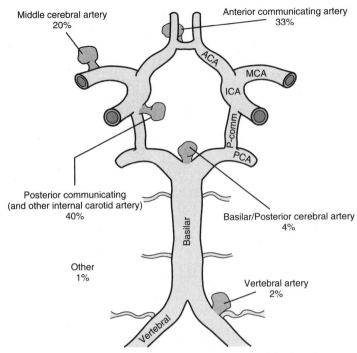

Figure 25-1 □ Most common sites of aneurysms. ACA, Anterior communicating artery; ICA, internal carotid artery; MCA, middle cerebral artery; PCA, posterior cerebral artery; P-comm, posterior communicating artery.

without substantial risk if cerebral vasospasm is present. Vasospasm is rare in the first 3 days, and it peaks around day 7. If, within the first 5 days after hemorrhage, an angiogram shows the aneurysm clearly and shows no vasospasm, surgery should be done within the following 24 hours. Transcranial Doppler ultrasonography is an effective means of monitoring vasospasm both preoperatively and postoperatively, checking for increases in flow velocity in the major vessels around the circle of Willis.

2. **Fluid management**

Patients with SAH are best managed in an intensive care unit. Abnormalities of fluid and sodium homeostasis after SAH favor free-water retention and sodium loss. The emphasis on fluid management is therefore on maintaining normal or increased intravascular volume using isotonic fluids and on avoiding all potential sources of free water. A pulmonary artery catheter may be helpful in assessing volume status, particularly when there is symptomatic vasospasm (Table 25–2).

Ischemic Stroke

Clinical Presentation and Diagnosis

Unlike SAH, both ischemic stroke and intracerebral hemorrhage (ICH) typically present with focal signs. The syndrome produced by infarction depends on the location of the lesion. Pain of any kind, including severe headache, is uncommon. One of the most difficult aspects of managing acute stroke patients is that focal symptoms, particularly minor ones, are often attributed by the patient to some nonneurologic cause and ignored. Visual changes may be interpreted as a need for new glasses. Sensory loss or weakness in an extremity may be brushed off as the result of lifting a heavy package or bumping into the door the day before. Transient symptoms (i.e., transient ischemic attack [TIA]) may portend stroke but may be identified as important only retrospectively (Box 25–1). Delay in treatment beyond the first several hours can result in a missed opportunity for acute intervention with a thrombolytic or neuroprotective agent. Despite an overlap in clinical syndromes among the various pathophysiologic stroke subtypes, one should try to identify the stroke subtype. The management algorithm for secondary prevention depends on the stroke mechanism. Four major categories of stroke mechanism are discussed.

Table 25–2 □ FLUID MANAGEMENT IN SUBARACHNOID HEMORRHAGE

Preoperative:	Normal (0.9%) saline at 80 to 100 ml per hour
Postoperative:	Normal saline at 80 to 100 ml per hour and 250 ml of 5% albumin IV every 2 hours for pulmonary artery diastolic pressure equal to or less than 14 mm Hg (or central venous pressure equal to or less than 8 mm Hg)
Postoperative, with symptomatic vasospasm:	500 ml 5% albumin IV over 30 minutes; if there is no response, raise systolic blood pressure with IV pressors until deficit resolves (to maximum of 200 mm Hg), then follow the postoperative hypervolemia protocol

Box 25–1. TRANSIENT ISCHEMIC ATTACKS

Transient ischemic attacks (TIAs) are defined as transient symptoms of vascular etiology that do not result in infarction. Although the standard clinical definition includes symptoms lasting up to 24 hours, most TIAs last from minutes to a few hours. The definition of TIA and stroke is further complicated by recent advances in brain imaging, which may identify a small infarction even when the stroke symptoms resolve within a day. **The clinical importance of TIA is highlighted by the high incidence of subsequent strokes.** Up to 50% of patients with TIA proceed to have an infarction within 5 years, if they are untreated. The most important etiology of TIA is high-grade carotid stenosis, producing hemodynamic failure or microemboli in the territory of the affected artery. Transient monocular blindness (TMB, amaurosis fugax) or a hemispheral syndrome such as unilateral weakness or sensory changes is a common presentation. Although TIAs may also arise from cardiac embolism or, rarely, from lacunar disease, the most important initial management step is to evaluate the internal carotid arteries, either with duplex Doppler ultrasonography or MR angiography. If stenosis greater than 70% is found, the patient should be considered for carotid endarterectomy. If no large-vessel stenosis is identified, the algorithm for investigating etiology of ischemic stroke should be followed. If no carotid stenosis or cardioembolic source is identified, **ASA 325 mg per day** is the first line of treatment.

Cardioembolic Stroke

Fifteen to 30% of strokes are embolic from a cardiac cause such as atrial fibrillation or valvular disease. The classic clinical presentation of cardioembolic stroke is of sudden deficit, maximal at onset. Syndromes more likely to be embolic include hemianopia without hemiparesis, pure Wernicke's aphasia, and ideomotor apraxia. Hemiparesis and forced gaze deviation suggest a large hemispheric or critical brain stem lesion, particularly if these signs are accompanied by decreased level of consciousness. Behavioral abnormalities such as aphasia or hemineglect without a gaze preference suggest smaller hemispheric lesions. CT and MRI scans that show a single cortical branch territory infarct are also consistent with an embolic source, because atheroma rarely extends into the surface vessels. Main stem branch occlusions are also often embolic, but local atherostenosis is also a possibility in such a setting. A potentially misleading scenario is one in which the initial CT scan shows a deep-lying lucency involving the internal capsule and basal ganglia approximately 2 to 3 cm in size, apparently sparing cortex, which can be misidentified as a large lacune. Often such instances are of embolic origin, involving several lenticulostriate branches of the middle cerebral artery after temporary occlusion of the middle cerebral stem, followed by rapid collateralization from anterior or posterior cerebral branches or recanalization of the occlusion with distal migration of the embolus. A right-to-left shunt, usually a patent cardiac foramen ovale, can be inferred when transcranial Doppler ultrasonography shows microbubbles in the intracranial vessels after injection of 10 ml of agitated saline in the antecubital vein. Contrast transesophageal echocardiography can usually locate the defect in the cardiac atrial wall. If atrial fibrillation is suspected but is not apparent on routine electrocardiogram (ECG), Holter monitoring may be useful.

Large-Vessel Stenosis

In 15% of cases, severe large-vessel atherosclerosis is present and appears to be responsible for the stroke, particularly when there is severe extracranial internal carotid artery stenosis or occlusion and a "distal field" lesion is imaged on CT or MRI as an infarct high over the convexity, spreading caudally from the border zone between arterial territories. The most common clinical profile of this type of infarct is fractional arm weakness (the shoulder is different from the hand). Male gender, hypertension, and diabetes mellitus appear significantly more frequently in this group than in patients with cardioembolic stroke. Intracranial atherosclerosis is more prevalent in non-Caucasian populations, whereas extracranial disease is more prevalent in Caucasians. Duplex Doppler ultrasonography readily delineates the severity of the internal carotid stenosis and shows high-velocity, turbulent flow. Transcranial Doppler ultrasonography often shows dampened pulsatility in the ipsilateral middle cerebral artery. Focal stenoses in the intracranial internal carotid artery (ICA) or other major intracranial vessels may also be documented by transcranial Doppler ultrasonography or MR angiography. Duplex Doppler ultrasonography in combination with MR angiography has generally replaced the more invasive traditional angiogram for evaluating extracranial or intracranial vessels.

Artery-to-Artery Embolus

In another 15% of all stroke patients, large-vessel atherosclerosis with less than hemodynamic stenosis (less than 80% occluded or with an ulcerated plaque) is detected when, radiographically, the infarct appears embolic. In such a setting, embolic fragments may have arisen from atherosclerotic lesions in the ICA. Distinguishing interarterial embolism from a possible cardioembolic etiology may be difficult. The former usually produces a smaller cortical infarct, however, and the latter is more often associated with a decreased level of consciousness and an abnormal initial CT scan.

Lacunar Stroke (Small-Vessel Disease)

Small, deep lesions in the subcortical white matter, the thalamus, the basal ganglia, or the pons accompanied by an appropriate clinical syndrome suggest lacunar disease, accounting for 15 to 20% of all strokes. Arteriolar wall lipohyalinosis, microatheroma, or even microemboli may produce the pathology. Although more than 70 syndromes have been reported with small, deep infarcts, the classic lacunar syndromes are *clumsy hand dysarthria, pure motor hemiparesis, ataxic hemiparesis, sensorimotor syndrome,* and *pure hemisensory loss.* All are typically characterized by an absence of cortical signs. CT scanning is positive in only 50% of lacunar stroke patients, with MRI increasing the yield substantially, especially in the hyperacute period. Asymptomatic lacunes (silent strokes) occur in up to 20% of patients over age 65. Hypertension is the risk factor most associated with lacunar infarction.

Other Etiologies

Despite efforts to arrive at a diagnosis, the cause of infarction in up to 40% of cases remains undetermined after the standard workup is completed. This may result from an inability to perform appropriate laboratory studies because of the patient's advanced age or comorbidity or because of unwillingness on the part of the physician or patient. It may also result from improper timing of tests, such as an angiogram performed after an embolus has cleared or CT or MRI done before the infarction appears. In many cases, however, appropriate testing done at the proper time produces normal or ambiguous findings. Some of these cases may be explained by *hypercoagulable states* from protein C or protein S deficiency, abnormal fibrinogen levels, or lupus anticoagulant or anticardiolipin antibody abnormalities. Other patients may have had emboli from severe *aortic arch atherosclerosis.* Pain in the neck, side of face, teeth, jaw, or retro-orbital area may indicate *vertebral or carotid artery dissection,* even without a history of neck trauma. Migraine, meningitis, arteritis, or inherited metabolic abnormality may explain rare cases. For the purposes of management, cases that cannot be categorized under one of the first four etiologies should be called "cryptogenic stroke." Additional diagnostic studies may be needed to secure a final diagnosis. Because of its grave prognosis, vasculitis of the central nervous system is discussed in Box 25–2.

Box 25–2. CEREBRAL VASCULITIS

Vasculitis is a rare cause of ischemic stroke. Infrequently appearing in the setting of a systemic collagen vascular disease such as polyarteritis nodosa, temporal arteritis, or Takayasu syndrome (aortic arch disease, pulseless disease), stroke may occasionally result from autoimmune disease restricted to the central nervous system. **Granulomatous angitis of the brain** is a rare condition that produces multiple small infarctions in the cortex and deep structures. The clinical presentation is usually one of fluctuating or stepwise progression of mental obtundation, with or without focal signs. CSF protein is elevated above 100 mg/dl and a pleocytosis of up to 500 mononuclear cells per mm^3 is common. The typical arteriographic appearance is of multiple segmental areas of arterial narrowing, often giving a "beaded" look. Clinical and radiographic data can be compelling in any given patient, but it is recommended that a brain and leptomeningeal biopsy specimen be obtained before embarking on the necessarily aggressive treatment regimen. The diagnosis is secured if there are multinucleated giant cells infiltrating arterial walls. Because of the multifocal nature of the disease, however, biopsy results may be negative in up to 50% of cases. Progression of encephalopathy or new focal signs in combination with new areas of arterial narrowing on angiography may be sufficient to begin treatment if the biopsy yields negative results initially. The usual treatment regimen includes high-dose steroids and pulse doses of an immunosuppressive agent such as cyclophosphamide for more than a year. The prognosis is poor overall, but occasionally there is functional restoration approximating previous levels.

Management

1. All patients with suspected stroke in which a deficit persists for more than 1 hour should undergo a CT or MRI head scan. Thrombolytic and neuroprotective protocols are largely experimental but promise to be in more widespread clinical use within a few years. Most hyperacute stroke treatment protocols require initiation of treatment in 3 to 12 hours.
2. If the clinical picture and CT or MRI appearances are consistent with a small or moderate-sized ischemic stroke, **heparin should be administered by intravenous infusion** until the stroke subtype is determined, maintaining a partial thrombo-

plastin time (PTT) of approximately 1.5 times control. This treatment may also be given if there is hemorrhagic infarction on brain imaging, *but only if the infarction is minor.*

3. If the stroke is large and disabling, there is greater risk of *hemorrhagic transformation*; brain imaging should be repeated 48 to 72 hours after stroke onset, and anticoagulation should be started only if hemorrhagic conversion has not occurred. If the clinical and imaging diagnosis is of intracranial hemorrhage, anticoagulants and antiplatelet agents should not be given.

4. *Investigation of stroke etiology* should focus first on cardioembolic sources and large-vessel atherothrombosis. Transthoracic echocardiography, carotid duplex Doppler ultrasonography, and transcranial Doppler ultrasonography should be performed in nearly all cases. MR angiography and transesophageal echocardiography may deliver a diagnosis when the aforementioned studies are inconclusive.

5. Stroke patients with recent myocardial infarction, atrial fibrillation, valvular disease, or intracardiac thrombus should be given **oral anticoagulants such as warfarin** for at least 1 year. The prothrombin time (PT) should be kept at 1.2 to 2.5 times the control value (International Normalized Ratio [INR] = 1.4 to 2.8). If there is atrial fibrillation, warfarin should be continued indefinitely, provided that reliable monitoring is available.

6. If the stroke is small, the heart is normal, and a duplex Doppler sonogram shows significant carotid stenosis (greater than 70%), intravenous heparin should be continued until the exact degree of stenosis has been determined by MR angiography. Digital subtraction or cut film angiography may be used in instances in which MR angiography is unavailable or MR angiography results are equivocal. Prophylactic *endarterectomy* for patients with greater than 70% stenosis should be undertaken as soon as possible. For patients with lesser degrees of stenosis, Doppler monitoring should be undertaken at intervals of 3 to 12 months to document those patients whose stenosis increases to greater than 70% and who then qualify for surgery. Patients in whom asymptomatic carotid stenosis greater than 60% is identified should be considered for endarterectomy, provided the operation is done at a center at which the perioperative morbidity and mortality is less than 3%. The benefit from endarterectomy compared to medical therapy is a 6% versus an 11% chance of stroke in 5 years for the asymptomatic carotid stenosis group, and a 9% versus 26% chance of stroke in 2 years for the symptomatic group.

7. If no cardioembolic source or operable carotid stenosis is identified, and if the patient is not considered at risk for hemorrhage, antiplatelet treatment with **aspirin 325 mg**

daily should be given as chronic outpatient therapy. **Ticlopidine 250 mg PO two times a day** may also be considered, particularly if the patient is female or aspirin therapy has failed. Close attention to the neutrophil count in the first 3 months is essential when using ticlopidine.

Intracerebral Hemorrhage

Clinical Presentation

Primary intracerebral hemorrhage (ICH) is defined as nontraumatic bleeding into the parenchyma of the brain. ICH accounts for approximately 15% of all strokes. Except for a higher frequency of headache and severe hypertension, the presentation of ICH may be identical to that for ischemic stroke occurring in the same location. Coma occurs with greater frequency, particularly when the hemorrhage is of larger volume, involves the brain stem, or dissects into the intraventricular space. Chronic hypertension is the most common cause of ICH and is presumed to result from rupture of the smallest penetrating arteries that have undergone degenerative changes such as lipohyalinosis, fibrinoid necrosis, and microaneurysm formation. Acute hypertension is present in 90% of the cases. Hypertension from sympathomimetics such as pseudoephedrine, amphetamines, or cocaine may also be seen. Hypertensive bleeds occur most commonly in the territory of small penetrating arteries, in the basal ganglia or thalamus (70%), in the brain stem (13%), or in the cerebellum (9%). In the 10% of cerebral hemorrhages that occur in the hemispheres, other causes must be suspected. The differential diagnosis of lobar ICH includes cerebral amyloid angiopathy (Box 25–3), primary or metastatic tumors (melanoma, choriocarcinoma, bronchiogenic carcinoma, or renal cell carcinoma), coagulopathies (disseminated intravascular coagulation, hemophilia, leukemia, thrombocytopenia, overdose of anticoagulant therapy), and vascular malformations.

Diagnosis

The cornerstone for diagnosis of ICH is neuroimaging. Both CT and MRI can detect fresh parenchymal blood in the hyperacute stage. Because the clinical presentation may be indistinguishable from ischemic stroke but the treatment strategies are quite different, any patient presenting with suspected ICH must undergo CT or MRI as soon as possible. In a patient under 60 years of age with a lobar hemorrhage of unclear etiology, an MRI with and without contrast material may disclose tumor or the abnormal vessels of a vascular malformation. For an arteriovenous malformation, cut film angiography would then be necessary to make a definitive diagnosis and plan for treatment.

Distinguishing between ICH and ischemic infarction with hem-

Box 25–3. CEREBRAL AMYLOID ANGIOPATHY

Cerebral amyloid angiopathy (CAA) results from the pathologic deposition of an amorphous eosinophilic amyloid material (that stains with Congo red) in small blood vessels of the cerebral neocortex and adjacent leptomeninges. CAA causes lobar hemorrhage in elderly adults with a mean age of 72. Recurrent hemorrhages are common. The amyloid protein precursor is a gene product from chromosome 21, stimulating interest about the role of amyloid in Down syndrome and Alzheimer's disease. The disease may occur as a familial trait or sporadically. Over 40% of patients with CAA have some degree of dementia. Hemorrhages are most common in the frontal and parietal lobes. MRI, particularly gradient echo sequences, will usually demonstrate multiple, old hemorrhages that may have been asymptomatic. No definitive treatment is currently available.

orrhagic conversion may present a challenge. ICH tends to have a denser, homogeneous appearance, whereas the hemorrhagic infarction is usually spotted or mottled. The location of ICH is more often subcortical, often in the deep gray matter, whereas hemorrhagic infarction, most often occurring in the setting of embolic arterial occlusion, usually involves the cortex and follows a branch artery territory. Intraventricular blood may be seen with ICH, particularly if the hemorrhage is in the thalamus or basal ganglia. Ventricular hemorrhage from embolic infarction does not occur. Significant mass effect may be present from the outset in ICH, whereas the mass effect from hemorrhagic infarction results from secondary edema formation, which peaks after 48 hours. The appearance of the hematoma on MRI follows a characteristic course from the acute to the subacute to the chronic stage (see Chapter 4). Coagulation studies (PT/PTT, platelet count) should be obtained at the time of diagnosis to rule out coagulopathy as a cause for the hemorrhage. Liver function tests should be obtained.

Management

1. **Correction of a coagulopathy** with administration of fresh frozen plasma may be necessary to terminate active bleeding in a patient with a coagulation disorder.
2. **Active control of blood pressure** to systolic levels of 140 to 160 mm Hg should be attempted with oral or intravenous antihypertensives. Unlike in ischemic infarction in which

reduction of blood pressure may result in decreased cerebral blood flow and consequent extension of infarction, reducing blood pressure in ICH may help prevent recurrent bleeding.

3. **Control of increased intracranial pressure** with pharmacologic measures and hyperventilation may allow the patient to pass through a critical phase until the hematoma begins to resolve. (See Chapter 13.)

4. **Placement of an intraventricular drain** may be necessary because intraventricular blood or direct compression of the cerebral aqueduct by a brain stem hematoma may cause obstructive hydrocephalus. If there is any clinical deterioration, a CT or MRI scan should be obtained to distinguish between hydrocephalus and worsening as a result of extension of the hemorrhage or edema.

5. Despite many surgical and medical series, indications for **surgical evacuation of a hematoma** have not been definitively established. When parenchymal hematoma threatens the life of a patient who was initially awake, surgical evacuation may be reasonable. The younger patient who is becoming progressively obtunded and has a large (greater than 30 ml) lobar hematoma may undergo CT-guided stereotactic or open evacuation of the clot. Cerebellar hematomas greater than 3 cm in diameter also appear to benefit from evacuation. For patients presenting in coma or for those with a stable neurologic deficit, surgery is unlikely to help.

26

MOVEMENT DISORDERS
Elan D. Louis

Movement disorders may be defined simply as *abnormal involuntary movements.* These movements are not the result of weakness or sensory deficits. Rather, they are the result of dysfunction of what may be defined anatomically as the basal ganglia or functionally as the extrapyramidal motor system.

The diversity of movement disorders can be overwhelming, with movements including those that are commonly known (tremors, tics) and those that are less familiar (dystonia, chorea, and hemiballismus). Despite this diversity, movement disorders may be conveniently categorized into two types:

1. *Hyperkinesias,* which are characterized by an excess of movement.
2. *Hypokinesias,* which are characterized by a paucity of movement.

Some basic principles should be kept in mind when first approaching a patient with a movement disorder.

■ BASIC PRINCIPLES

1. Take time to **observe** the patient. Some movements may be quite elaborate. At this point, do not make interpretations or think about treatment.
2. **Describe** what you see. Do not label anything yet. For example, note that "the eyes seem to be intermittently squeezing closed" or that "there are rapid jerking movements of the left arm every 5 seconds."
3. **Classify** the movement as a hyperkinesia or a hypokinesia, as defined earlier.
4. **Give the movement a name** (e.g., tremor, chorea). The list of different types of abnormal movements (in Step 4, p. 328) provides a glossary of terms. Read each term and its definition and try to decide which of these terms best describes what you have seen.
5. **Diagnose a specific disease** after naming the movement. For example, both tremor and bradykinesia are features of Parkinson's disease.
6. Finally, think about the appropriate **treatment.** Table 26–1 lists the medications and dosages for treatment of movement disorders.

Table 26–1 □ MOVEMENT DISORDER MEDICATIONS AND DOSAGES

Medication	Dose	Condition Treated
Amantadine (Symmetrel)	100 to 300 mg per day (two to three times a day)	Parkinson's disease
Baclofen (Lioresal)	10 to 80 mg per day (three times a day)	Dystonia
Bromocriptine (Parlodel)	7.5 to 30 mg per day (three to four times a day)	Parkinson's disease
Carbamazepine (Tegretol)	300 to 1200 mg per day (three to four times a day)	Dystonia
Clonazepam (Klonopin)	1 to 10 mg per day (two to three times a day)	Tics
Clonidine (Catapres)	0.2 to 1.0 mg per day, divided	Tics
Diazepam (Valium)	2 to 10 mg per day, divided (two to three times a day)	Dystonia
Haloperidol (Haldol)	1 to 10 mg per day (two to three times a day)	Tics, chorea
Levodopa/carbidopa (Sinemet)	100 to 2000 mg per day, divided	Parkinson's disease
Methazolamide (Neptazane)	50 to 100 mg per day (four times a day)	Essential tremor
Penicillamine (Cuprimine)	250 to 1000 mg per day	Wilson's disease
Pergolide (Permax)	0.75 to 3.0 mg per day (three to four times a day)	Parkinson's disease
Pimozide (Orap)	2 to 10 mg per day, divided	Tics, chorea
Primidone (Mysoline)	100 to 2000 mg per day (three to four times a day)	Essential tremor
Propranolol (Inderal)	40 to 240 mg per day (three to four times a day)	Essential tremor
Reserpine	0.5 to 8 mg per day (three to four times a day)	Tics, chorea
Selegiline (Eldepryl)	5 to 10 mg per day (two times a day)	Parkinson's disease
Trientine (Syprine)	750 to 1250 mg per day (two to four times a day)	Wilson's disease
Trihexyphenidyl (Artane)	1 to 100 mg per day (three to four times a day)	Parkinson's disease

The most common error is for students to skip straight to diagnosis and treatment. It is important first to **observe, describe, classify, and name.**

The remainder of this chapter will follow the above six-step outline.

Step 1: Observe

Inform the patient that you are going to watch his or her movements and then *just observe the patient.* Some patients may be self-conscious and may try to inhibit their movements, particularly if these are embarrassing. If this is the case, ask the patient to allow the body to behave naturally and not stop any movements. Sometimes, you may need to ask the patient to perform certain maneuvers that will bring out the movement (e.g., writing may bring out a tremor, walking may bring out a dystonic foot movement). Some movements may be elaborate, and the period of observation may be lengthy before you get a sense of a pattern or before you can fully describe what you see.

Step 2: Describe

Try to describe the movements. This is not easy. In fact, neurologists find it easier to use gestures, rather than words, when describing a movement.

Some descriptions may be straightforward. For example, you might describe Mr. H.'s movements in the following way: "The right side of Mr. H.'s face twitches every 5 seconds." Other descriptions may be elaborate. For example, you might describe Mrs. R.'s movements as follows: "Mrs. R.'s neck remains completely hyperextended, and once every minute, there is a rapid, violent movement in the opposite direction, so that the head is completely anteroflexed for a brief moment."

Avoid describing Mr. H. as having hemifacial spasm and Mrs. R. as having torticollis. These are not descriptions. These are diagnoses.

Step 3: Classify

It is important to classify the movement as a hyperkinesia or a hypokinesia. This is the easiest step. One caveat is that some patients may simultaneously exhibit both types of movements. For example, a patient with Parkinson's disease may have a tremor (hyperkinesia) as well as bradykinesia (hypokinesia).

Step 4: Give the Movement a Name

The following is a list of different types of abnormal movements. Movements in **bold** letters are the hypokinesias; all others are hyperkinesias. The essential element of each movement is *italicized.*

Name of Movement	Definition or Description
Akathisia	A subjective *feeling of inner restlessness* that is relieved by movements. The movements are stereotypic and complex and convey restlessness (e.g., squirming, crossing and uncrossing legs, rocking back and forth, and pacing).
Asterixis	Sudden periods of *cessation of muscle contraction* best seen when the patient's arms are extended in front, as if stopping traffic.
Athetosis	Slow, *sinuous, writhing* movements, usually of the distal parts of the limbs.
Ballismus	Wild *flinging, flailing* movements that represent large-amplitude proximal choreiform movements. Ballismus is often unilateral (hemiballismus).
Bradykinesia	Movements that are either *slow* or of *diminished frequency* or of *diminished amplitude.*
Chorea	*Semipurposeful flowing* movements that flit from one part of the body to another in a continuous and random pattern.
Dyskinesia	A general term for any excessive movement. The term dyskinesia is often used as an abbreviation for "tardive dyskinesia" (repetitive oral movements often seen in patients taking certain psychiatric medications).
Dystonia	*Twisting* movements that are often *sustained* for variable periods of time.
Freezing	Brief episodes (usually lasting several seconds) during which a motor act is temporarily blocked or halted. Walking is the motor act that is most commonly affected.
Myoclonus	Sudden, brief shock-like *jerks.*
Myokymia	*Quivering* or rippling of muscle.
Rigidity	Muscle tone that is increased on passive motion. Distinct from spasticity, it is present equally in all directions of movement (i.e., both in flexors and in extensors).
Tachykinesia	Movements or speech characterized by *continuous acceleration* or loss of amplitude.

| Tics | *Repetitive, stereotypic* movements or sounds that are *suppressible* and that *relieve a feeling of inner tension.* |
| Tremor | *Regular, oscillatory* movements that may be present at rest or with action. |

Step 5: Diagnose a Specific Disease

Parkinson's Disease

Parkinson's disease was first described by James Parkinson in 1817.

Types of Movements

The types of movements involved in this disease are tremor, rigidity, bradykinesia, freezing, and tachykinesia. The *tremor* of Parkinson's disease is most commonly a *rest tremor.* This means that the tremor is present when the arms are resting in the patient's lap or when they are hanging at the patient's side. One way to bring out a rest tremor is to ask the patient to walk. The *rigidity* is often called *cogwheel* rigidity because it may have a ratchet-like quality. The *bradykinesia* is characterized by a decrease in the frequency of movements (diminished blink frequency, few facial expressions, or *masked facies*) and by slowness of movement, with loss of amplitude. *Postural reflexes,* lost later in the disease, may be tested by performing the *pull test.* Stand behind the patient and pull him or her backward. A normal response is for the patient to take one or two steps back without falling. Always stand behind the patient in the event that you need to catch him or her! *Freezing* is most commonly seen as *start hesitation* or *turning hesitation.* Walking in narrow, cramped quarters may bring on freezing. *Tachykinesia* may take the form of rapid accelerating speech *(tachyphemia)* or rapid accelerated walking *(festination).*

Diagnostic Tests

Parkinson's disease is a clinical diagnosis. The cardinal features are tremor, rigidity, bradykinesia, and loss of postural reflexes. Lumbar puncture (LP), electroencephalogram (EEG), computed tomography (CT), and magnetic resonance imaging (MRI) are nonspecific. The deoxyglucose position emission tomography (PET) scan may show increased uptake in the region of the basal ganglia.

Treatment

Levodopa-carbidopa (Sinemet) 100 to 2000 mg per day of levodopa, with administration of individual doses ranging from every 2 to 3 hours to two times a day.

Bromocriptine (Parlodel) 7.5 to 30 mg per day, divided, three to four times a day.

Pergolide (Permax) 0.75 to 3.0 mg per day, divided, three to four times a day.

Amantadine (Symmetrel) 100 to 300 mg per day, divided, two to three times a day.

Trihexyphenidyl (Artane) 1 to 10 mg per day, divided, three to four times a day.

Selegiline (Eldepryl) 5 to 10 mg per day, divided, two times a day.

Benign Essential Tremor

Many cases of benign essential tremor are very mild, and the symptoms are often mistaken as part of normal aging.

Types of Movements

The movement involved is tremor. The tremor of benign essential tremor is most commonly an *action tremor*. It is present when the patient holds his or her arms extended in front of the body and is often present with tasks such as writing, pouring water, and touching the finger to the nose.

Diagnostic Tests

Essential tremor is diagnosed on the basis of the clinical features described above. Other causes of similar tremor, including hyperthyroidism and certain medications (e.g., lithium or valproate), should be ruled out. The diagnosis may be confirmed by computerized tremor analysis with accelerometry.

Treatment

Propranolol (Inderal) 40 to 240 mg per day, divided, three to four times a day.

Primidone (Mysoline) 100 to 2000 mg per day, divided, three to four times a day.

Methazolamide (Neptazane) 50 to 100 mg per day, divided, two to four times a day.

Huntington's Disease

Huntington's disease was first described by George Huntington in 1872.

Types of Movements

Chorea and dystonia are common features of the disease. The *chorea* of Huntington's disease may involve the face, tongue, limbs, or trunk. It is often exacerbated by anxiety or stress and may be brought on by asking the patient to close the eyes, hold the arms extended in front of the body, and count backward or perform simple arithmetic. Although *dystonia* and *tics* may also be present, these features are less common. The dystonia may take the form of fist clenching, shoulder elevation, or foot inversion during walking. Another feature of Huntington's disease is *motor impersistence* (inhibitory pauses occurring during voluntary motion that account for the "milkmaid grips" seen when hand grasp is tested). Patients with Huntington's disease do not have only involuntary movements. Psychiatric features (depression, psychosis) are very common in this disease, as are cognitive problems (mild to severe) and changes in personality, with prominent disinhibition.

Diagnostic Tests

Because the disease is transmitted in an autosomal dominant manner, a family history is an important feature of the diagnosis. One should rule out other causes of chorea including hyperthyroidism, use of anticonvulsants, and Sydenham's chorea. The abnormal gene, on the short arm of chromosome 4, consists of an abnormally long CAG repeat fragment. The CT or MRI scan may show atrophy of the caudate nuclei.

Management

In many cases, the movements are not bothersome to the patient, and the psychiatric manifestations are often the focus of treatment. However, treatment for the movements might consist of

Haloperidol (Haldol) 1 to 10 mg per day, divided, two to three times a day.

Reserpine 0.5 to 8 mg per day, divided, three to four times a day.

Idiopathic Torsion Dystonia (Dystonia Musculorum Deformans)

This illness is characterized by twisting dystonic movements.

Types of Movements

The illness usually begins in childhood and has a progressive course. The *dystonia* often involves the foot initially and is most apparent with certain actions but not with others (e.g., intermittent spasmodic inversion of the foot while walking but not while running or walking backward). Although the dystonia initially consists of twisting *movements* with action, sustained dystonic *postures* at rest become apparent eventually.

Diagnostic Tests

The diagnosis is based on clinical history and examination. It should be distinguished from other secondary or symptomatic causes of dystonia (e.g., Wilson's disease, Hallervorden-Spatz disease) and from adult-onset dystonia. The latter usually runs a more benign course and begins in adulthood with involvement of the neck, eyes, or hand, but it rarely involves the leg. The gene for idiopathic torsion dystonia, the DYT1 gene, is located on the long arm of chromosome 9 and is inherited in an autosomal dominant manner with a penetrance as low as 30%.

Management

Trihexyphenidyl (Artane) 1 to 100 mg per day, divided, three to four times a day.

Baclofen (Lioresal) 10 to 80 mg per day, divided, three times a day.

Diazepam (Valium) 2 to 10 mg per day, divided, two to three times a day.

Carbamazepine (Tegretol) 300 to 1200 mg per day, divided, three to four times a day.

Botulinum toxin (Botox) injected into selected muscles several times per year.

Tourette's Syndrome

Tourette's syndrome was first definitively described by Gilles de la Tourette in 1885.

Types of Movements

Tics are characteristic of Tourette's syndrome. They may be *simple motor tics* (eye blinking, eyebrow raising), *complex motor tics* (head shaking, wrist shaking), *simple phonic tics* (throat clearing, grunting), or *complex phonic tics* (uttering words). *Coprolalia* (uttering obscenities) and *echolalia* (repeating sounds or words) are examples of the latter. As with most tics, these are voluntarily suppressible for brief periods and may vary in intensity over time.

Diagnostic Tests

The diagnosis is clinical. This is a disorder that begins in childhood with both motor and phonic tics. Coprolalia is not an essential feature of the diagnosis.

Management

Clonazepam (Klonopin) 1 to 10 mg per day, divided, two to three times a day.

Pimozide (Orap) 2 to 10 mg per day, divided.

Haloperidol (Haldol) 1 to 10 mg per day, divided, two to three times a day.

Reserpine 0.5 to 8 mg, divided, three to four times a day.

Clonidine (Catapres) 0.2 to 1.0 mg per day, divided.

Wilson's Disease

Wilson's disease was first described by Samuel Alexander Kinnier Wilson in 1912.

Types of Movements

The movements are protean. Tremor, rigidity, bradykinesia, dystonia, and chorea are all seen in this disease, and one or more of these movements may be present. A *parkinsonian form* of the illness may be characterized by rest tremor, rigidity, or bradykinesia. A *pseudosclerotic* form of the illness is associated with a *wing-beating tremor* (a large-amplitude, flapping, violent tremor that is present when the shoulders are abducted, elbows are flexed, and fingers are facing each other). *Dystonia* and *chorea* may also be present. Dysarthria occurs frequently and may progress to anarthria. Psychiatric manifestations (anxiety, depression, psychosis) are a common feature of the illness.

Diagnostic Tests

The diagnosis is based on clinical history and examination and is supported by the presence of Kayser-Fleischer rings (ring-shaped copper deposits in the cornea), low serum ceruloplasmin level, abnormalities in liver function tests, or hepatitis. Lesions in the basal ganglia may be seen on an MRI scan. The gene pWD is located on the long arm of chromosome 13.

Management

Penicillamine (Cuprimine) 125 to 1000 mg per day.
Trientine (Syprine) 750 to 1250 mg per day, divided, two to four times a day.

Miscellaneous Disorders

This section briefly discusses those movements from the list in **Step 4** that were not discussed under specific diseases.

Akathisia is most commonly seen as a side effect of certain psychiatric medications.

Asterixis, usually seen bilaterally in the arms, is most commonly a feature of toxic/metabolic states such as liver or renal failure. Patients are often encephalopathic.

Athetosis may appear in a variety of neurologic disorders ranging from cerebral palsy to paroxysmal kinesiogenic choreoathetosis. Athetotic movements may merge with chorea (choreoathetosis).

Ballismus, most commonly unilateral (hemiballismus), is usually the result of a stroke in the contralateral subthalamic nucleus.

Myoclonus may occur anywhere in the body, including palatal myoclonus and ocular myoclonus. Myoclonus may be the result of anoxic ischemic injury (Lance-Adams syndrome), birth injuries, degenerative disorders (Ramsay Hunt syndrome), infections, tumors, strokes, or even medications (levodopa). Hiccups are a physiologic form of myoclonus.

Myokymia, most commonly seen in facial muscles, is often due to pontine lesions, particularly plaques in multiple sclerosis or pontine gliomas.

APPENDIX A–1

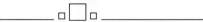

MUSCLES OF THE NECK
AND BRACHIAL PLEXUS

Muscle	Action to Test	Roots	Nerve
Deep neck	Flexion, extension, rotation of neck	C1, C2, C3, C4	Cervical
Sternocleidomastoideus	Rotation of head to contralateral shoulder	XI, C2, C3	Spinal accessory
Trapezius	Elevation of the shoulders	XI, C3, C4	Spinal accessory
Diaphragm	Inspiration	C3, C4, C5	Phrenic
Serratus anterior	Forward shoulder thrust	C5, C6, C7	Long thoracic
Rhomboideus minor	Adduction and elevation of scapula	C4, C5	Dorsal scapular
Levator scapulae	Elevation of scapula	C4, C5	Dorsal scapular
Supraspinatus	Abduction of arm (0 to 90 degrees)	**C5,** * C6	Suprascapular
Infraspinatus	Lateral arm rotation	**C5,** C6	Suprascapular
Deltoideus	Abduction of arm (>30 degrees)	**C5,** C6	Axillary
Teres minor	Medial arm rotation	C4, C5	Axillary
Biceps brachii	Flexion of supinated forearm	**C5,** C6	Musculocutaneous
Brachialis	Flexion of pronated forearm	C5, C6	Musculocutaneous
Teres major	Medial rotation and adduction of arm	C5–C7	Subscapular
Latissimus dorsi	Adduction of arm	C6, **C7,** C8	Thoracodorsal
Flexor carpi ulnaris	Ulnar flexion of hand	C7, **C8,** T1	Ulnar
Flexor digitorum profundus (ulnar part)	Flexion of distal phalanx of fingers 4 and 5	**C8,** T1	Ulnar
Adductor pollicis	Adduction of thumb	C8, T1	Ulnar
Abductor digiti minimi manus	Abduction of little finger	C8, T1	Ulnar
Flexor digiti minimi brevis manus	Flexion of little finger	C8, **T1**	Ulnar
Interossei	Abduction (dorsal) or adduction (palmar) of fingers	C8, T1	Ulnar
Lumbricales 3 and 4	Flexion of proximal phalanges and extension of two distal phalanges (fingers 4 and 5)	C8	Ulnar
Flexor digitorum superficialis	Flexion of middle phalanx fingers 2 to 5, flexion of hand	C7, **C8,** T1	Median

Muscle	Action	Nerve root	Nerve
Pronator teres	Pronation of forearm	C6, C7	Median
Flexor carpi radialis	Radial flexion of hand	C6, C7	Median
Palmaris longus	Wrist flexion	C7, C8, T1	Median
Abductor pollicis brevis	Abduction of thumb metacarpal	C8, **T1**	Median
Flexor pollicis brevis	Flexion of proximal phalanx of thumb	C8, **T1**	Median
Opponens pollicis	Opposition of thumb	C8, **T1**	Median
Lumbricales 1 and 2	Flexion of proximal phalanx and extension of distal phalanges (fingers 2 and 3)	C8, **T1**	Median
Flexor digitorum profundus (radial part)	Flexion of distal phalanx of fingers 2 and 3; flexion of hand	C7, **C8**	Median (anterior interosseous nerve)
Flexor pollicis longus	Flexion of distal phalanx of thumb	C7, **C8**	Median (anterior interosseous nerve)
Triceps brachii	Forearm extension	C6, **C7**, C8	Radial
Brachioradialis	Forearm flexion (with thumb pointing upwards)	**C6**, C7	Radial
Extensor carpi radialis	Radial hand extension	**C6**, C7	Radial
Supinator	Forearm supination	**C7**, C8	Radial
Extensor digitorum	Extension of hand and phalanges of fingers 2 to 5	**C7**, C8	Radial (posterior interosseous nerve)
Extensor carpi ulnaris	Ulnar hand extension	**C7**, C8	Radial (posterior interosseous nerve)
Abductor pollicis longus	Abduction of thumb metacarpal	**C7**, C8	Radial (posterior interosseous nerve)
Extensor pollicis brevis and extensor pollicis longus	Thumb extension and radial wrist extension	**C7**, C8	Radial (posterior interosseous nerve)
Extensor indicis	Index finger extension and hand extension	**C7**, C8	Radial (posterior interosseous nerve)

*Boldface letters indicate primary innervation.

APPENDIX A–2

MUSCLES OF THE PERINEUM AND LUMBOSACRAL PLEXUS

Muscle	Action to Test	Roots	Nerve
Iliopsoas	Hip flexion	L1, **L2**,* **L3**	Femoral and L1, L2 and L3
Sartorius	Hip flexion and lateral thigh rotation	L2, L3	Femoral
Quadriceps femoris	Leg extension	L2, **L3, L4**	Femoral
Adductor longus	Thigh adduction	L2, **L3,** L4	Obturator
Adductor brevis	Thigh adduction	L3, L4	Obturator
Adductor magnus	Thigh adduction	L2, L3, L4	Obturator
Gracilis	Thigh adduction	L3, L4	Obturator
Obturator externus	Thigh adduction and lateral rotation	L3, L4	Obturator
Gluteus medius and gluteus minimus	Thigh abduction and medial rotation	**L4, L5,** S1	Superior gluteal
Tensor fasciae latae	Thigh abduction	L4, L5	Superior gluteal
Gluteus maximus	Hip extension	**L5, S1,** S2	Inferior gluteal
Biceps femoris	Knee flexion (and assistance with thigh extension)	L5, S1, S2	Sciatic (trunk)
Semitendinosus	Knee flexion (and assistance with thigh extension)	L5, S1, S2	Sciatic (trunk)
Semimembranosus	Knee flexion (and assistance with thigh extension)	L5, S1, S2	Sciatic (trunk)
Tibialis anterior	Foot dorsiflexion and inversion	L4, **L5**	Deep peroneal
Extensor digitorum longus	Extension of toes 2 to 5 and foot dorsiflexion	**L5,** S1	Deep peroneal
Extensor hallucis longus	Great toe extension and foot dorsiflexion	**L5,** S1	Deep peroneal
Extensor digitorum brevis	Extension of toes	**L5,** S1	Deep peroneal
Peroneus longus and peroneus brevis	Foot eversion (and assistance with plantar flexion)	**L5,** S1	Superficial peroneal
Tibialis posterior	Foot plantar flexion and inversion	**L5,** S1	Tibial
Flexor digitorum longus	Foot plantar flexion and flexion of toes 2 to 4	S2, S3	Tibial
Flexor hallucis longus	Foot plantar flexion and flexion of terminal phalanx of great toe	S1, S2	Tibial
Gastrocnemius	Knee flexion and ankle plantar flexion	**S1** (S2)	Tibial
Soleus	Ankle plantar flexion	**S1** (S2)	Tibial
Perineal muscles and sphincters	Voluntary contraction of the pelvic floor	S2, S3, S4	Pudendal

*__Boldface__ letters indicate primary innervation.

339

APPENDIX A–3

BRACHIAL PLEXUS

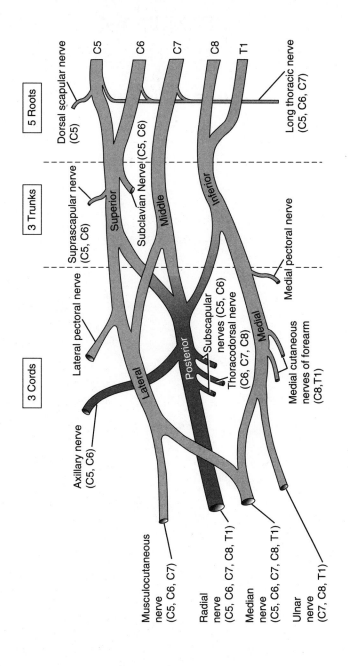

341

APPENDIX A–4

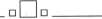

LUMBAR PLEXUS

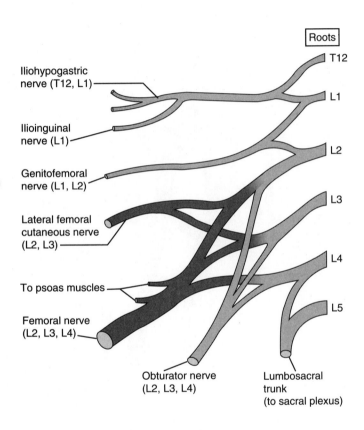

Roots

T12

L1

L2

L3

L4

L5

Iliohypogastric
nerve (T12, L1)

Ilioinguinal
nerve (L1)

Genitofemoral
nerve (L1, L2)

Lateral femoral
cutaneous nerve
(L2, L3)

To psoas muscles

Femoral nerve
(L2, L3, L4)

Obturator nerve
(L2, L3, L4)

Lumbosacral
trunk
(to sacral plexus)

SENSORY DERMATOME MAP

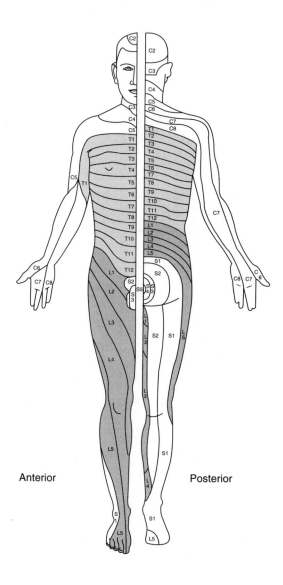

Anterior

Posterior

APPENDIX A-6

□ ▢ □

MINI MENTAL STATE EXAMINATION

Patient: _____

Date __/__/__

Examiner: _____

	Normal Score*
Younger Patients	28–30
Older Patients	24–30
(*Score = number correct)	

Instructions: Say to the person "I would like to ask you some questions to check your memory and concentration. Some questions may be easy and some may be difficult." Record the patient's response, where applicable, and darken one circle to indicate correctness of each response.

	Patient's Response	Incorrect	Correct
1. What is today's date?	_____	⓪	①
2. What is the year?	_____	⓪	①
3. What is the month?	_____	⓪	①
4. What is the day of the week?	_____	⓪	①
5. What season is it?	_____	⓪	①
6. What is the name of this place?	_____	⓪	①
7. What floor are we on?	_____	⓪	①
8. What town or city are we in?	_____	⓪	①
9. What county (district, borough, area) are we in?	_____	⓪	①
10. What state are we in?	_____	⓪	①

	Patient's Response	Incorrect	Correct
11. Say, "I am going to name three objects. After I have said them, I want you to repeat them. Remember what they are because I am going to ask you to name them again in a few minutes. Then say "apple," "table," "penny" clearly and slowly, about one second for each. Score the first try. Repeat the objects until the patient can repeat all three, for up to three trials.	"Apple"	⓪	①
	"Table"	⓪	①
	"Penny"	⓪	①
12. Say, "I am going to say a word and ask you to spell it forward and backward. The word is WORLD. First can you spell it forward? Now spell it backward." Repeat if necessary, and help the patient to spell WORLD forward. Indicate and score the first five letters of the backward spelling.	1st _____	⓪	①
	2nd _____	⓪	①
	3rd _____	⓪	①
	4th _____	⓪	①
	5th _____	⓪	①
13. Show the patient a wristwatch and ask "What is this called?"	"Watch"	⓪	①
14. Show the patient a pencil and ask "What is this called?"	"Pencil"	⓪	①
15. Say, "I would like you to repeat a phrase after me. The phrase is 'No ifs ands or buts.' " Allow only one trial.		⓪	①
16. Say "I'm going to give you a piece of paper. When I do, take the paper in your right hand, fold the paper in half, and then put the paper on your lap." Read the full statement, then give him or her the paper. Do not repeat or coach.	Takes paper in right hand	⓪	①
	Folds paper in half	⓪	①
	Puts paper on lap	⓪	①

	Patient's Response	Incorrect	Correct

17. Hold the piece of paper that reads "Close your eyes," so the patient can see it clearly. Say "Read the words on this page, then do what they say." Score correct only if the patient actually closes his or her eyes.

                     ⓪   ①

18. Ask "What were the three objects I asked you to remember?"

   "Apple"   ⓪   ①
   "Table"   ⓪   ①
   "Penny"   ⓪   ①

19. Give the patient a blank piece of paper and say "Write a complete sentence on this piece of paper." It is to be written spontaneously and must contain a subject and a verb to be correct. Correct grammar and punctuation are not necessary.

                     ⓪   ①

20. Show the page with the intersecting pentagons and say "Here is a drawing. Draw this same drawing on this same page." Two five-sided figures must intersect to form a four-sided figure, and all angles must be preserved. Tremor and rotation are ignored.

                     ⓪   ①

CLOSE YOUR EYES

A

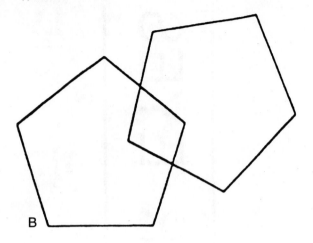

B

APPENDIX B

ON-CALL FORMULARY: COMMONLY PRESCRIBED MEDICATIONS IN NEUROLOGY

Acetazolamide (Diamox) (Chapters 12 and 15)

Indications	Pseudotumor cerebri
Actions	Diuretic that is thought to reduce cerebrospinal fluid (CSF) volume, and intracranial pressure
Side effects	Paresthesias, tinnitus or hearing dysfunction, anorexia, nausea, vomiting, diarrhea, polyuria
Dose	500 mg PO two times a day

Amantadine (Symmetrel) (Chapter 26)

Indications	Parkinson's disease
Actions	Antiviral agent that also increases dopamine release, blocks dopamine reuptake, and stimulates dopamine receptors
Side effects	Livedo reticularis, ankle edema, confusion, hallucinations, insomnia
Comments	More effective for akinesia and rigidity, less effective for tremor; best used for 6 months to a year as monotherapy in patients with mild to moderate Parkinson's disease; may delay need for initiation of levodopa
Dose	100 to 300 mg PO two times a day

Amitriptyline (Elavil) (Chapters 15 and 18)

Indications	Peripheral neuropathy, dysesthesias, migraine prophylaxis, antidepressant
Actions	Inhibitor of membrane pump responsible for uptake of norepinephrine and serotonin, anticholinergic effects; unknown mechanism for action on neuropathy and migraine
Side effects	Drowsiness, paresthesias, urinary retention, dry mouth, constipation, blurred vision, confusion, cardiac conduction block, arrhythmias

349

Comments	Sedative effect may limit use for migraine and neuropathy to evening doses
Dose	25 to 75 mg every day at night time for migraine and peripheral neuropathy; up to 150 mg daily in divided doses may be required for antidepressant effect

Azathioprine (Imuran) (Chapter 16)

Indications	Myasthenia gravis (long-term management)
Actions	Immunosuppressant
Side effects	Leukopenia, thrombocytopenia, nausea, vomiting, increased secondary infection risk
Comments	Adequate immunosuppression is reflected by mild decrease in white blood cell count and increase in mean corpuscular volume
Dose	100 to 250 mg PO per day

Baclofen (Lioresal) (Chapters 22 and 26)

Indications	Dystonia, spasticity of multiple sclerosis
Actions	γ-aminobutyric acid agonist, antispasmodic
Side effects	Confusion, sedation, increased muscle weakness
Comments	Can be given via intrathecal pump for severe cases
Dose	10 to 20 mg three times a day

Bethanechol (Urecholine) (Chapter 22)

Indications	Urinary retention due to neurogenic atonic bladder
Actions	Cholinergic agonist that stimulates parasympathetic muscarinic receptors
Side effects	Cramps, nausea, diarrhea, lacrimation, hypotension, sweating
Comments	Antidote for overdose is atropine 0.6 mg IV
Dose	10 to 50 mg PO three to four times a day

Botulinum toxin (Botox) (Chapter 26)

Indications	Focal dystonia, blepharospasm
Actions	Neuromuscular blocking agent
Side effects	Increased muscle weakness

Comments	Antibody-mediated tolerance may develop over time
Dose	1.25 to 2.50 units per injection site

Bromocriptine (Parlodel) (Chapters 21 and 26)

Indications	Parkinson's disease, neuroleptic malignant syndrome
Actions	Dopamine agonist
Side effects	Nausea, headache, dizziness, fatigue, vomiting
Comments	May delay the need for levodopa
Dose	2.5 mg to 10 mg three times a day

Capsaicin (Zostrix) (Chapter 18)

Indications	Painful peripheral neuropathy
Actions	Topical analgesic; probable substance P mediator in sensory neurons
Side effects	None significant
Comments	Now available without prescription
Dose	0.025% or 0.075% cream, apply topically three to four times a day

Carbamazepine (Tegretol) (Chapter 5)

Indications	Partial and generalized seizures, trigeminal neuralgia
Actions	Reduces polysynaptic responses and blocks post-tetanic potentiation; action on tregeminal neuralgia unknown
Side effects	Double or blurred vision, dizziness, vertigo, gastrointestinal upset, diarrhea, rare agranulocytosis, syndrome of inappropriate antidiuretic hormone, Stevens-Johnson syndrome
Comments	Half-life of 10 to 35 hours; drug levels needed for anticonvulsant use are 4 to 12 μg/ml; raises levels of phenytoin, lowers levels of valproate
Dose	300 to 1200 mg daily in divided doses three to four times a day; usual starting dose is 200 mg three times a day

Clonazepam (Klonopin) (Chapter 26)

Indications	Tourette's syndrome, tics
Actions	Benzodiazepine sedative-hypnotic drug

Side effects	Sedation
Comments	May be habit forming
Dose	1 to 10 mg per day, divided, two to three times a day

Cyproheptadine (Periactin) (Chapter 15)

Indications	Migraine prophylaxis
Actions	Serotonin and histamine antagonist
Side effects	Dizziness, drowsiness, decreased coordination
Comments	Second line of therapy; contraindicated with monoamine oxidase inhibitors, closed-angle glaucoma, pyloric or bladder obstruction
Dose	4 to 8 mg PO three times a day

Dantrolene (Dantrium) (Chapter 21)

Indications	Neuroleptic malignant syndrome
Actions	Direct-acting skeletal muscle relaxant
Side effects	Pulmonary edema, thrombophlebitis
Comments	Approved by Food and Drug Administration for use in malignant hyperthermia; use in neuroleptic malignant syndrome described in medical literature
Dose	1 to 10 mg/kg IV every 4 to 6 hours

Dexamethasone (Decadron) (Chapters 6, 8, and 24)

Indications	Spinal cord compression, neoplasm or abscess in the central nervous system (CNS) with mass effect
Actions	Anti-inflammatory agent
Side effects	Peptic ulcer disease, sodium and fluid retention, hypertension, hyperglycemia, myopathy, impaired wound healing, avascular necrosis of femoral or humeral heads, endocrine abnormalities
Comments	Reduces vasogenic edema but not cytotoxic edema
Dose	For spinal neoplasm: 100 mg IV bolus; for intracranial mass: 6 mg IV every 6 hours

Diazepam (Valium) (Chapters 5 and 9)

Indications	Seizures, anxiety, alcohol withdrawal
Actions	Benzodiazepine sedative-antianxiety agent

Side effects	Sedation, hypotension, respiratory depression, paradoxical agitation
Comments	May be administered IV, IM, or PO; patients with history of benzodiazepine use or ethanol abuse may have cross-tolerance, requiring higher doses; habit forming with chronic use
Dose	For ongoing seizure or status epilepticus: 5 mg IV push, with repeats every 5 minutes up to 20 mg; for agitation, anxiety, or ethanol withdrawal: 2 to 10 mg PO or IV every 3 to 4 hours.

Diphenhydramine (Benadryl) (Chapter 19)

Indications	Acute drug-induced dystonic reaction, insomnia
Actions	Antihistamine and anticholinergic
Side effects	Drowsiness, dizziness, dry mouth, urinary retention
Comments	Avoid use in elderly, confused patients: may have CNS side effects
Dose	For dystonic reaction: 50 mg IV or IM, may repeat after several minutes; for insomnia: 25 to 50 mg PO per day at night

Divalproex sodium (Depakote) (Chapter 5)

Indications	Partial or generalized seizures
Actions	Anticonvulsant
Side effects	Nausea, weight gain, hair loss, tremor, hepatitis, agranulocytosis, thrombocytosis, Stevens-Johnson syndrome
Comments	Therapeutic range is 50 to 100 $\mu g/ml$; increases levels of carbamazepine and phenytoin
Dose	250 to 1000 mg PO four times a day

Donepezil hydrochloride (Aricept) (Chapter 19)

Indications	Alzheimer's disease
Actions	Cholinesterase inhibitor
Side effects	Nausea, diarrhea
Comments	May promote GI bleeding in patients with peptic ulcer disease
Dose	5 mg to 10 mg PO per day

Edrophonium (Tensilon) (Chapter 16)

Indications	Evaluation for myasthenia gravis
Actions	Short-acting anticholinesterase (cholinergic action)
Side effects	Nausea, bradycardia, arrhythmias
Comments	Atropine 0.4 mg should be kept at the bedside to reverse adverse cholinergic side effects
Dose	2 mg IV test dose, then 8 mg IV after 45 seconds

Ergotamine (Dihydroergotamine or D.H.E. 45 IV or IM injection; with caffeine: Cafergot, Wigraine) (Chapter 15)

Indications	Migraine (abortive therapy)
Actions	Alpha-adrenergic/serotonin antagonist; cranial vasoconstrictor
Side effects	Precordial tightness, myalgias, paresthesias, nausea
Comments	D.H.E. 45 may require pretreatment with metoclopramide 10 mg IV or IM and promethazine 50 mg IV as antiemetic; contraindicated in complicated migraine or patients with coronary artery disease
Dose	1 tablet PO at onset, then repeat every 30 minutes up to 6 tabs; alternatively, 1 suppository PR, may repeat one time; D.H.E. 45: 1 mg IV or IM, repeat in 1 hour if needed

Ethosuximide (Zarontin) (Table 5–5)

Indications	Absence seizures
Actions	Anticonvulsant
Side effects	Drowsiness, gastrointestinal (GI) upset, anorexia, headache, dizziness
Comments	Pediatric population
Dose	250 mg PO per day (ages 3 to 6), 500 mg PO per day if over 6 years of age

Felbamate (Felbatol) (Chapter 5)

Indications	Monotherapy or adjunctive therapy in partial seizure or secondarily generalized seizure
Actions	Anticonvulsant
Side effects	Aplastic anemia, hepatotoxicity, anorexia, headache, insomnia, somnolence

Comments	Second line medication; drug interactions: reduces carbamazepine levels but increases toxic metabolite, therefore doses of carbamazepine, as well as phenytoin, must be reduced
Dose	400 mg PO three times a day, taper up to 3600 mg per day; in pediatric patients: begin 15 mg/kg per day

Fludrocortisone (Florinef) (Chapter 17)

Indications	Orthostatic hypotension
Action	Potent mineralocorticoid
Side effects	Volume overload, congestive heart failure, hypertension, edema
Comments	The lowest possible effective dose should be used
Dose	0.1 mg PO one to three times per day

Fosphenytoin (Chapter 5)

Indications	Status epilepticus
Actions	Anticonvulsant
Side effects	Nystagmus, ataxia, cardiac arrhythmias, hypotension
Comments	IV form of phenytoin
Dose	15 mg/kg IV load infused at 50 mg per minute

Gabapentin (Neurontin) (Chapter 5)

Indications	Adjunctive therapy in adult epilepsy
Actions	Anticonvulsant
Side effects	Somnolence, dizziness, ataxia, fatigue, nystagmus
Comments	Second line medication for epilepsy; may be effective for painful peripheral neuropathy
Dose	Taper up to 300 mg PO three times a day over a few days; may taper up to maximum 3600 mg per day

Glycopyrrolate (Robinul) (Chapter 16)

Indications	Control of secretions in myasthenia gravis or bulbar amyotrophic lateral sclerosis
Actions	Anticholinergic (antimuscarinic) agent

Side effects	Anticholinergic: decreased sweating, urinary retention, tachycardia, blurred vision
Dose	1 to 2 mg PO three times a day

Haloperidol (Haldol) (Chapters 9 and 26)

Indications	Psychosis, acute agitation, Tourette's syndrome, Huntington's disease
Actions	Antipsychotic neuroleptic butyrophenone
Side effects	Sedation, extrapyramidal effects (acute or with chronic use), galactorrhea, jaundice, neuroleptic malignant syndrome
Comments	Extrapyramidal effects may occur acutely or with chronic use
Dose	For agitation or acute psychosis: 2 to 10 mg IM, may repeat every hour; for chronic agitation or psychosis: 0.5 to 2 mg PO two to three times a day

---

Heparin (Chapters 7, 12, and 25)

Indications	Acute embolic or progressing stroke, transient ischemic attack
Actions	Antithrombin effect; acts in conjunction with antithrombin III
Side effects	Hemorrhage, thrombocytopenia
Comments	Monitor aPTT, usually to a target of 1.5 to 2 times control
Dose	20,000 units in 500 ml D5W at 20 ml per hour (800 units per hour maintenance, no bolus)

Immune globulin (IVIG) (Chapters 16 and 21)

Indications	Guillain-Barré syndrome (GBS), chronic inflammatory demyelinating polyneuropathy (CIDP)
Actions	Immunosuppressive
Side effects	Renal failure, aseptic meningitis, anaphylaxis
Comments	Hydrate patient well to avoid renal toxicity
Dose	For GBS: 0.4 g/kg IV per day for 5 days; for CIPD 0.4 g/kg IV weekly

---

Interferon beta-1b (Betaseron) (Chapter 22)

Indications	Relapsing-remitting multiple sclerosis (MS)
Actions	Antiviral, immunoregulatory agent

Side effects	Injection site pain and inflammation, influenza-like symptoms, headache
Comments	Reduces frequency and severity of MS episodes
Dose	0.3 mg (9.6 million IU [one vial]) SC every other day

Levodopa-Carbidopa (Sinemet, Sinemet CR) (Chapter 26)

Indications	Parkinson's disease
Actions	Levodopa is converted to dopamine in the basal ganglia; carbidopa inhibits dopamine production (dopa decarboxylation) in the periphery
Side effects	Dyskinesias: dystonia, chorea; confusion, paranoia
Comments	Dosing highly dependent on clinical response; top number denotes milligrams of carbidopa, bottom number denotes milligrams of levodopa; controlled-release preparation (CR) may mediate on/off changes; available in 10/100, 25/100, 25/250, and 50/200 (CR)
Dose	Start with 25/100 tablets three times a day, taper up as clinically indicated

Lamotrigine (Lamictal) (Table 5–5)

Indications	Adjunctive therapy for adult epilepsy
Actions	Anticonvulsant
Side effects	Dizziness, ataxia, nausea, vomiting, somnolence, headache
Comments	Second line medication; dose must be reduced with concurrent phenytoin, carbamazepine, or phenobarbital; no concurrent valproic acid
Dose	Start 50 mg PO per day for 14 days, then 50 mg two times a day for 14 days, up to 150 mg to 250 mg two times a day

Lorazepam (Ativan) (Chapters 5 and 9)

Indications	Ongoing seizure or status epilepticus, anxiety
Actions	Benzodiazepine sedative, anxiolytic; anticonvulsant
Side effects	Drowsiness, respiratory depression
Comments	Habit forming
Dose	For ongoing seizure: 2 to 4 mg IV push, repeat

once after 10 to 20 minutes; for anxiety 0.5 to 2 mg PO two times a day

---

Mannitol (Osmitrol) (Chapter 13)

Indications	Increased intracranial pressure
Actions	Osmotic diuretic
Side effects	Hypotension, dehydration, hyponatremia, hyperosmolar renal tubular damage, CHF exacerbation
Comments	Rebound intracranial hypertension with prolonged administration; monitor serum osmolality, electrolytes
Dose	0.25 to 1.0 g/kg of 20% solution (20 g per 100 ml), repeat every 4 to 6 hours

---

Meclizine (Antivert) (Chapter 14)

Indications	Benign positional vertigo, labyrinthitis
Actions	Antihistamine
Side effects	Drowsiness, dry mouth, blurred vision
Comments	Efficacy in about 50% of patients
Dose	12.5 to 25 mg PO three times a day

Methylprednisolone (Solu-Medrol) (Chapters 12, 15, and 22)

Indications	Traumatic spinal cord injury, multiple sclerosis exacerbation, inflammatory optic neuritis, pseudotumor cerebri
Actions	Anti-inflammatory/immunosuppressive agent
Side effects	Peptic ulcer disease, sodium and fluid retention, hypertension, hyperglycemia, myopathy, impaired wound healing, avascular necrosis of femoral or humeral heads, endocrine abnormalities
Comments	Stronger mineralocorticoid effect than dexamethasone or prednisone
Dose	For multiple sclerosis and inflammatory optic neuritis: 1 g IVSS per day for 10 days, followed by prednisone taper; for traumatic cord injury: 30 mg/kg IV bolus over 15 minutes, then 45-minute pause, and then 5.4 mg/kg per hour continuous IV infusion over next 23 hours; for pseudotumor cerebri: 250 mg IVSS four times a day

Methysergide (Sansert) (Chapter 15)

Indications	Migraine prophylaxis
Actions	Serotonin antagonist
Side effects	Retroperitoneal and pleuropulmonary fibrosis, nausea, vomiting, drowsiness, insomnia, hallucinations
Comments	Should not be used for 2 to 6 months after 6 months of use
Dose	2 mg PO one to three times a day

Midazolam (Versed) (Chapters 5 and 16)

Indications	Agitation while on ventilator, refractory status epilepticus
Actions	Short-action benzodiazepine sedative-hypnotic
Side effects	Drowsiness, respiratory depression, hypotension
Comments	Rapid acting, with very short half-life
Dose	For sedation: 1 to 2 mg IV/IM every 30 to 60 minutes; for status epilepticus: 0.1 to 0.3 mg/kg IV push load, then maintenance of 0.05 to 0.4 mg/kg per hour

Midodrine (Pro Amatine) (Chapter 17)

Indications	Orthostatic hypotension
Actions	Alpha receptor agonist
Side effects	Supine hypertension, paresthesias, pruritus
Comments	Last dose should be given no later than 6 PM to avoid nocturnal supine hypertension
Dose	10 mg PO three times per day

Naloxone (Narcan) (Chapter 6)

Indications	Suspected narcotic coma
Actions	Narcotic antagonist
Side effects	Nausea, vomiting, may precipitate withdrawal in narcotic addicts
Comments	Reversal of narcotic coma may wear off after 1 to 2 hours
Dose	0.4 to 2.0 mg IV, IM, or SC every 5 minutes to a maximum dose of 10 mg

Oxybutynin (Ditropan) (Chapter 22)

Indications	Bladder spasticity (detrusor dysynergia), e.g., in multiple sclerosis
Actions	Smooth muscle antispasmodic, antimuscarinic
Side effects	Palpitations, decreased sweating, dry mouth, dizziness, urinary retention, constipation
Comments	Contraindicated in patients with obstructive uropathy
Dose	5 mg PO two to three times a day

Pemoline (Cylert) (Chapter 22)

Indications	Narcolepsy, abulia after brain injury, attention deficit disorder
Actions	CNS stimulant
Side effects	Insomnia, anorexia, weight loss, seizure, dyskinesias, hallucinations, rare aplastic anemia
Comments	Contraindicated in patients with impaired hepatic function
Dose	18.75 mg PO every day, taper weekly as indicated up to maximum of 75 mg per day

Penicillamine (Cuprimine) (Chapter 26)

Indications	Wilson's disease
Actions	Copper chelator
Side effects	Lupus-like rash, polyarteritis, leukopenia, thrombocytopenia, epigastric pain, nausea, diarrhea, nephrotic syndrome, tinnitus, neuropathy
Comments	May precipitate myasthenia gravis
Dose	125 to 1000 mg per day, divided, two to four times a day

Pentobarbital (Chapter 5)

Indications	Status epilepticus, increased intracranial pressure
Actions	Anticonvulsant, sedative
Side effects	Respiratory suppression, sedation, hypotension
Comments	EEG monitoring indicated; hypotension may require pressors
Dose	5 to 20 mg/kg IV load, 1 to 3 mg/kg per hour maintenance

Pergolide (Permax) (Chapter 26)

Indications	Parkinson's disease
Actions	Dopamine agonist
Side effects	Nausea, headache, dizziness, fatigue, vomiting
Comments	May delay onset or reduce required dose of levo-dopa
Dose	0.75 to 3.0 mg per day, divided, three to four times a day

Phenobarbital (Chapter 5)

Indications	Epilepsy, status epilepticus
Actions	Anticonvulsant
Side effects	Sedation, respiratory suppression, hypotension, behavioral changes, hyperactivity
Comments	For chronic therapy, therapeutic range is 20 to 40 μg/ml; lowers levels of phenytoin, carbamazepine, and valproate
Dose	For status epilepticus: 20 mg/kg IV load infused at 100 mg/min; for epilepsy 60 mg PO two to three times a day; for pediatric patients: 3 to 6 mg/kg per day

Phenytoin (Chapter 5)

Indications	Epilepsy, status epilepticus
Actions	Anticonvulsant
Side effects	Nystagmus, ataxia, gingival hyperplasia, hirsutism, cardiac arrhythmia
Comments	For chronic therapy, therapeutic range is 10 to 20 μg/ml; lowers levels of carbamazepine and valproate and increases or decreases phenobarbital level
Dose	Typical maintenance dose is 300 mg every day at night

Pimozide (Orap) (Chapter 26)

Indications	Tourette's syndrome
Actions	Piperidine antipsychotic
Side effects	Dry mouth, sedation, dyskinesias, akinesia, behavioral effects, prolongation of QT interval
Comments	None

| Dose | Start with 1 mg PO two times a day, up to 2 to 10 mg per day in divided doses |

Primidone (Mysoline) (Chapters 5 and 26)

Indications	Generalized tonic-clonic epilepsy, essential tremor
Actions	Anticonvulsant
Side effects	Ataxia, vertigo, nausea, anorexia, vomiting, irritability, sedation
Comments	Second line of therapy; metabolized to phenobarbital
Dose	Start with 100 to 125 mg PO once a day, taper up to 250 mg three to four times a day

Prednisone (Chapter 12)

Indications	Temporal arteritis
Actions	Anti-inflammatory agent
Side effects	Peptic ulcer disease, sodium and fluid retention, hypertension, hyperglycemia, myopathy, impaired wound healing, avascular necrosis of femoral or humeral heads, endocrine abnormalities, increased susceptibility to infection
Comments	Initiate therapy as soon as diagnosis is suspected to avoid irreversible visual loss
Dose	100 mg PO per day, tapered slowly to alternate-day therapy over several weeks

Propantheline bromide (pro-Banthine) (Chapter 16)

Indications	Control of secretions in myasthenia gravis
Actions	Antimuscarinic agent
Side effects	Anticholinergic: decreased sweating, urinary retention, tachycardia, blurred vision
Comments	None
Dose	15 mg PO four times a day

Propranolol (Inderal) (Chapters 15 and 26)

Indications	Benign essential tremor, migraine prophylaxis
Actions	Nonspecific beta-adrenergic blocker
Side effects	Hypotension, bradycardia, bronchospasm, may mask symptoms of hypoglycemia, impotence

Comments	Avoid use in asthmatics and diabetics
Dose	For tremor: 40 to 240 mg PO per day, divided, three to four times a day; for migraine 20 to 40 mg per day

Pyridostigmine (Mestinon) (Chapter 16)

Indications	Myasthenia gravis
Actions	Acetylcholinesterase inhibitor
Side effects	Excess salivation, pulmonary secretions, diarrhea
Comments	Muscarinic side effects controlled by glycopyrrolate or propantheline bromide
Dose	Start at 30 mg PO three times a day, up to 120 mg every 3 to 6 hours

Riluzole (Rilutek) (Chapter 21)

Indications	Amyotrophic lateral sclerosis
Actions	Glutamate antagonist
Side effects	Malaise, abdominal pain, nausea, dizziness, circumoral numbness, liver function abnormalities
Comments	May extend survival 60 to 90 days and delay time to intubation; avoid use in patients with liver dysfunction
Dose	50 mg PO two times a day

Selegiline (Eldepryl) (Chapter 26)

Indications	Parkinson's disease
Actions	Monoamine oxidase B inhibitor: antioxidant
Side effects	Nausea, dizziness, confusion, hallucinations
Comments	Thought to slow progression of disease
Dose	Taper up to 5 mg PO two times a day

Sumatriptan (Imitrex) (Chapter 15)

Indications	Migraine (abortive therapy)
Actions	Selective serotonin agonist
Side effects	Coronary vasospasm, tingling, flushing, tightness in jaw, neck, and chest, dizziness, injection site reaction
Comments	Contraindicated in patients with coronary artery disease

Dose	6 mg SC, may repeat in 1 hour, maximum 12 mg per day, 6 doses per month; 25 mg PO, may repeat up to 100 mg in 2 hours

Tacrine (Cognex) (Chapter 19)

Indications	Alzheimer's disease
Actions	Reversible cholinesterase inhibitor
Side effects	Nausea, vomiting, diarrhea, abdominal pain, fatigue, agitation, confusion
Comments	May improve cognitive scores in some patients
Dose	Start 10 mg PO three times a day, tapering up to 30 mg three times a day

Thiamine (Chapters 5 and 9)

Indications	Coma, thiamine deficiency neuropathy
Actions	Enzymatic cofactor in oxidative metabolism (thiamine pyrophosphate)
Side effects	None
Comments	Give with glucose in setting of coma to prevent Wernicke's encephalopathy
Dose	For coma: 100 mg IV push; 100 mg PO or IM for 3 days

Tissue plasminogen activator (t-PA) (Chapters 7 and 25)

Indications	Hyperacute ischemic stroke
Actions	Thrombolytic
Side effects	Intracerebral hemorrhage
Comments	Must be given within 3 hours of stroke onset; increases chance of full recovery or minimal residual deficit at 3 months by 33%; patients with hemorrhage, recent head injury, prior stroke, or marked hypertension, or those on anticoagulant therapy should be excluded
Dose	0.9 mg/kg IV (10% IV push, then infuse the remaining 90% over 1 hour), maximum dose 90 mg

Trihexyphenidyl HCL (Artane) (Chapter 26)

Indications	Parkinson's disease, idiopathic torsion dystonia
Actions	Anticholinergic
Side effects	Visual blurring, dry mouth, urinary retention

Comments	May be effective in treating parkinsonian tremor; botulinum toxin has largely replaced anticholinergics for the treatment of focal dystonias
Dose	1 to 15 mg PO per day, divided, three to four times a day

Warfarin (Coumadin) (Chapters 7 and 25)

Indications	Stroke prophylaxis
Actions	Inhibits vitamin K–dependent clotting factors
Side effects	Hemorrhage, rash
Comments	Used for secondary stroke prevention in cardio-embolic stroke and in large vessel atherosclerosis when antiplatelet therapy has failed; used for primary stroke prevention in atrial fibrillation; close monitoring of prothrombin times (PT or International Normalized Ratios [INRs]) required
Dose	Begin with 4 mg PO per day, with dose adjusted according to target PT/INR

INDEX

Note: Page numbers in *italics* refer to illustrations; page numbers followed by b refer to boxed material, and those followed by t refer to tables.

Abdomen, in amnesia/dementia evaluation, 231
in delirium evaluation, 112
in dizziness/vertigo evaluation, 168
in gait failure evaluation, 136
in head injury evaluation, 125
in pain syndrome evaluation, 219–220
Abdominal reflexes, in neurologic examination, 22
Abducens (VI) nerve, in neurologic examination, 15–16
Abductor digiti minimi manus muscle, testing, roots, and innervation of, 336t
Abductor pollicis brevis muscle, testing, roots, and innervation of, 337t
Abductor pollicis longus muscle, testing, roots, and innervation of, 337t
Abscess(es), brain, 289–292
bacterial, 289–290
epidural, 291
spinal cord compression from, 99
Absence (petit mal) seizures, 62t
Acetazolamide, for pseudotumor cerebri, 185
information summary on, 349
Acetylcholine receptor antibodies, in myasthenia gravis diagnosis, 199
Acetylcholinesterase inhibitors, for myasthenia gravis, 200
Acoustic neuromas, 309–310
evoked potentials in, 46
Acquired immunodeficiency syndrome (AIDS). See also *HIV* entries.
neurologic complications of, 295–297
Activity, in acute stroke management, 96

Acute disseminated encephalomyelitis, 278
Acute necrotizing hemorrhagic encephalomyelitis, 278
Acyclovir, for facial (Bell's) palsy, 256
for herpes encephalitis, 293
for herpes zoster infection, 223
Adamantiades-Behçet syndrome, 280–281
Adductor brevis muscle, testing, roots, and innervation of, 339t
Adductor longus muscle, testing, roots, and innervation of, 339t
Adductor magnus muscle, testing, roots, and innervation of, 339t
Adductor pollicis muscle, testing, roots, and innervation of, 336t
Adenoma(s), pituitary, 310–311
binocular visual loss from, 145
Adventitial movements, in amnesia/dementia evaluation, 233
Adventitious movements, in neurologic examination, 18
Afferent pupillary defect, in neurologic examination, 16
in vision disturbance evaluation, 148
Age, in neurologic history, 6
Agitation, treatment of, 114–115, 238
AIDS (aquired immunodeficiency syndrome). See also *HIV* entries.
neurologic complications of, 295–297
AIDS dementia complex, treatment of, 239
Airway, in acute stroke evaluation, 84–85
in head injury evaluation, 125
in head injury management, 128
in headache evaluation, 177

367